WELL-GROUNDED

WELL-GROUNDED

GROUNDED

The Neurobiology of Rational Decisions

KELLY LAMBERT

Yale

UNIVERSITY PRESS

New Haven and London

Published with assistance from the Mary Cady Tew Memorial Fund.

Yale University Press books may be purchased in quantity for
educational, business, or promotional use. For information,
please e-mail sales.press@yale.edu (U.S. office) or sales@yaleup.co.uk
(U.K. office).

Set in Janson type by Integrated Publishing Solutions,
Grand Rapids, Michigan.
Printed in the United States of America.

Library of Congress Control Number: 2018936848
ISBN 978-0-300-20730-9 (hardcover : alk. paper)

A catalogue record for this book is available from the British Library.
This paper meets the requirements of ANSI/NISO Z39.48-1992
(Permanence of Paper).

10 9 8 7 6 5 4 3 2 1

To Dr. Craig Howard Kinsley (1954–2016)
Colleague, Friend, Knowledge Enthusiast

His passion for behavioral neuroscience continues to influence his former colleagues and students . . . it certainly continues to influence my thoughts about the wonders of the brain

Contents

Acknowledgments   ix

INTRODUCTION   I

1. The Brain's Contingency Calculator: The Secret of
   Our Success   6
2. The Brain's Output: Behavior's Many Forms   26
3. The Human Brain: An Embarrassment of Riches   48
4. Building the Brain's Contingency Circuit   73
5. When Life Distorts the Contingency Filters   95
6. Fine-Tuning the Contingency Calculators:
   Well-Grounded Lessons from Rats, Comedians,
   and Triple-Crown Horse Owners   122
7. Parenting: Time to Recalculate Life's Contingencies   150
8. Calculating Effective Strategies for Treating
   Mental Illness   182
9. Getting Down to Business: Putting the Contingency
   Calculators to Work   211
10. Stretching the Contingency Limits: New and
    Imagined Realities   232

EPILOGUE   Redefining Prosperity—From Strategic
           Champagne Bubbles to Accurately Perceived
           Life Affordances   255

Notes   261
Index   285

Acknowledgments

THE CONTENT IN THIS book is an amalgamation of the fascinating research of countless neuroscientists who have contributed to the scientific literature. Working in various contexts, these neuroscientists have provided the scientific information that serves as a backdrop for the evolving science of adaptive neuroscience and healthy brain functions. Because these science stories are complex and dynamic, I am indebted to the generosity of two giants in the field of behavioral neuroscience, Bryan Kolb (University of Lethbridge) and Don Stein (Emory University), for their informed and insightful comments. Although lingering mistakes will no doubt be found in this book, their comments were extremely valuable, saving me from unwanted detours and misinterpretations. John Salamone (University of Connecticut) also provided valuable feedback about specific neurochemical sections.

I am also indebted to multiple individuals for taking the time to allow me to interview them, including but not limited to: Penny Chenery, Judge Robert Francis, Judith Cochrane Gilman-Hines, Mike Lacey, Sheri Storm, and Kate Tweedy. My former and current undergraduate students, too many to name here, have also contributed to the scientific stories introduced throughout the chapters of this book. I have most certainly benefited from having the distinct honor of working with these students over the past three decades. I have also been fortunate to have worked with many amazing collaborators at several different institutions through the years. I received support from my former colleagues and staff in the Psychology and Biology

Departments at Randolph-Macon College and, most recently, at the University of Richmond. The support I received from the Macon and Joan Brock Neuroscience Professorship, and the generous donations of Pepper and Stuart Laughon and others at Randolph-Macon College, contributed to the *experiential capital* necessary for this writing endeavor, as did research support from the National Institute of Mental Health and the National Science Foundation.

Not surprisingly, this book required me to work above and beyond my "real" job as a professor, and I thank my family for understanding the required long hours, especially during weekends, while working on this project. My daughters, Lara and Skylar, have accepted that their rat-and-brain-loving mother is a little different than other moms. My own brain has most certainly been enriched and restructured by having them in my life, and I have included a few of our adventures in this book! My very supportive husband, Gary, has spent countless hours listening to my various ideas about brain bubbles and contingency calculations—his insight and many editing sessions were critical for the development of this manuscript.

Finally, the transition of my ideas about distorted brain bubbles into an actual book is the result of my stellar colleagues in the world of publishing. I will always be indebted to Katherine Ellison, an accomplished author and valued friend, who convinced me years ago that I could write a book for mainstream audiences—giving me the opportunity to extend my classroom to a larger audience. My agent, Michelle Tessler, has once again done a wonderful job of listening to my initial ideas and providing informed feedback necessary to transform those ideas into a viable proposal. My editor at Yale University Press, Jean Thomson Black, was extremely patient as I navigated my way through the many challenges of completing this neuroscience story, all the while providing support and valuable feedback to keep me working toward the finish line. Michael Deneen has had the difficult job of keeping the manuscript in the appropriate order and format in his role as an Editorial Assistant. I appreciate his professionalism and patience guiding me through this process.

Finally, I would be remiss if I neglected to acknowledge the core contributors to my own experiential capital. I am thankful for a minimally micromanaged childhood that allowed curiosity to guide my neural development in the backyards and backwoods of Alabama, as well as for family members who encouraged me to follow my passion to learn more about brains and behavior even though a career in higher education and academics was far from their perception of the norm. I am also grateful for many professors who, in addition to providing the building materials for my neuroscience career, planted the seeds of curiosity that continue to make neuroscience fascinating after all these years. As I submit this final draft manuscript, I am thinking about the most recent batch of beautifully stained neural tissue in my laboratory—and I can't wait to work with my wonderful postdoctoral fellow, Molly Kent, and my current student investigators to learn more about how the brain adapts to life's many challenges.

Introduction

IN EIGHTEENTH-CENTURY GREAT BRITAIN, merchants were enthusiastic about a new opportunity to "earn" money. The South Sea Company was created by Parliament in 1711 to facilitate trading among the South Seas and parts of America. The appearance of financial markets during this time represented a new way for the brain to experience a return on investments. Whereas in the past, acquired resources were more closely tied to an investment of personal effort typically involving some form of physical labor, the new financial investments and market schemes seemed to bypass such work. Less work, more money: perfect! After several years the South Sea Company gained an impressive corporate presence, boasting a market capitalization that exceeded 200 million pounds.

Amid the apparent success of the South Sea Company, Archibald Hutcheson, an attentive lawyer and economist, spotted a potential problem, or "bulge," as he called it. He warned investors that the valuations of the South Sea shares were unrealistic—that their intrinsic value was inflated. It turned out that Archibald was onto something. The irrational mania behind the South Sea Company's apparent success led to what was later described as an *asset bubble*. The lack of relevant experience of the company's board of directors was just one of many reasons for the eventual bursting of the bubble in 1720—resulting in the first international market crash.[1]

Fast-forward three centuries to the present, and asset bubbles and market crashes remain a threat in the brave new world of financial markets. In 1996, Alan Greenspan, chair of the Federal Reserve at the time, warned that *irrational exuberance*, similar to that observed in the South Sea crash, was artificially escalating asset values, leading once again to false assumptions about the true intrinsic value of such assets.[2] This didn't stop the inflated intrinsic value of real estate in the United States that peaked in 2006 and led to the bursting of the housing bubble two years later. It appeared that, in order to avoid bubble assets leading to crashes in the financial market, a close connection between real and perceived asset values had to be maintained.

As a behavioral neuroscientist, I am constantly looking for trends that characterize the ways mammals navigate their complex habitats to survive and thrive in a world filled with endless uncertainties. With so many choices, where do animals invest their time, energy, and resources? In many ways, the keys to our personal survival "markets" are similar to the financial markets. Similar to our desire to achieve maximal financial returns on minimal financial investments, we search for ways to experience maximal emotional highs with minimal emotional investments. Who could argue with such a successful formula? Indeed, such emotional success stories also sometimes appear to be *almost too good to be true* . . .

My own scientific journeys, mostly with clever rats, have emphasized the importance of allowing our neural processing capacity to maintain relevant and meaningful connections with the outside world. If either the brain or the environment strays too far from its natural context, this elegant, complex system gets a little wonky, requiring recalibration to reestablish optimal brain-behavior baselines. If allowed to go unchecked, our brains start to assign inaccurate values to behavior and aspects of the world around us—sometimes with deadly results. Perhaps the most extreme example of such an emotional crash is found in individuals who take psychoactive drugs to achieve emotional highs that nature reserved for reinforcing life's most valuable investments such as eating, sex, social relationships, and personal achievement. When these relevant behaviors are bypassed by taking drugs for shortcuts to euphoria, we lose the ability to assess the true intrinsic value of more natural elements of the world around us and, consequently, artificially inflate the value of drugs. A drug-induced high is irrational exuberance incarnate. Of course, in the case of addiction, the results can be even more devastating than the financial market crashes. In the most unfortunate cases, the distorted valuation assigned to these drugs of choice can completely shut the body down, tragically ending in death. This distortion of reality represents a form of neural propaganda, as incoming information representing the authentic environment that we depend on for our minute-to-minute survival is altered from its original form. Regardless of whether the end result is viewed as positive or negative, the distortion itself is the primary interest of this book.

Thus, when the return on investments in either the financial or the emotional markets seems to be too good to be true, there is a very good chance that this is exactly the case. Ideally, left to our own devices, we self-correct these distortions, or miniature asset bubbles, to recalibrate mismatches between our effort and emotional payoffs. If following a new diet plan doesn't result in actual weight loss, we move on to a different diet or at least stop following the ineffective diet. Thus, it is important that our past experiences accurately inform future experiences. If brain bulges or bubbles lead to distorted realities that impair future decisions, then our well-being, broadly defined, is compromised.

In addition to drug use, another lifestyle context that lends itself to such distortions is that of celebrity. Exorbitant paydays, lavish lifestyles, and unconditional praise from social contacts stray so far from any form of reality that the neural networks begin to get confused about the actual intrinsic value of once highly regarded life assets such as putting in a hard day's work, developing meaningful social relationships, and enjoying Mom's legendary lasagna. Under the spotlight of celebrity, some individuals lose their ability to fine-tune neural responses to respond to new challenges in life, often requiring an intervention of sorts.

Despite celebrities' vulnerability to distortions of reality, the barrage of entertainment "news" featuring the varied lifestyles of the rich and famous suggests that some of these individuals are opting for noncelebrity, reality-based lifestyles. Billionaire businessman Warren Buffett, for example, still lives in the same unpretentious house that he purchased approximately a half-century ago for $30,000. Shortly after moving her family into the White House, former First Lady Michelle Obama expressed the importance of maintaining a sense of normalcy for her daughters, Malia and Sasha. She announced to the ninety-five members of the White House residence staff that her daughters were responsible for continuing the chores they had been doing in Chicago—including making their own bed, cleaning their room, and clearing their plates from the table after eating. Michelle Obama emphasized that an understanding of a working household should be a familiar, not foreign, concept to her daughters. "Don't spoil them, spoil mom!" was her running joke with the staff.[3]

Such compensatory efforts to maintain realistic connections with one's environmental context likely provide a dose of prevention against the onset of emerging emotional asset bubbles that may contribute to a host of mental illnesses. Later in this book we will contrast this reality-based approach to celebrity status with Michael Jackson's approach of enhancing his celebrity brain bubble by building the most unrealistic home and retreat imaginable. He called it "Neverland," and it was complete with a menagerie of exotic pets including a chimpanzee with the somewhat prophetic name of "Bubbles."[4]

Regardless of our social status, profession, or geographic location, one of the most certain aspects of life is that it is filled with uncertainties. Even when we are consciously living a grounded, self-recalibrating lifestyle, we encounter an endless stream of choices and decisions. As we make decisions throughout our lives, the choice with the highest payoff is not always clear. Our relevant and meaningful interactions with the world around us, our life backstories, build our response inventories so that we enhance our odds of experiencing those coveted emotional payoffs as opposed to heading toward the emotional crashes. In fact, our impressive brains are nature's ultimate payoff for effectively interacting with our changing world; new challenges and experiences literally build new neuronal connections. Could it be that our most prized asset, our brain's ability to draw from real-life experiences and determine optimal decision choices, is compromised by our insatiable desire to find shortcuts to life's rewards?

Our journey in this book will compare the contemporary societal view of prosperity—obtaining resources with minimal energy investments—to scientific research emphasizing lifestyle practices associated with the richest brain responses. Not unlike the valued stock market index updates, among the brain's most valued assets are the ever-changing neural networks, a neural market index of sorts, that constantly update new and relevant information about our surrounding world. If there is indeed a disconnect between societal and neural perspectives of prosperity, how can we generate a more authentic view of prosperity that will maximize optimal returns on our emotional and physical investments? Similar to our quest for sustainable lifestyles to preserve our planet, we should be just as motivated to identify sustainable lifestyles for preserving our sanity—and even happiness. Such lifestyles enable us to understand which responses produce the most desirable immediate and future outcomes. Spoiler alert: to my knowledge there's no way to avoid the occasional encounter with brain bulges or emotional asset bubbles as we progress through life, but, with a little vigilance and a few lifestyle adjustments, we can hedge our bets against future brain bubble bursts and emotional crashes.

In the chapters that follow, influences on our behavioral output will be considered from both expected and unexpected perspectives. Since current neuroscience research has confirmed that the brain is the foundation of our behavioral, cognitive, and emotional responses, a close examination of the brain is necessary for this journey. Although the celebrated philosopher René Descartes contributed valuable information to many scientific areas, his dualistic ideas about the mind and body representing separate independent entities are not embraced by contemporary neuroscientists and informed mental health practitioners today.[5] Thus, far from a dualistic approach, a discussion of our brain's responses in this book is, in reality, a discussion of our responses in general—no different than looking under the hood of a car to determine how the engine influences its performance on the road.[6] Meaningful, well-grounded experiences allow our brains to maintain accurate filters to determine optimal life outcomes, ensuring that our highs are based on rational, as opposed to irrational, exuberance. As tempting as living a fairy tale–like affluent existence may be, you will learn that the brain feeds on more grounded life experiences just as the stomach needs real food, and lungs need real air. Although it is fun to stray from reality for brief interludes, the best advice is to simply *Keep It Real!*

CHAPTER ONE

The Brain's Contingency Calculator
The Secret of Our Success

con·tin·gen·cy (/kən'tinjənsē/). Noun: A future event or circumstance that is possible but cannot be predicted with certainty.[1]

THE HUMAN BRAIN IS unmatched in its complexity and competence. How, then, can it run off the rails so often? Too frequently, we predict one outcome only to be disappointed when our contingency calculation is off and the desired outcome doesn't appear. With such an impressive brain on board, how do individuals such as Michael Jackson (as described in the Introduction), who had so many resources at his fingertips, make decisions that lead to their ultimate demise? When it becomes apparent that a disease has invaded our body, we take cautionary measures to rid our system of the life-threatening condition. Distorted realities, a neural disease of sorts, creep into our neural networks and compromise the brain's distinct survival advantages. This condition is often disguised in the form of celebrity, privilege, poverty, religion, politics, or psychoactive drugs—any means of warping our perspective of reality can become our most feared silent killer. Indeed, one of the most debilitating consequences of diseases we refer to as psychiatric illnesses is the dangerous distortion of reality.

Our view of prosperity in contemporary Western societies with creature comforts such as lush surroundings and various personal services to avoid physical effort may suffocate our neural functions. Consequently, it is time to recalculate our perception of prosperity from the perspective of healthy brain functions. Although we begin this chapter with a discussion of the critical genetic foundation of our impressive nervous system, we ultimately have to look beyond our genome to the world we interact with every day. Our ability to navigate and survive in a continuously changing world requires a nervous system that is changing in tandem with a dynamic world. Thus, we are able to maintain a truly prosperous brain—accompanied by neural, as opposed to financial, assets—only by remaining tuned into the world around us.

Maintaining active interactions with our external surroundings keeps our experiential stockpiles at healthy levels, producing neural prosperity in the form of a sense of competency and achievement. As 16-year-old Florida high school student Benjamin Stern declared after receiving an investment from Mark Cuban, owner of the professional basketball team Dallas Mavericks, on the popular TV show *Shark Tank*, "It's like winning the lottery! But better, you earned it." According to my interpretation of the neuroscience literature, this hard-working entrepreneurial teen's experience represents one of our brain's most successful moments—a contingency calculation payoff. He got a job at 14 so he could pay the costs of launching a business aimed at producing water-soluble shampoo packaging to help end the stream of discarded plastic bottles that currently end up in landfills each year.[2] As we will learn throughout this book, such grounded individuals accumulate valuable information and experiences that enable them to calculate the most accurate contingencies leading to desired payoffs.

Beyond the Genome

Few scientific achievements rival the sequencing of the human genome. When former president Bill Clinton announced at a much-anticipated press conference in the summer of 2000 that the human genome had been sequenced, the excitement in the room and throughout the scientific community was palpable. "This is the most important, most wondrous map ever produced by humankind . . . Humankind is on the verge of gaining immense new power to heal," Clinton boasted as he conveyed the exciting news.[3]

The final sequencing of the 3 billion base pairs serving as the building blocks for human DNA was arguably the most ambitious scientific achievement in history. According to some, it even exceeded putting humans on the moon. The scientific community now possessed sequencing data for the approximately 23,000 genes serving as the blueprint for humanity. With this accomplishment, the formula for life, or the distinct formula for humanity, had been revealed.

Or had it? Now that well over a decade and a half has passed since the announcement, scientists from various biomedical disciplines are quick to admit that the gains from this scientific breakthrough have been slower to materialize than initially anticipated. Although the biological sciences clearly have benefited from the genome by seeing advancements in areas such as the technology associated with genetic sequencing, the benefits have been less visible in clinical medicine. Even though specific genes have been identified as posing risks for various diseases, the cures for diseases mentioned by President Clinton are, years later, still *in development*. After the excitement died down, it was obvious that the formula for humankind was much more complicated than could be conveyed by sequences of the nucleotide bases defining our genes. The DNA script was obviously important, and there is no denying its scientific contribution, but it has become clear that this script represents only one component of the distinctive formula for humankind.

Obviously, additional essential ingredients for nature's recipe for humanity are necessary to provide more information about how specific nucleotide bases lead to healthy and happy lives. To aid in the search for these distinguishing characteristics, the goal of this book is to shift the spotlight to the workings of evolution's most crowning achievement—the human brain—and how it determines optimal actions to produce desired outcomes that are linked to health and survival. By exploring the brain's responses in various circumstances we will come closer to understanding the signature characteristics of human success. With enhanced understanding comes enhanced accountability of how we treat our brains throughout our lives. As we learn more about our optimal functioning capacity, we become equipped to generate buffers against the emergence of mental illness, avoiding lifestyle and environmental hazards as we navigate through the journey of life. We also gain an enhanced understanding of the associations between our actions and their consequences as we build experiential stockpiles, or *contingency capital*, that enable us to live more fulfilling lives. Having multiple past experiences with dogs, for example, will inform your decision of how to interact with the unfamiliar dog approaching you and your toy poodle at the park.

Not all contingency strategies are informed and productive. Twentieth-century cartoonist Rube Goldberg provided delightful images of incredibly complex inventions designed to allow us to passively achieve even the simplest of outcomes such as swatting a fly. In Goldberg's "Self-Operating Napkin" invention, the desired outcome of wiping one's face while eating is the product of a complex sequence of events dependent on several individual contingencies (Figure 1). Such an effort is indeed comical when presented in cartoon format. In real life, however, we are increasingly relinquishing control over our life contingencies when we bypass the more traditional responses that lead to the targeted outcomes. Would the fictional self-operating napkin contraption compromise one's ability to wipe his or her own face when this invention wasn't available? If we have depended on a dog walker for that previously mentioned toy poodle, do we lose our ability to respond to a menacing dog in an effective way? Our ability to generate accurate contingency calculations gets rusty and distorted as we progress through a lifetime of taking shortcuts and opting for the most passive responses leading to desired outcomes. Considering that we need to generate accurate predictions throughout our lives, we need to avoid rusty contingency calculating neural networks at all costs.

In this book, the importance of our past experiences in predicting life's uncertain outcomes, or life-contingencies, will be discussed. It should become increasingly clear that the outcomes in our lives are often contingent on our experience-guided actions. Different

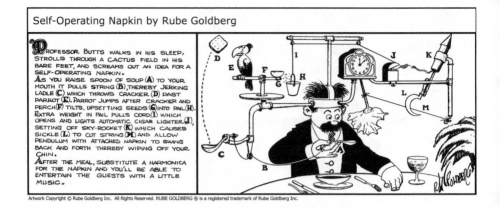

Figure 1. Outsourcing Contingency Calculations. *Twentieth-century cartoonist Rube Goldberg entertained audiences by depicting passive-response contingency scenarios to accomplish various mundane tasks such as wiping one's face with a napkin, swatting a fly, or squeezing toothpaste on a toothbrush. Although it seems bizarre to construct such a complex invention to avoid making the simple response of wiping your face with a napkin (as shown in this cartoon), humans are increasingly inventing ways to avoid traditional responses to produce both essential and desired resources for our well-being. It is interesting to consider whether adapting to such passive responses will compromise our ability to make smart decisions and effective responses in the future. (Artwork Copyright © and TM Rube Goldberg Inc. All Rights Reserved. RUBE GOLDBERG ® is a registered trademark of Rube Goldberg Inc. All materials used with permission. rubegoldberg.com)*

from mere probability calculations, finely tuned contingency calculations require us to have some skin in the game. The backlog of experiences becomes an important compass to guide us through the many uncertainties we face throughout our lives. You merely need data to generate accurate actuary tables to predict the life spans of various demographic groups; however, personal experiences with past outcomes are required to determine if someone has friendship potential or if your training program is the best to catapult you to a winning position. Put another way, our behavioral choices become more informed as we pay attention to the outcomes of our past experiences. Life experiences leading to contingency capital help us

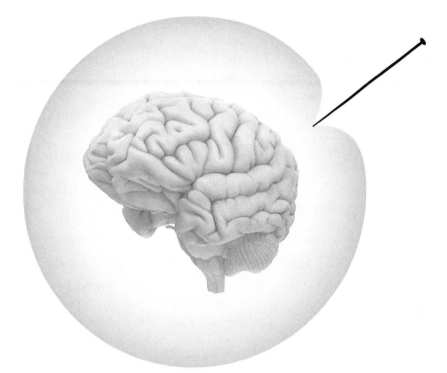

Figure 2. Bursting Brain Bubbles. *It's important to burst distorting brain bubbles through authentic contingency testing before they distort reality in ways that make us more vulnerable to the emergence of mental illness.*

generate rational outcome plans providing protection against the irrational exuberance that creates brain bubbles and the emotional crashes that often accompany them (Figure 2).

Decoding the Brain

Throughout time the brain has been a difficult nut to crack. In some ironic form of a metaphysical hoax, only the brain can decipher the brain. As far back as three thousand years ago, humans must have associated the organ inside the head as important for behavior. When individuals acted in bizarre ways, holes were drilled through their skulls, a process known as trepanning, in order to release the

mischievous "spirits." Even with this early start, progress to decipher the brain's output has been slow. With so many disciplines
interested in the brain and its functions, including philosophy, biology, psychiatry, psychology, and neuroscience (just to name a
few), progress in this area has likely suffered from having too many
academic cooks in the kitchen, each with unique brain recipes and
perspectives.

At this point, many of you may be thinking, *Wait a minute, but
we do know a lot about the brain—and this information has been around
for a long time.* After all, in the fourth-century BC, Hippocrates
stated the functions of the brain quite succinctly and eloquently when
he wrote:

> Men ought to know that from nothing else but the brain
> come joys, delights, laughter and sports, and sorrows, grief,
> despondency, and lamentations. And by this, in an especial
> manner, we acquire wisdom and knowledge, and see and
> hear and know what are foul and what are fair, what are bad
> and what are good, what are sweet and what are unsavory. . . .
> And by the same organ we become mad and delirious, and
> fears and terrors assail us . . . All these things we endure
> from the brain when it is not healthy . . . In these ways I am
> of the opinion that the brain exercises the greatest power in
> the man.[4]

I agree that this was an incredibly insightful statement for the
time; in fact, I include it on the first page of my Clinical Neuroscience course syllabus each year. Although the statement is informative, it is far from definitive and falls short of providing useful information about maintaining healthy brains possessing the capacity to
maximize opportunities. What could distort the "wisdom and knowledge" Hippocrates spoke of? And what factors transformed a healthy
brain into one that was "mad and delirious?" For the most part,
neuroscientists are still searching for these answers.

Other organs of the body have been easier to figure out. Although there was much speculation about the function of the heart
prior to the seventeenth century, with one popular view that it was
the seat of consciousness, the question was answered when William

Harvey identified its function as a pump that distributes blood through-out the body.[5] This basic understanding paved the way for many dis-coveries and treatments in cardiovascular medicine. Unfortunately, the brain lacks such a definitive eureka moment. For much of the twentieth century, Freud and his lingering subjective ideas distracted everyone with his fantasy-style theories about unconscious motives, superegos, and psychosexual stages of development, none of which were especially appropriate for empirical scientific investigation. Even so, important brain discoveries were made beginning in the nineteenth century. Beautiful and intricate cells and networks were introduced to the scientific community, along with critical clues about their complex mechanisms of operation. Nobel prizes were won as these key structures and descriptive elements were identi-fied, but the big picture about the ultimate and most critical output of this organ remained elusive.

There were, however, credible glimpses into the brain's primary currency and functions. Above and beyond regulating basic physio-logical systems, the emergence of behaviorism in the new discipline of psychology around the turn of the twentieth century added a new perspective for brain enthusiasts.[6] The important works of the behav-ioral pioneers, including Ivan Pavlov, John B. Watson, E. L. Thorn-dike, and B. F. Skinner, were published in the scientific literature. Given that there was no real mention of the brain's involvement in these unique behavioral research programs, the ties between the brain and behavior were somewhat ignored by these pioneers, especially by Skinner. Even today, as behavioral investigations have become more sophisticated, and neuroscience techniques are allowing re-searchers to peer into every nook and cranny of the brain, the estab-lishment of the brain's true identity remains a mystery. As discussed later in the book, revisiting the insightful findings of the behavioral pioneers, with their findings strategically considered in the context of relevant neuroscience, provides valuable clues about the most im-portant functions of the brain.

The lack of understanding about the brain's outputs and func-tions is seen most clearly in the area of mental illness. Whereas technological advances have been matched with treatment advances in virtually every other medical area, this is not the case for mental illness. In fact, I am always embarrassed when I lecture about the trajectory of mental illness treatments because the lack of progress is so very sad for the many people suffering from some form of it. Indeed, Thomas Insel, former director of the National Institute of Mental Health, noted that although the medical community can celebrate drastic reductions in many medical conditions—for example, in the past half-century, mortality rates in children diagnosed with leukemia have been reduced by a whopping 85 percent, and, affecting a larger portion of the population, mortality from cardiovascular disease has decreased by 63 percent—this has not been the case for mental illness.[7] Major depressive disorder, a condition associated with intense emotional pain and significant personal and societal costs, has experienced no decrease in prevalence. According to the World Health Organization, depression has risen to the unenviable status of being one of the world's most disabling medical conditions.[8] As I so often say to my students, this lack of progress for patients suffering from mental illness is *unacceptable*. We have to be more strategic in our attempt to decode the brain and its critical functions if there is to be any hope of reversing the rising rates of mental illness.

The Brain's Unique Behavioral Apps

The heart pumps blood, the lungs pump air, the stomach pumps food, and the brain, well, it is clearly more than just a pump. I suppose it can be argued that brains pump ions and neurochemicals, but that description falls short of truly identifying its most important functions. Actually, the brain carries out multiple levels of functions, not the least of which is directing those aforementioned pumps to keep our bodies alive and functioning. If the brain stem stops working, an automated artificial mechanical life support system is necessary to keep a person alive. But beyond the physiological basics, the mammalian brain has a few more tricks up its sleeve. In the case of the human, it recruits approximately 86 billion neural cells to choreograph strategic movements and complex behaviors that enhance our survival on many levels.

Complex behavior, perhaps the most unique output of the brain, distinguishes mammals from their reptilian cousins. Although the popular advertising icon—the Geico gecko—appears to be highly intelligent as it dispenses advice about the best insurance to purchase, real world reptiles exhibit very simple behavioral responses as they reflexively navigate through their environments. Put a lizard in front of a mirror and it will continually attack itself, reflexively responding to the sight of its approaching reflection with an inability to read the surrounding environment and discern that its responses are meaningless. As mammals arrived on the evolutionary scene, the brain invested in increased real estate and tools to acquire new behaviors and make real-time decisions that maximize survival. Considering that approximately 84 percent of the 20,000-plus genes in the human genome are expressed in the brain—a structure that represents only 2 percent of our body's weight yet consumes 20 percent of its resources—there is little doubt that the brain is an integral component of the formula, or blueprint, for humankind.[9]

As a behavioral neuroscientist who has been teaching and conducting research for nearly three decades, I frequently think about why it has taken so long to unlock the many mysteries surrounding the brain. As mentioned above, the brain's functions have been formally contemplated since the early Greeks, yet real progress has been, at best, hit or miss. Although stellar progress has been made in the field of neuroscience, these developments have to be assessed in various contexts and in various species to reveal critical information about understanding the brain's functions sufficiently to enable mental illness to be treated effectively. The brain doesn't function in a vacuum; thus, an understanding of how the brain influences behavior in various contexts is key to understanding the effectiveness of its functions. Just as a cardiologist often prescribes aerobic activity to treat an ailing heart, it is important for people to engage in relevant behaviors to maintain mental health. But what exactly are these brain-healthy behaviors?

The importance of behavior in mental health has become increasingly clear as my students and I have developed rodent models requiring certain behavioral strategies to cope with stress, the precursor for many varieties of mental illnesses. In one behavioral model we refer to as the *effort-based reward* model, rats are required to produce physical effort to earn their food treats. More specifically, the group of rats known as the contingent-trained rats spend a mere six minutes a day engaged in strategic actions, in this case going out in my laboratory "fields" to dig up coveted Froot Loops cereal in order to build connections between their actions (digging) and outcomes (eating yummy Froot Loops). The results indicate that, compared to their noncontingent rat counterparts who don't have to work for their rewards, these working rats have enhanced emotional resilience, an ability to bounce back in challenging times that may serve as a buffer against the onset of mental illnesses such as depression. This rodent model serves as a reminder of the importance of building strong associations between our actions and subsequent outcomes.[10]

From a survival perspective, the relationship between our actions and outcomes has changed drastically throughout human evolution. Our ancestors needed to remain vigilant about responses leading to important resources or the avoidance of harm, actions that are less critical in many but not all areas of our contemporary world. Decisions to try a novel, possibly poisonous, new food, or track a particular wild and dangerous animal for dinner, or move camp to an unknown area, have been replaced with decisions about which take-out food to order, which songs to download on our playlist, and whether or not we should tweet about our friends' latest social faux pas. Of course, there are still areas across the world that require a high level of vigilance for survival, but this scenario has changed for more affluent societies. Considering that we generally have the same brains as our ancestors, one has to wonder about the consequences of these drastic changes and if these changes have an influence on the increasing rates of mental illness.

If we stop to think about it, no one should be surprised that the sequencing of the genome has been so slow to benefit those suffering from mental illness. Aside from neurological diseases such as Alzheimer's and Parkinson's, which have been associated with modified proteins and neurochemicals, mental illnesses—schizophrenia, depression, anxiety disorders, etc.—are thought to be associated with multiple factors and aren't likely to be associated with a single gene dictating the production of a particular protein. In its current state, the sequenced genome is comparable to a map that includes streets and highways but no destination points such as cities or states, and no landscapes such as mountains, oceans, rivers, deserts, or forests. The map would need to be painstakingly matched with these interesting sites to maximize its value. Accordingly, the human genome, comparable to a map of the world of humankind, has to be matched with neural and behavioral functions, and associated emotions and thoughts, before we can begin the journey to develop genetic-based treatments for mental illnesses such as obsessive-compulsive disorder or depression.

Representing a positive move in the direction of mapping critical information onto the genome maps, Harvard geneticist George Church launched an ambitious project, the Personal Genome Project, in 2007. Whereas the first human genome that was sequenced cost the National Institutes of Health (NIH) $3 billion, the costs have dropped considerably, pushing closer to a mere $1,000 per person. The purpose of the Personal Genome Project is to sequence the genomes of thousands of individuals, collecting blood, saliva, and skin cell samples from each volunteer and, relevant to this discussion, personal information about behavior and lifestyles. These data should yield a more accurate map of exactly how genes influence behavior and when specific genes, in the context of certain lifestyle variables, pose the most risk for an individual. As this information is unearthed, a systematic analysis of behavioral functions will enhance the value of this sea of personal information.[11]

To keep up with medical advancements and offer hope for the prevention and treatment of mental illness, it is becoming increasingly clear that behavior needs to be systematically investigated to bring the most valuable information to the mental health table. Beyond the salivating dogs and pecking pigeons described by Pavlov and Skinner, respectively (and discussed in the next chapter), the brain's ability to process the relationship between our actions and their consequences for various competing responses is a critical behavioral strategy for survival and life success. The scientific literature uses the terms *action-outcome contingencies* and *response-outcome contingencies* to refer to the important relationship between behavior and its consequences, so they are both used in this book. Regardless of the specific term, calculating the probability of desirable outcomes is important in many areas of mental health and neuroscience. One relevant area is the fascinating and broadly defined field of neuroeconomics. Should you play another hand at the blackjack table or leave with your current winnings? Should you sell your house now or wait for the market to improve? Should you enroll little Bobby in toddler T-ball or wait until he's a little older? Our ability to maintain healthy *contingency calculators* in order to respond to life's uncertainty in the most strategic manner, therefore, is critical for mental health and well-being—and may be a contender for one of the critical functions of the brain. Hearts pump blood, lungs pump oxygen, and brains pump contingencies to churn out the most adaptive behavioral responses possible.

Camouflaged Contingencies

There are certain situations in nature where camouflage is desired. A moth that blends in with the bark on a tree and an insect that looks like a twig on a branch are critical adaptations for surviving when a predator passes by. However, if certain factors mask contingency outcomes, so that critical causes for targeted outcomes are not apparent, this represents a lost learning opportunity. If eating a certain type of berry leads to sickness, we need to know about it; if making a facial gesture alienates a potential friend, we need to know about it; if using a specific study strategy leads to failure on a test, we need to know about it. The possession of accurate, real-time, authentic information about the effectiveness of our responses is essential for the brain's maintenance of accurate contingency calculators.

Although we strive to strengthen personal traits—our speed, strength, and knowledge—we don't seem to mind if we compromise our ability to assess the accuracy of our contingency processors. Too often, instead of investigating reasons why our decisions lead to failure, we're quick to rule out personal responsibility by focusing on other factors such as a fellow worker's incompetence, a health issue, or just bad luck. We often protectively hide the reasons for success and failure from our children by telling them that *everyone is a winner* or that they should not pay attention to a friend who always beats them in a relay race. Individuals with financial privilege can be quick to hire others to strategically address contingencies for them (e.g., financial investors, interior designers, life coaches for day-to-day activities), allowing their own contingency calculators to become atrophied. And, perhaps worst of all, in the pretenses of helping individuals gain mental competency or mental health, many vulnerable individuals are prescribed medications that often mask real-world contingencies so that their emotions are more manageable. Most tragic was the mid-twentieth-century use of frontal lobotomies, a literal frontal attack on the brain's critical contingency processors, in an attempt to tame behavioral and emotional responses that were viewed as unacceptable. Could it be that several of our approaches to treating mental illness could just as easily be perceived as techniques that *create* mental illnesses due to their contingency-masking effects? And, does this line of thinking explain why cognitive and behavioral therapies that focus on the patient's ability to gain control over desired and authentic action-outcome contingencies have excellent success rates, oftentimes reaching 100 percent success, with no side effects? The answer is a resounding YES.

Accurate contingency calculators are also camouflaged by incorrectly associating actions with outcomes. This is typically done when the outcome is of extreme importance to an individual who, out of desperation to control the outcome, fabricates inaccurate causal actions. It has always amazed me that a cognitively complex human brain could conclude that wearing a certain pair of socks or touching certain body parts in a particular sequence would increase the chances of getting a great hit or throwing a perfect pitch in baseball. Nonetheless, it is difficult to see a professional baseball game without seeing public displays of these faulty contingencies, better known as superstitious behaviors. This is not to pick on baseball players—we are all susceptible to this contingency bias as we use our favorite pen to take a test or wear lucky underwear to an interview. As long as these behaviors are situation-specific and don't take the place of the actual actions leading to the desired outcomes (practicing baseball to prepare for the upcoming season, studying for a final exam, researching a company prior to an interview), they appear to pose little threat to mental health.

If the crowning glory of the human brain is the ability to effortlessly evaluate potential response outcomes in order to select the most adaptive option, then the healthiest brains are those that continue to monitor these contingencies throughout life. Brains that continue to be "grounded," in that they are able to read the most relevant aspects of a situation and incorporate pertinent past contingencies to make the most informed decisions, maintain the most impressive contingency calculators. Instead of running from, avoiding, or denying failure, we should analyze our inevitable mishaps just as a football team gathers to review the game it just played in an attempt to understand the most strategic responses that will lead to a desired outcome in subsequent games. Learning from our failures, at times, is even more important than learning from our successes—as failures offer critical information for recalibrating our contingency calculators.

Amy Bastian, director of the Motion Analysis Laboratory at Johns Hopkins School of Medicine, has learned that the brain's recognition of motor errors, something she calls error-driven learning, is critical for rehabilitation following a stroke. Patients who experience poststroke paralysis on one side of the body typically stride unevenly, making their walking pattern inefficient. Bastian's team uses a split-belt treadmill that allows the walking pace for each leg to be programmed separately to adjust the stride of each leg to help facilitate rehabilitation of the paralytic leg. But making small adjustments and instructing the patient to take shorter or longer steps to make their gait more symmetrical didn't produce meaningful results. Perhaps the team's efforts in attempting to prevent the patients from experiencing mistakes and falls was backfiring. If the treadmill was adjusted, however, so that gait asymmetry was exaggerated and patients therefore made obvious mistakes, their nervous system was then prompted to make the necessary corrections to produce a more symmetric gait. In a recent talk given at the Society for Neuroscience meeting, Bastian emphasized the importance of these patients "owning the error correction" in order to achieve improvements in their natural walking gaits. Thus, in this case, the brain needs to be aware of the error in the behavioral output in order to make the neural adjustments to reestablish symmetrical walking gaits. Although this is a very specific form of behavioral output, it raises concerns about our desire to mask errors as our children are learning certain skills.[12]

No Math Required

Although the words *contingency* and *calculator* conjure up images of probability theories and equations, mathematical ability is not necessary to calculate contingencies accurately. After all, our brains solve physics equations each time we catch a ball, clear a hurdle, or swing a golf club. We are most often unaware of the complicated equations brewing in our minds when we execute these actions. Our unawareness of our neural physics computations is perfectly fine; as long as a skill is practiced, precise calculations allow us to execute relevant skills almost effortlessly. In a similar manner, individuals who are always testing the water and exploring different outcomes are building impressive contingency libraries, or contingency capital, to consult in future scenarios characterized by uncertainty.

Of course, if one possesses mathematical skills, they can be put to good use when contingencies involve the actions of other people. Nobel Prize–winning mathematician John Nash proposed his Equilibrium Theory addressing how the most successful social decisions incorporate the probable actions of others. As famously depicted in the biopic of Nash, *A Beautiful Mind*, if all the men in a bar ask the woman patron deemed the "prettiest" out on a date, they will block each other's actions. In this case, the smartest move is to ask the second-most desirable woman out and avoid rejection. This is a simplistic example (and is one that is far from politically correct), but it clearly illustrates Nash's ideas about strategic responses produced by a hyperawareness of contingencies. And Nash put his contingency testing to the ultimate test when, after being diagnosed with schizophrenia, he eventually opted to forgo the traditionally prescribed antipsychotic medication as he continued to work in his office at Princeton University, where he solved his beloved mathematical theorems, keeping him grounded in the moment as he did this work. Eventually, amid the threatening hallucinations and delusions, a rational John Nash began to emerge as he became better and better at differentiating between imagined and actual response-outcome contingencies.[13] Thus, math skills are not required to enhance contingency calculators although, as discussed later in the book, knowledge of math and/or statistics can serve as a contingency prosthetic of sorts in facilitating the most sophisticated contingency calculations. Beyond the use of mathematics, however, the essential requirement for predicting future outcomes is maintaining relevant contingency capital through continued interactions with the environment and people around us. Instead of memorizing probability formulas, your time is better served living life—to its fullest! Being engaged and active, pushing the limits of the world around us, and exploring the unknown are all prime training grounds for establishing and fine-tuning the contingency calculators that differentiate humans from other mammals, even other opportunistic mammals.

Home Free! Or Are We?

Many creatures have amazing abilities that surpass those of humans. Your dog can detect the smell of another dog long before your brain registers those molecules, a honeybee can see shades of light that don't even register in your perceptual world, and snakes can detect infrared thermal radiation that can be detected by humans only by using special military devices. So, when it comes to sensory detection, humans fall short in many areas. However, it is difficult to compete with humans' sophisticated cognitive abilities. Humans and chimpanzees share about 96 percent genetic similarity (lower than originally thought), yet somewhere in the remaining 4 percent lie genetic codes leading to vast differences in cognitive abilities. Although the cognitive abilities of chimps are impressive, there is no real comparison to humans. Our ancestors' ability to navigate the tough decisions in life to find food, resources, and companionship in changing environments, all the while avoiding multiple threats, may have led to the human brain's impressive capabilities. Our human ancestors' constant contingency-testing enabled their brains to expand and transform their habitats (for better or worse!). Chimps forage for food and build nests, but they don't transform their environments.[14] One simply has to compare the exploding human population to the protected sanctuaries for dwindling populations of chimpanzees to gain insight into which species made more strategic responses ensuring their survival and success—that is, so far . . .

As previously mentioned, for many populations across the world our environment is very different from our ancestors' world—the habitat that nurtured our cognitive genius. Relatedly, a question that keeps me up at night is whether our cushy contemporary world, the shining product of our ancestors' impressive contingency calculators, is actually *compromising* our distinctive cognitive abilities. Could the brains that created a world allowing more passive and disengaged responses, accompanied by less dependence on contingency calculations for survival, actually compromise the cognitive ability of future generations? Are we domesticating our own brains? If so, will the continuing evolution of the human brain lead to smaller brains as observed in other animals? Or, will our health be affected in other ways? Psychologists such as University of Waterloo's James Danckert have conducted research on boredom—the absence of available outcome/response opportunities. It turns out that individuals who are bored are more likely to suffer from depression, attention deficit/hyperactivity disorder, and even cardiovascular disease.[15] Creating lifestyles that remove the brain's ability to calculate the most strategic responses may seem desirable but could lead to toxic boredom that creates rusty contingency calculators. These are all interesting experimental questions that are being explored at this very moment in our own brains. Evolution is a dynamic process that allows organisms to adapt to changing environments. It is never *done*. Even though the human brain is, at the time, generously stocked with brain cells and intricate networks, the complexity pendulum could swing a different way in the absence of environmental pressures. Perhaps we should all have that intelligence test now before it's too late.

Coming Attractions

The themes described in this introductory chapter will be elaborated in subsequent chapters to build a case that we need to engage in relevant contingency calculation exercises to maintain a sense of control over our environment and, accordingly, make the best decisions for our well-being. In a sense, these real-time calculations are a form of mental push-ups that build cognitive muscles for the challenges ahead and help us avoid life's potential brain bubbles leading to distortions of reality, emotional crashes, and the onset of a host of psychiatric illnesses. Our world has become increasingly complex, but this technologically driven environment may not be the healthiest backdrop for our brains. Many of us work long hours, feeling stress associated with career-related competition and promotions, but the potential outcomes are very different than those of our ancestors. When was the last time "avoid predators" was on your daily to-do list? Further, our technologically advanced society allows us to bypass many types of action-outcome scenarios that even our grand-parents encountered. Authentic, grassroots contingency experiences such as building our homes, growing our food, and preparing our meals each day are becoming less and less visible to our experience-craving brains. We can't let our contemporary "advanced" society shut down our contingency calculators that got us this far.

In the chapters that lie ahead, a formal introduction to the scientific study of behavior will be provided so that you will fully appreciate the brain's ability to generate healthy responses. The brain's contingency networks will also be explored before learning more about how various life situations such as privilege, poverty, and psychoactive medications can distort action-outcome contingencies. An enhanced understanding of the importance of accurate contingency calculations provides an interesting explanatory framework for variables identified by the Gallup polling organization as core elements for success in the workplace such as employee knowledge of a manager's expectations (i.e., outcomes) in their employment settings. The role of contingency forecasting in the treatment of various mental illnesses is an important application of accurate contingency calculators and will also be discussed. Of course, history can rewrite action-outcome contingency formulas, and this is often demonstrated in the excessive number of awards doled out each year—awards that don't always correctly associate actions with outcomes. The notion that our contingency calculators can be fine-tuned will also be considered in case studies which will inform us about varying types of contingency calculating abilities and career success. A glimpse of how the brain equips itself in perhaps one of the most dramatic turns of the contingency tables—that is, the arrival of a child—will also be explored. Protecting and caring for a person in addition to oneself obviously complicates contingency calculators. Our brains' predisposed tendency to search for adaptive action-outcome associations will also be considered in understanding how sham treatments can actually lead to healing, a phenomenon known as the placebo effect. On a lighter note, the phenomenon of make-believe contingencies will be discussed in the form of superstitions, creativity, and imagination. Finally, tips about avoiding the *contingency conundrum*—that is, using our calculated contingencies to avoid environmental traps that lead to compromised neural abilities—will be presented in the final chapter.

My hope is that this book will facilitate awareness about how our brain's never-ending processing of past and current experiences provides a valuable experiential backstory and distinct advantage for responding to unavoidable uncertainty throughout our lives. Once you are enlightened about this well-kept secret, you will be better equipped to opt for responses that lead to the most meaningful and desirable outcomes. Ironically, allowing our brains to *keep it real* by remaining grounded in real-life contingencies is the most effective strategy for translating your dreams into realities.

CHAPTER TWO

The Brain's Output
Behavior's Many Forms

I'M NOT PROUD OF the responses that emerge when I walk into a movie theater. Although I am typically overanalytical, these cognitive systems seem to momentarily shut down as I move toward the concession line in a zombie-like fashion to purchase popcorn. I'm perfectly aware of all the reasons this is NOT a smart choice—the popcorn is overpriced, too salty, excessively fattening and, when carefully scrutinized, probably shares more similarities with cardboard than with an actual food source. None of this seems to matter, however, as I anticipate sitting in the dark theater escaping into the movie's narrative and experiencing this sensory-rich gastronomical pleasure.

By all accounts, my snack choice in the movie theater represents perhaps the most unsophisticated decision-making in my entire cognitive-behavioral inventory. Similar to the reflexive responses displayed by the mirror-fighting reptile described in Chapter 1, my neural circuits also act in a reflexive, non-reflective manner in this movie theater context. In defense of the lizard, its brain is not nearly as complex as the human brain. The reptile brain is characterized by strongly imprinted reflexive responses that typically lead to the location of food, mates, and the successful defense of highly valued territories. The truth is that this works just fine for the lizard. Whereas

I can describe my reptilian-like reflexive behavior driving me toward the overpriced popcorn, I offer no excuses—it's the guilty pleasure that I have consciously elected to continue from my childhood—and I enjoy every crunch. But what happens in the movie theater needs to stay in the theater. Outside of this context, when faced with more sophisticated decisions with varied outcomes, I need to employ more brain power to make the most adaptive decisions.

As a behavioral neuroscientist, I have been fascinated by *all things behavior* since my undergraduate days at a small liberal arts institution, Samford University, in Birmingham, Alabama. As I began learning about the efforts of the ancient Greeks, enlightened philosophers, physiologists, and, ultimately, the behavioral psychologists and neuroscientists, my fascination grew. I couldn't learn enough about the formal and systematic analysis of behavior in whatever form it was presented. Three decades later, my enthusiasm to learn more about how the brain generates its moment-by-moment responses is as strong as ever, even though progress in this area has been slow at best. In this chapter, we'll retrace the steps of the past and current behavioral pioneers as we try to make sense of how our brains churn out complex behavioral output in various scenarios.

Behavioral Science Comes into Its Own

More than a thousand years ago, the Roman physician Galen predicted that organized behavioral responses were the product of some form of interactions between hypothesized nerves and the body's muscles. This idea lay dormant for several centuries as the causes of behavioral output were focused on more spiritual phenomena such as demons and spirits, far from a systematic, objective study. Finally, in the seventeenth century, René Descartes brought the potential study of behavior back to the forefront by suggesting that it could indeed be approached from a physical, rather than mystical, approach. But it appeared that even Descartes was cautious about suggesting that complex behavior could be the subject of scientific inquiry, as he suggested that the more complex behaviors existed outside the boundaries of scientific inquiry.[1]

It took another couple of centuries—to the early twentieth century—before an accidental discovery by Russian physiologist,

Ivan Pavlov, would enable pioneers in the new discipline of psychology to get the behavioral ball rolling.[2] Whereas the subjective workings of the mind were positioned in the academic wheelhouses of philosophers and religious scholars, Pavlov's reputation as a respected physiologist appeared to catapult the study of behavior into a more objective, scientific realm. In the midst of his Nobel Prize–winning research focusing on the physiology of the digestive system, Pavlov made a critical step toward being able to predict the behavior of his canine subjects. When the dogs became aware of approaching caretakers bringing their food, their behavior started to reorganize as it would in the actual presence of food. The small tubes that had been implanted in their mouths to monitor the amount of saliva produced when food was placed in the dog's mouth revealed the production of saliva to these predictive signals. That is, the dogs started salivating in anticipation of the food being in the mouth. Although Pavlov wasn't focused on behavioral output at the time, he saw that this reflexive-like behavioral response could explain some of the mysteries surrounding behavioral output. If two environmental events, in this case hearing the caretakers' footsteps and the presentation of a food bowl, were associated in the mental workings of an animal, the presentation of either one would prompt a response. The dogs started salivating when food was presented, but also when the sounds predicting the presence of food were detected. To use a human example, if a loud clap of thunder makes you wince in fear, and you know that lightning always precedes this thunder, you will also wince in response to the lightning in anticipation of the oncoming loud clap of thunder. The formulas for this basic type of learning known as classical conditioning were simple, but they were formulas nonetheless—bringing the topic of behavior into a more scientific context.

    In the United States, the discipline of psychology, defined today as the scientific study of behavior and mental processes, had stalled around the turn of the twentieth century. Although William James, often referred to as the father of U.S. psychology, had contributed the well-known *Psychological Principles* textbook, the discipline lacked the desired rigor of the more traditional sciences such as chemistry and physiology.[3] German physiologist Wilhelm Wundt, dubbed the father of psychology (from a more global perspective), emphasized the subjective technique known as introspection that required human subjects to report their inner feelings verbally.[4] No surprise that this methodological approach was viewed as lacking in scientific rigor. Further, Wundt's goal was to determine the elements of consciousness, also viewed as a subjective endeavor at the time. In fairness to Wundt, the tools of the future, such as functional magnetic resonance imaging (fMRI) scans that could more objectively record the workings of the brain and various mental states, were unavailable to these pioneers. Consequently, the discipline of psychology continued to float around philosophy, physiology, education, and religion departments . . . struggling to establish its own scientific identity.

In the eyes of the Southern charismatic psychologist James B. Watson, Pavlov was a game changer. In his famous talk, "Psychology as the Behaviorist Views It," Watson preached the virtues of the systematic study of behavior as introduced by Pavlov.[5] Instead of subjective personal stories that characterized Wundt's introspective approach, more objective data in the form of actual numbers could be entered into the lab journals—the delay in seconds to respond to stimuli, the volume of saliva produced, and the number of associations necessary to establish conditioning—all constituted objective observations that looked like science more than philosophy. Finally, it appeared that behavior could be studied under the auspices of the natural sciences such as biology, chemistry, and physics. Even though Pavlovian conditioning focused on simple, reflexive responses, Watson argued that this work transformed the discipline of psychology from the mystical to the empirical. In his position of authority at Johns Hopkins University, Watson began to sell Pavlov's approaches to the emerging discipline of psychology. He was influential for a short time until a scandalous affair with one of his graduate students became "viral" after being made public in newspaper articles across the country, prompting his abrupt dismissal from academia.

Others in the field of psychology also published varying ideas about the more scientific pursuit of behavior at the onset of the twentieth century. Columbia psychologist E. L. Thorndike introduced the classic "puzzle boxes," in which cats were placed in a small crate and challenged to solve the problem of how to open a door to get to a desired food reward.[6] Which response would lead to the desired outcome? This was done by seemingly random trial and error efforts until eventually the cat stumbled upon the response that opened the door, giving the cat access to the food reward. For example, the cat may have inadvertently stepped on a lever that was attached to a pulley that opened the door. When this happened, the next attempts were more predictable and efficient as the cat appeared to be learning the correct response (stepping on the lever) that led to the desired food. Thorndike dubbed this phenomenon the "Law of Consequences," or "Law of Effect," to capture the idea that consequences drove the production of specific behaviors. The use of the term *law* added to the more scientific appearance of the new science of behavior. As you will learn throughout this book, hard and fast laws are few and far between when it comes to the study of behavior. Although this has been a frustrating issue for behaviorists trying to build a respected science of behavior, contemporary scientists from multiple and diverse disciplines are beginning to appreciate that behavioral flexibility is one of nature's most impressive behavioral engineering achievements in enhancing the survival probability of our species. But we're getting ahead of the story . . .

Harvard-trained psychologist B. F. Skinner carried the behaviorism torch in the mid-twentieth century by conducting research in an area he described as "radical behaviorism" to distinguish himself from psychologists interested in the subjective inner workings of the mind.[7] Skinner was interested in how an environmental event influenced an animal's response. His version of behaviorism focused on stimulus-response associations as opposed to the stimulus-stimulus associations characterizing Pavlov's behavioral approach. A cockroach running across your kitchen floor (stimulus) may prompt you to stomp it with your shoe (response), and if this response resulted in killing the cockroach (desired outcome), the cockroach stomping response will likely be repeated upon future cockroach encounters. Thus, Skinner spoke of animals achieving successful contingencies when they exhibited the correct response to the correct stimulus to produce the desired consequence.[8] In his lab, the rats pressed levers in small arenas known as Skinner Boxes. He emphasized the importance of reinforcers and even schedules of reinforcers in understanding behavioral outcomes. As it emerged, this type of learning became known as operant conditioning, as the animal "operated" on its environment.[9] Psychologists clamored around these new scientific ideas, and the introduction of new science-sounding terms such as schedules of reinforcement, response outcomes, associative learning, and response engineering seemed to move the discipline a little closer to gaining scientific respect. Or, did it?

Skinner was a brilliant scientist and writer but, even with this acknowledged insight, his version of behavioral science lacked a critical element . . . umm . . . the BRAIN. He expressed his disinterest in the workings of the "black box" and any mention of personal and subjective mental properties, and made the executive decision to ignore the one organ that drove the very executive functions he wanted so desperately to understand. A few steps forward, a few steps backward.

It would be inaccurate to suggest that no one was exploring the role of the brain in psychological concepts such as learning during the mid-twentieth century. Among the pioneers was physiological psychologist Karl Lashley, who was hired by Harvard University at one point in his career after the search committee members concluded that he fit their criterion of being the best psychologist in the world. Lashley reminded the discipline of psychology that the brain had to be factored into any explanations of behavior. He was the first to admit, however, that this was easier said than done— especially with the rather crude methodological tools he had at his fingertips. After many valiant attempts to locate the specific brain area responsible for forming memories—the "engram"—he had to declare it simply didn't exist in the specific form he originally envisioned. Alternatively, memory formation was a product of "mass action" of the cerebral cortex, with the brain's organization playing an important role in achieving complex functions.[10] Lashley was a bit ahead of his time—as the technology advanced in the field of neuroscience, the intricate workings of the brain in learning, memory, and problem-solving would become undeniable.

Acknowledging Behaviorism's Dirty Little Secrets

In addition to being a bit extreme and simplistic, the early behaviorism theories and laws faced additional challenges. When the new behaviorism truths were taken for various test drives outside of the controlled context of the laboratory, the behaviors were a little less predictable. Experimental psychologist John Garcia of the Univer-

sity of California, Berkeley, found that, contrary to laboratory predictions, virtually no training was necessary to associate two stimuli,
or "events," when one of the stimuli made an animal sick.[11] He discovered this when water paired with radiation was avoided by rats
after a single trial. This was different from the observation that several trials were necessary for Pavlov's version of behavioral conditioning. If you have ever suffered from food poisoning you have also
been a subject of this one trial conditioning known as conditioned
taste aversion. Even though you know that the sushi made you sick
only because it had gone bad, you will never eat that type of sushi
again. Obviously, there were some types of learning that nature
couldn't leave to either chance or training persistence.

Additionally, the fixed "stamped in" behavior that was ultimately
conditioned in Thorndike's puzzle boxes would often become less
stamped in as animals started to tweak the responses after they had
become well established. They would go off-task and fiddle with
other aspects of the cage, acting less like the optimized robots predicted by the behaviorism theories. Yes, the animals showed improvement—they were learning—but they also seemed to be looking for new ways to produce favorable outcomes. This drives us crazy
in my own lab. My students will spend weeks training animals until
they flawlessly navigate a maze or obstacles to achieve their coveted
Froot Loop rewards. Then, at that critical moment, as the student
researchers start recording data during the test trials (when the data
count and will determine the likelihood of publishing the results),
the animals often appear distracted. The students have described
their responses as "goofing off" or getting bored with the same way
of doing the task. It's as if they tell themselves, "I've got this so
there's no rush . . . the Froot Loop will always be in the baited
well . . . why rush and be placed back in my laboratory cage, the trial
is three minutes and I want to be out of my cage the entire time."
Forgive my anthropomorphism in giving the rats a human voice,
but you see my point. These new behavioral trends are interesting
and confirm that the rats are indeed a pretty good model for studying human behavior, especially the behavior of children in a classroom, but not a great one for that manuscript or endless stream of
grant proposals necessary to obtain funds to conduct the research.

I'm not the first behavioral scientist to get frustrated with so-called trained animals. Exceptions to Skinner's behaviorism rules were publicly described in a famous article written by two of his former graduate students, Keller and Marion Breland, who by that time were a married team.[12] When they used Skinner's operant conditioning to train animals for commercials and other forms of entertainment, the conditioning didn't always stick. The Brelands thought they had successfully trained raccoons to put coins in the bank for a bank television commercial until the raccoons started taking the coins to their water bowl, appearing to wash them, before dropping them in the bank. Of course, this trick would have been even cuter with pigs placing coins in a piggy bank, so they trained the pigs on this task. After successfully demonstrating the desired behavior they, like the raccoons, added their own twist. Instead of immersing their coins in water, they started rooting them around on the floor. These training hiccups were referred to as instinctual drifts and were embraced by comparative psychologists and ethologists, who easily discerned that naturally evolved responses were interfering with the acquired learning response patterns: raccoons naturally forage by searching for food in water, while pigs naturally forage by rooting around in dirt. It was a battle of the behaviors!

Then there were the animals who responded when there was no apparent stimulus evoking a response. What was behind the burst of play in a puppy sitting in a completely quiet room? Or the sudden performance of a unique song by a child sitting motionless in the backseat of his parent's car? What could the puppy and the child be responding to? What was the triggering stimulus? How could a child perform a behavior (singing an impromptu song) she had never encountered? According to the behaviorists, all of our responses were the product of training and rehearsal. Could innovation be taught or conditioned? Maybe. When I recently took my comparative animal behavior students to the Dolphin Research Center in Grassy Key, Florida, I was impressed to learn that the trainers declared that they had conditioned the dolphins to perform a new trick each time they gave them the hand signal for the behavior *innovate*. Can innovation be shaped and trained? Regardless of the answer, it was clear that these observations would muddy the waters for the extreme behaviorism views.

Irrespective of whether innovative responses can be conditioned, we routinely respond to stimuli in novel ways that don't appear to be easily explained by classical or operant conditioning. In a famous study thought to demonstrate the sudden emergence of insight in an animal's behavioral repertoire, German psychologist Wolfgang Kohler created a new problem scenario to determine if chimpanzees could solve it without being trained to do so.[13] After introducing the chimps to a cage with a banana hanging from the top, out of reach, he also threw in a few crates and a long stick. These chimps made behavioral psychology headlines when they stacked the crates together, climbed on top of them, and knocked down the bananas with the stick. And this was nothing compared with what the '80s television protagonist MacGyver could do to escape from various predicaments to save both his life and many others' lives week after week. Need to diffuse a bomb with string and Silly Putty? No problem! Although the laboratory behaviorists loved their training charts and tables, it was becoming apparent that behavior didn't always follow the training rules.

Although it was unclear whether and to what extent innovative responses were the product of training, they were most definitely the product of the brain. I agree with Karl Lashley that, even though the tools for investigating the brain were unsophisticated at the time, the brain should have been incorporated into the behaviorism formulas from the beginning. Pavlov was the exception because he claimed that the cerebral hemispheres were responsible for complex behavior.[14] Further, the early behaviorists' quest for understanding the most predictable animal behaviors led them a bit astray. If all behavior was as predictable and inflexible as indicated by the early behavioral findings, we would be extremely limited in our lifestyle options, never able to respond to novel challenges and move to more attractive scenarios. Life is more accurately represented by having multiple contingencies at our fingertips, not a single bar to press.

Another line of research that threatened the rigorous rules of the behaviorists was the famous developmental work conducted by Harry Harlow. If behavior is driven by external reinforcers, why did the rhesus monkeys in his experiments spend more time climbing on the soft, cuddly surrogate monkey mothers than on the cold, wire surrogate monkey mothers that provided their milk? Shouldn't the milk reward drive the response and keep the monkeys on the wire surrogates longer? No, the young motherless monkeys spent more time on the surrogate that offered no visible external reinforcers. Harlow declared that he had shifted from his previous focus on learning to that of love.[15] As discussed in Chapter 7, parenting and social bonds incorporate important internal rewards that were ignored by the extreme behaviorists.

And then there's the fact that we're not clones—we each respond a bit differently to the same environmental events. How did this factor fit in radical behaviorism ideas? Even though individual differences weren't emphasized in the classic behavioral theories, there was no denying their existence.[16] Nineteenth-century Dutch psychologist F. C. Donders provided clues about the lack of predictability of various behaviors when he reported the first evidence of individual differences, as opposed to individual consistencies, in reaction times. In this case, astronomers watching the same star cross a certain position in the sky each reported that it did so at a different time. Donders realized that this inconsistency was the result of the astronomers' differing reaction times. In subsequent brilliant experiments, for example, he found that reaction times were longer when subjects were presented with two buttons, each with a signaling light directing the participant toward the correct button to press, than when they were confronted with only a single button. With this work, Donders was one of the earliest scientists to measure choice and decision-making objectively. Another nineteenth-century pioneer, German physiologist Gustav Fechner, attempted to formalize the introspection process by introducing the term *just noticeable difference*, referring to the amount of change needed to appear in a stimulus (e.g., brightness of a light) before it could be noticed as qualitatively different by the subject. As you may predict, individual differences existed in this perceptual work as well, probably fueled by varying sensitivities in the sensory systems of study participants. On the surface, these methodological innovations appeared to focus more on mental as opposed to behavioral processes, but at the end of the day sensory perceptions, decision-making speed, and behavioral execution all had a common denominator—the brain—that was demanding to be a respected player in this new discipline.

Although to the tried-and-true behaviorists it was the research equivalent of opening Pandora's box, there was no going forward with understanding behavior unless the brain's role in behavioral and mental processes could be understood. In retrospect, Skinner may have been smart to avoid all the confusion of incorporating the brain in his explanation of the production of behavioral output, as the brain's role was anything but simple. But it was becoming clear that gaining the most accurate information about the critical role of behavior in maintaining an animal's survival involved learning more about how neural systems choreographed real-time and relevant behavior, regardless of its form.

Understanding Behavior: Thinking Inside the Box

Although the behavioral pioneers are to be commended for providing methods to bridge the gap between philosophical and physiological approaches to behavior, the early approaches focused on the simpler behavioral outputs . . . more reflexive than reflective. Or, in the words of Nobel Prize–winner Daniel Kahneman, responses that were the result of *fast*, as opposed to *slow*, thinking.[17] This trend started well before Pavlov, as Descartes described a simplistic sensory input–motor output algorithm. At one level, this view is right on the money. If you touch a hot stove your sensory neurons will deliver a message of heat, pain, and discomfort to your central nervous system, which will quickly divert the message to the appropriate nerve cells that will allow you to instantaneously remove your finger before your skin starts sizzling. Sensory information in; motor response out. This needs to be a fast response to avoid extensive tissue damage. In fact, this superfast response doesn't even require the involvement of your brain—your spinal cord can manage such simplistic situations.

Neuroscience pioneer Charles Sherrington's description of the mechanism of the brain's information processing supported this simple idea of neural functions. The term *synapse*, literally *to clasp*, was introduced by Sherrington to refer to a tiny gap between two nerve cells filled with neurochemicals that selectively activated certain responses of neighboring brain cells. This work earned Sherrington a shared Nobel Prize in 1932 and served as a template that further reinforced the idea of simple incoming messages being connected with simple motor responses in a reflexive, predictable way.[18]

And the early behavioral work also reinforced the simplistic nature of behavioral output. Pavlov's psychical reflex, Thorndike's problem-solving laws, and Skinner's iconic graphs of various reinforcement schedules all began to paint a simple mechanical picture of the inner workings of the black box.

If only life's choices were so simple. Once you move beyond rats in cages, it's more difficult to respond reflexively when several choices are simultaneously presented in the real world. Even the mundane task of selecting toothpaste from the dozens of options on the drug store shelf appears to involve a different form of learning and neural connections than described by the behavioral and neural pioneers. And toothpaste is simple in the relative scheme of our life decisions. What about deciding on a life partner? Whether or not to have a baby? The right career path? Or, perhaps more important than any other decision . . . whether life is worth living? Once the response moves from simple to complex and from predictable to unpredictable, the decision-making/behavioral output story starts to get much more complicated, regardless of what those early psychology textbooks told us about behavior.

During the 1990s, researchers in the field of neuroeconomics set out to understand how the brain arrived at the hard decisions in life. Whereas the early behaviorists tried to separate themselves from the subjective inner workings of mental processes, these brave new scientists embraced these challenges. For good reason, in order for behaviorism to establish relevance beyond training animals in laboratory tasks or circus tricks, the field needed to merge with other areas such as cognitive science and economics to produce more relevant answers about how and why the brain produces one behavior over another. In a refreshing new approach, New York University's Paul Glimcher and his colleagues focused the light on just what was happening inside the black box that Skinner tried so hard to avoid.[19] To accomplish this, the neuroeconomics pioneers created very different tasks. Instead of emphasizing a clear-cut response that leads to certain rewards, experimental scenarios were characterized by ambiguity and uncertainty. Further, with the use of the new and improved brain imaging tools of the late twentieth century, the inner workings of the brain were front and center in this new behavioral approach.

Rhesus monkeys were a popular subject in these early neuro-economics studies. Addressing the real-world observation that the actual association between certain stimuli and rewards is sometimes ambiguous (should I order the pasta or the seafood tonight?), this observation was mimicked in a laboratory setup in which monkeys were presented with ambiguous tasks. For example, the monkeys were trained to associate the movement of dots in a specific direction (right vs. left) on a visual screen with a juice reward. To step up the complexity, these animals were ultimately presented with a screen displaying what appeared to be chaotically moving dots moving both right and left. There was also a small coherent group of dots, however, moving in a particular direction among the more chaotic action. As the monkeys integrated the incoming visual information with past reinforcement, cells in the cortical area that controlled eye movements were activated, as well as brain cells that this area regularly communicates with—an area known as the posterior parietal cortex.[20] This was definitely more complicated than pressing a bar when a light came on in a Skinner Box!

Far from the earlier, more reflexive behavioral studies, neuro-economics approaches force the animal to strategically evaluate information to make the most informed response. Eventually, the group of dots is identified so the correct response can be made. But, again, in the real world there may not be enough presenting evidence to determine a clear preference about optimal responses, even though our brain seems to search for reasons to make certain responses. In situations when the brain can't detect distinguishing features between different options, there are ways of tipping the scales in a specific direction. Neuroscientist Read Montague, currently at the Virginia Tech Carilion Research Institute, and his colleagues presented a taste test to human subjects before peering into their brains via fMRI scans. The subjects were asked to choose between two popular sodas, Coke and Pepsi.[21] However, they didn't know which was which. With the missing identifying information (a red or a blue soda can, for example), the brain scans revealed no indication that it could tell the difference between these two sodas through mere taste discrimination. However, when the all-too-familiar branding information was presented in the form of a Coke or Pepsi can prior to the presentation of the soda, the scans suddenly exhibited a different activation pattern. As the majority of subjects now claimed to prefer the Coke sample over the Pepsi sample, a section of the prefrontal cortex known for its role in executive functions, as well as an area involved in memory, lit up. This type of research targeting the inner workings of the "black box" prior to engaging in certain behaviors allowed Montague to visualize the neural correlates of persuasion. All of a sudden, the once celebrated "laws of behavior" were becoming much more complicated. Clearly, the brain's response to environmental clues has a huge impact on the responses we make minute by minute throughout the day.

So, as you listen to two political candidates to determine who best represents your political beliefs, brain areas such as the posterior parietal cortex (above your ear area) and prefrontal cortex (behind your eyes), both components of the outer layer of the brain known as the neocortex, are likely activated as your neural system determines who deserves your vote. More information about neuroeconomics and specific brain areas that help us navigate the uncertainty in our lives will be discussed in Chapter 4. Even with an increasing awareness of the brain's complexity in determining responses in specific situations, there's evidence that the brain often takes advantage of shortcuts in the form of habits when ambiguity shifts toward certainty.

Brain Habits

As we repeat familiar behaviors and they lead to familiar and predictable results, the amount of brain scrutiny necessary for behavioral output begins to diminish. When I first started driving, I'm quite certain that my cortical areas were buzzing as I carefully processed incoming information to determine when I needed to begin accelerating to pass a car before merging onto the exit ramp, or just how much time I had before a yellow light turned red. Today, the neural energy devoted to those decisions has been downgraded as I have become a more experienced driver. But more experience isn't always the perfect solution for adaptive behavioral output. Although my driving has become more consistent and reliable through the years as I have gained valuable experience, my relaxed demeanor and daydreaming may make me more vulnerable than I was as a newbie driver with my hands clenching the wheel. As behaviors morph from awkward, insecure responses to choreographed habits, there's a costly shift in attention—a trade-off for expertise. But, of course, there's a benefit for developing these habits.

MIT neuroscientist Ann Graybiel has spent her distinguished career disentangling habits from goal-directed behavior to determine exactly which brain areas manage the shift from goal-seeking behaviors in their early learning phases to more reflexive habits.[22] The benefits of habits are obvious. Once you figure out certain behavioral patterns, you don't need to devote so much of the brain's energy toward that tried and true behavioral experience. Whereas you may have had to think about all the aspects of preparing an omelet the first several times you made one, after a while, you shift to habit mode and proceed through the steps in a somewhat robotic fashion. The saved neural energy can be devoted to other tasks such as having a conversation with someone or thinking through the next day's activities while you're cooking the omelet.

As depicted in Figure 3, Graybiel's research suggests that a large cluster of brain structures in the central portion of the brain, known collectively as the basal ganglia, facilitates the shift from learning mode to what many refer to as being on "automatic pilot." In the early stages of learning a task, the lower portion of this brain structure is engaged as you try to figure out how everything works. This lower, or ventral, area is positioned close to a brain area viewed simplistically as the goal-directed pleasure center of the brain known as the nucleus accumbens (a more thorough, contemporary consideration of this brain area will be covered in Chapter 6). The signature neurochemical of this structure, dopamine, helps to guide the exploratory behavior, accentuating the important aspects of the new response. But once the exploration is complete and the new environmental context has been mastered, the upper section of the basal ganglia begins to take over. This shift in brain area reflects a shift in attention as less attention and scrutiny are involved once you have mastered the task and proceed with the more automated response. This may explain why you didn't notice the eggshells that managed to find their way into the omelet mixture.

Although efficiency is often desired, it is easy to see how habits can lead us to dangerous and undesired predicaments. The minute

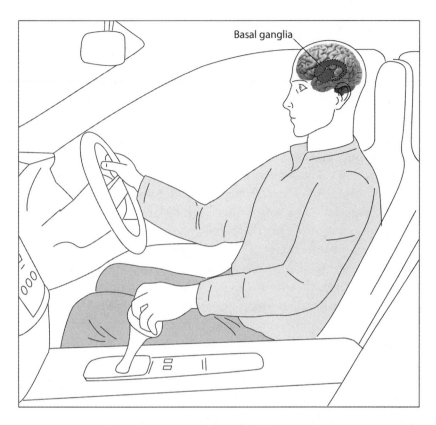

Figure 3. Basal Ganglia Drives Habitual Behavior. *The large collection of structures in the center of the brain collectively known as the basal ganglia plays an increasingly important role as behaviors shift from requiring attention to a more reflexive response mode. Although reflexive responses appear more efficient on the surface, the lack of attention in habitual responding may lead to accidents when performing tasks for which we feel we have gained mastery and competence, such as driving, cooking, etc. (Image by Bill Nelson)*

we let our evaluative guard down, we become more vulnerable to the inevitable curve balls life throws our way. As your brain is on automatic pilot reviewing the conversation you plan to have with your boss later that morning, you may not notice the car that speeds through the red light or the child that suddenly runs into the street to retrieve a ball. Thus, it is advisable to remain as vigilant as possible even when going through the mundane motions of life. And you can imagine how important it is to keep the basal ganglia–enforced habit mode at bay when performing something more than a mundane task. You definitely don't want your surgeon lapsing into habit mode and not noticing he left those forceps beside your lung before closing you up. Key Dismukes, previous chief scientist for human factors research at NASA, conducted research confirming that, considering the number of mistakes that take place in the airplane cockpit when pilots go on a basal ganglia mode of automatic pilot, you definitely don't want your actual pilot lapsing into habit mode. Even with a multitude of enforced checklists, it's difficult to keep the brain on task, especially in a world filled with distractions. Consequently, Dismukes, along with his colleagues, wrote *The Multitasking Myth* to convey the vulnerability of a brain attempting to multitask in dangerous situations.[23] Even though we have illusions that we are effective multitaskers, there are plenty of cases in which, even when performing simple routines, our so-called multitasking leads to tragedy. Perhaps the most gut-wrenching examples of our behavioral vulnerabilities are seen in the cases of parents who, absorbed in the routine of driving or taking in the groceries, forget that their child is also in the car, a deadly error in extreme temperatures. It's inconceivable that we could ever be that distracted, but there are plenty of unfortunate child deaths to prove us wrong.

On a lighter note, this lesson was brought to my attention about two decades ago, when I attended the annual meeting of the Southern Society for Philosophy and Psychology. As a speaker took the podium to describe his research, he opened with a bizarre story of a habit gone wrong. He shared that he brushed his teeth prior to the talk but noticed—after it was too late—that he was brushing his teeth with Preparation H, a popular hemorrhoid medication packaged similarly to toothpaste. He earnestly conveyed that he wasn't sure of the impact of ingesting Preparation H orally, so he felt compelled to announce this prior to his talk should he suffer a dire reaction during his presentation, necessitating a call to emergency medical technicians. For him, the product labeling on the tube and the funny taste as he swished the Preparation H through his teeth and around his mouth failed to break the habitual routine his basal ganglia had created for tooth brushing, even though something was off. Such a response can be explained by our knowledge of the neural circuits underlying habitual responses. His decision, however, to share this embarrassing information to a room full of professional colleagues who wondered about potential unsanitary places the tube had been is a little more difficult to explain. It's not clear which brain area we should blame for that interesting behavioral output known as a faux pas.

What's a Shrew to Do?

In many cultures people can find food virtually anywhere they look. For these individuals it's difficult to imagine a time when their ancestors lived with a constant awareness of hunger and looming starvation. For those of an earlier era, a majority of their cognitive power would certainly have been devoted to searching and securing food, a response known as *foraging* behavior. In fact, researchers have dedicated a lot of time to determining optimal foraging strategies that yield the most valuable food payoffs for a diverse array of animals. Skinner can also be credited for his early foraging research (laboratory-style) with his varying schedules of reinforcement. Outside of the constraints of a laboratory, if an animal has to direct a lot of energy toward chasing or capturing a food source that has minimal nutritional content, this particular strategy typically doesn't qualify as an optimal foraging strategy. However, if this is the only available food source, then it quickly becomes an optimal foraging strategy. We now know many factors that contribute to the most optimal foraging strategies. Energy expenditure, safety, consistency of availability, richness of nutritional content, and competition are just a few factors that affect a food payoff. Throughout evolution, the need to sharpen probability skills to determine optimal food searching strategies bolstered the complexity of the brain.

Take the common shrew, for example. Yes, that tiny rodent with an aardvark-like pointy nose and little beads for eyes that is prevalent across Europe. Weighing about the same as just two or three pennies, it has to pretty much consume its weight in food each day to survive. With an extremely high metabolic rate and excessive energy loss due to its very small body, these little mammals have to eat every couple of hours to avoid certain death—and they can't order out! Even though it's not clear how much awareness shrews have of their precarious situation and looming death, their nervous system is tuned into foraging possibilities since they are always just one meal and a couple of hours from death.[24]

The shrews' ongoing metabolic crisis leaves little room for foraging errors. Not only do they need to expend minimal energy for a calorie payoff, they need to be careful not to become a meal for predators such as owls or foxes. And, can you imagine what the added pressure of a female having a litter of energy-demanding pups does to this precarious metabolic formula? Scientists have taken advantage of the shrew's dire feeding situation to learn more about behavioral output in the form of risk-taking and decision-making by altering the yield of multiple potential feeding sights in the lab. For example, in one study shrews were given a choice between a food bowl that always delivered one piece of food, yummy mealworms in this case, or a food bowl that delivered two pieces of food, but just half of the time. The shrews opted for the safe consistent payoff source of one reward for each visit. However, after the researchers removed both food options from the cage for a while, the shrews opted for the riskier payoff of two pieces of food as their hunger increased.[25] This is an example of an environmentally induced brain switch that directed the animals toward different outcome contingencies to optimize the caloric payoff. Yes, the shrews are unknowingly engaging in some advanced probability calculations.

Perhaps these complex food searching strategies help explain a long-standing brain mystery. Whereas a human's brain typically makes up 2 percent of its body weight, the shrew's brain makes up a whopping 10 percent. In fact, across the *entire* animal kingdom no animal sports a higher brain-to-body ratio than the tiny shrew. We now know that intelligence and cognitive complexity are influenced by more than just the ratio of brain weight to body weight but, even so, the generous size of the shrew brain has never made a lot of sense. What's up with having such a large brain? Even though I've yet to come across any evidence of impressive intellectual abilities in these animals, it may be that the shrew's ongoing food crisis requires a specialized form of uber-cognitive sophistication for problem-solving in these specific foraging scenarios. Or maybe, since they lack the ability for impromptu problem-solving, they need to store more information about how to habitually respond to these foraging scenarios, and they need more space—kind of like needing a larger brain suitcase because they don't have a very sophisticated way of packing their neural tissue. Regardless of the function of their larger brain, it is possible that the urgency with which the shrew has to locate food every two–three hours requires a larger than usual investment in neural machinery than brains found in larger mammals with less energy loss and lower metabolic rates. These unassuming little animals may represent the foraging savants of the animal kingdom.

That's a Head-Scratcher!

Earlier in this chapter, Pavlov's research studies designed to detect predictions in behavioral output were described. Animals learned that a light presaged the presentation of food, and, after sufficient training, they prepared to receive food every time the light was presented. As groundbreaking as these studies of classical conditioning were, it has been pointed out in this chapter that, unless you live in a world of perfect predictions, the relevance of this observation goes only so far. In actuality, the most predictable feature of our lives is the unpredictable nature of life's events.

Later in his career, one of Pavlov's assistants, N. R. Shenger-Krestovnikova, designed a study to determine just how disruptive uncertainty could be in certain situations. In this experimental prelude to future neuroeconomics studies, she trained dogs to respond to a circle to receive desired food. The animals also learned that responding to an oval shape never resulted in receiving the desired food. So, when a circle and an oval were presented together, the dogs knew to respond to the circle to get the food. Then the task got tricky. The oval was morphed so that it started to look more and more like a circle and completely confused the dogs. You may think that, in the big scheme of life contingencies, this wasn't a very big deal for the dogs. According to Pavlov's description, the dogs thought otherwise.

> The whole behavior of the animal underwent an abrupt change. The hitherto quiet dog began to squeal in its stand, kept wriggling about, tore off with its teeth the apparatus for mechanical stimulation of the skin, and bit through the tubes

connecting the animal's room with the observer, a behavior which never happened before.[26]

Animal behaviorists refer to behaviors observed in unexpected situations as displacement behaviors. Humans do this as well. When presented with a perplexing situation with no clear-cut answer, we may scratch our heads or tap a pen on our leg. Regardless of what the conflicting situation is, it's unclear how scratching your head or tapping a pen may help you solve the problem. If we want to depict uncertainty in a PowerPoint presentation, we use an avatar of a human form scratching its head and circumscribed by question marks. Scratching your head can certainly fill a purpose if your scalp suddenly itches, but seems somewhat displaced in situations characterized by uncertainty.

These observations provide convincing evidence that displaced behaviors are a marker of a brain that is struggling with contingency formulas—unable to determine the consequences of making a specific response. But, interestingly, this displaced, seemingly dysfunctional behavior may ultimately have a function of allowing us to respond in a somewhat familiar way (pacing, scratching, etc.) to calm our anxiety and enable us to push through the uncertainty to arrive at the best response. At times, however, even with the boost of a therapeutic head-scratching, our circumstances keep our contingency calculators from making accurate responses. Life contexts such as poverty, celebrity, psychoactive drugs, emotional and physical abuse, and impaired neural functions can result in contingency deficiencies that ultimately manifest themselves in the form of psychiatric illnesses such as obsessive-compulsive disorder, posttraumatic stress disorder, and depression.[27] We'll learn more about these maladaptive responses to uncertainty in Chapter 8.

It's interesting to consider that an aspect of these contingency calculations may be an empirical basis for what philosophers call *free will*. The philosophers who served as the precursors for the field of psychology considered free will as something unique to humans, somehow separate from the natural forces that influence other functions. The brain's calculations of the consequences of responses could be considered as a more natural interpretation of free will in that these brain-based calculations, determined most often by past experiences, influence individual responses. Given this complexity, it's unlikely that two people will respond to similar situations in exactly the same way. Consequently, "free will" is a more accurate description of flexible and informed behavioral output than the "fixed will" in the form of predicted responses that seemed to be proposed by the early behaviorists.[28]

As interesting as the discussion of philosophical terms such as free will may be, we'll turn next to a discussion of the inner workings of the brain—the control center for contingency calculations. In order to learn about the most effective production of contingency calculations, it's important to understand more about the organ that facilitates the production of these strategic moves. This will get us one step closer to preventing emerging brain bubbles as we understand more about the neural response patterns that lead to the most adaptive behavioral and desirable outcomes.

CHAPTER THREE

The Human Brain
An Embarrassment of Riches

LTHOUGH MANY MYSTERIES PERSIST about the brain's functions, the pace at which neuroscientists have been stockpiling information inventories of the brain's physical characteristics is mind-numbing. In the past half-century,
rapidly evolving sophisticated methodologies have allowed neuroscientists to investigate the brain in numerous ways, taking us light
years beyond the old-fashioned studies in which scientists would
damage a brain area in an animal model and observe its impact or,
when working with humans, wait until natural damage was done before assessing its effects.[1] Using these crude techniques, researchers
could associate certain brain areas with basic abilities such as aggression or hunger, but those unsophisticated methodological techniques
provided little in the way of explaining how or why these effects were
observed. Using contemporary techniques ranging from genetic manipulations to imaging the brain in real-time, researchers have generated massive volumes of data.

Existing in today's tsunami of neuroscience information, we have
difficulty imagining a time when virtually nothing was known about
the brain. However, that was essentially the status of the field as recently as the late eighteenth century. No objective and reliable data
were available to promote even informed speculation; the method-

ological disadvantages positioned the discipline of brain science behind more objective and established disciplines such as physics and
mathematics. At least researchers were focusing on the correct body
organ, the brain. Although the earliest methods were crude, the acknowledgement that the brain was the sole organ of the body associated with thoughts, behavior, and emotions—a bold premise
introduced by Hippocrates in the fourth-century BC—was quite a
triumph in itself. But now that the brain was the target of investigation, scholars had virtually no idea what turned it on and what maintained its critical functions. In this chapter, current knowledge about
operating the brain's circuits will be discussed, a necessary detour
from our discussion of behavioral outcomes. Subsequent chapters,
however, will return behavior and sharpened contingency calculations to the forefront.

Brain Imaging through the Centuries

When attention was first directed toward the brain, this three-and-
a-half-pound organ was viewed as nothing more than a pile of mush.
Not until the insightful discovery of a specific "brain stain" in the
latter part of the nineteenth century was an outline of the cells contained within the brain's mushy tissue first revealed. Italian scientist
Camillo Golgi discovered this brain staining technique, hoping to
learn more about how the brain pulled off its impressive feats. Sadly,
Golgi failed to see what was right before his eyes and didn't quite
catch the individual nature of these brain cells. In Spain, Santiago
Ramon y Cajal studiously examined brain tissue stained with Golgi's
new stain and accurately discerned that it consisted of individual
cells as opposed to the continuous network that Golgi had described
(as depicted in Figure 4, brain tissue stained with Golgi's famous stain
from my neuroscience laboratory). Together, Cajal and Golgi were
awarded the Nobel Prize in 1906.[2]

At a Society for Neuroscience meeting about a decade ago I
couldn't resist indulging in one of my favorite guilty pleasures—
visiting a historical book booth managed by John Gach, a knowl-
edgeable book collector who specialized in original volumes related
to brain and behavior. The book that "spoke" to me on this visit was
J. Batty Tuke's *The Insanity of Over-Exertion of the Brain*, published in

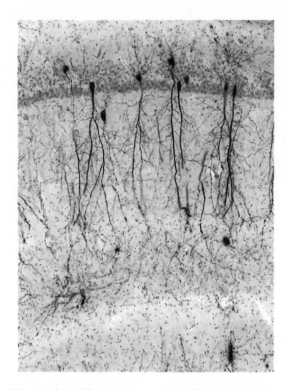

Figure 4. Distinctly Different Neuronal Cells. *Although he created the "brain stain" that provided the first glimpse of individual brain cells, Camillo Golgi's own brain held on to his current thoughts about the cells being continuous in form. It took the fresh perspective of Santiago Ramon y Cajal to see that the cells, known as neurons, were distinctly different. Subsequent research, however, would need to be conducted before scientists understood how these individual cells communicated. (Photo courtesy of Lambert Neuroscience Laboratory, University of Richmond)*

1894.[3] This book chronicled a series of lectures delivered to the Royal College of Physicians of Edinburgh in which Tuke attempted to persuade the medical audience that the key to understanding psychiatric illness was understanding the inner workings of the brain. But the pièce de résistance was the beautiful colored frontispiece of this old book—a foldout drawing of layers of brain cells known as neurons, seemingly all connected like river tributaries. This was likely the first introduction of these odd little cells in an English publication. The conference attendees and readers of Tuke's book were indeed in for a treat as they absorbed the intricate details and majestic beauty of the mushy brain tissue. Over a century later, as I held this book in my hands, I marveled at this picture and convinced myself that, regardless of the price, its home was on my bookshelf.

Once the characteristics of neurons were described, it was important to learn more about how they were clustered and positioned throughout the brain. Long before functional MRIs were around to take high resolution images of the brain in real time to match brain areas with seemingly specific functions such as listening to music or solving calculus problems, one of my favorite brain pioneers, Franz Joseph Gall, started mapping out brain functional images in the early part of the nineteenth century. Gall was so passionate about understanding the brain's components that he refused to let a little detail such as not having the proper equipment to generate the images hold him back. His limited accumulated knowledge of the human brain and limitless imagination seemed to be sufficient for the task. He proposed that specific clusters of brain cells manifested themselves in bulges on the outside layer of the brain, known as the cortex, and the size of these bulges was directly proportional to the abilities of the person. These weren't bulges in the figurative sense of the word as suggested in the Introduction; they were proposed as literal skull and brain bulges, or bumps. The bump for keeping track of time, for example, was larger in individuals with a keen sense of time and smaller in those who were perpetually running late. After Gall partnered with a colleague with an entrepreneurial spirit, Johann Spurzheim, his imaging project was rebranded as *Phrenology*, and examiners were trained in the United States to assess individuals before hiring them for various jobs.[4] Eventually, the lack of any supporting evidence (i.e., actual brain bumps) halted the progress of Phrenology, but the pursuit of learning about specific brain components and associated functions persisted.

Today we can place human subjects in large scanners and track brain activity when they are asked to engage in various activities. These functional magnetic resonance imaging (fMRI) scans provide beautiful colorful images depicting the most active areas of the brain during specific tasks. This human brain imaging research, coupled with the more precise laboratory work with animal models, has provided valuable information about the various working parts of the brain. Although more questions remain unanswered than answered, we know the basic brain areas involved in behavioral responses such as sleep, alertness, fear, language, decision-making, vision, hearing, hunger, and movement. From an evolutionary perspective, nature has retained a basic template in the brain production department. The rat brains that I most often work with, for example, have all the same basic parts as human brains, but, as we'll discuss later in the chapter, there are some unique differences between the two.

In addition to fMRI scans, technological advances in neuroscience have yielded several additional exciting techniques, such as tensor diffusion imaging, that highlight connections between brain areas. These connections are sometimes called "white matter" due to the cellular insulation that is pearly white. Further, CLARITY, a technique developed by Karl Disseroth at Stanford University, washes away the brain's fat tissue, leaving it clear so that specific areas can be stained in a "whole" brain.[5] According to Harvard neuroscientist Jeff Lichtman, who is using a technique to generate 3-D reconstruction of neurons, the challenge with the new imaging techniques is the sheer magnitude of data the techniques are generating. A case in point is his own research mapping the neural connections in a mouse brain. Working with a tiny slice of brain tissue the size of a grain of salt has produced a hundred terabytes of data. For comparison, a hundred terabytes would hold the data of approximately 25,000 high definition movies.[6] Considering that this massive amount of data characterizes such a small amount of mouse brain tissue, it is beyond our imagination to consider the amount of data produced by analyzing an *entire* mouse brain or, heaven help us, a human brain, which is 3,000 times larger than the mouse brain! Although this research is exciting, we are far from translating it into meaningful therapeutic approaches for maintaining the healthiest brains.

As previously mentioned, the barrage of neuroscience research over the past century has pointed to certain brain areas associated with general functions, sometimes known as localization of function. For example, in the simplest of categorizations, the hippocampus, Latin for sea horse, has been associated with learning and memory; the amygdala has been associated with fear; the thalamus is a relay station of sorts and is involved in many basic functions; the cingulate cortex is involved in responses involving both emotional and cogni-

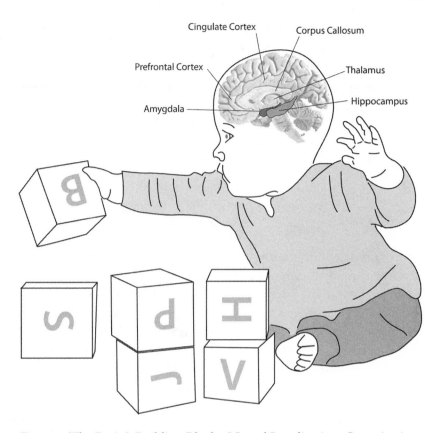

Figure 5. The Brain's Building Blocks: Neural Localization, Organization, and Integration. *As response opportunities become more complex, such as in play, many brain areas work together to integrate sensory systems, movement, emotions, and decision-making to generate the appropriate behavioral response. The hippocampus, amygdala, and cingulate cortex are often considered part of the brain's emotional (or limbic) system, the prefrontal cortex is important for our most sophisticated decisions, and important sensory and motor information is routed through the thalamus. There are two cerebral hemispheres sitting on top of a single brainstem; these hemispheres are integrated through the corpus callosum. (Image by Bill Nelson)*

tive components, and the prefrontal cortex is critical for carrying out executive functions. As seen in Figure 5, these areas work together in a healthy developing brain to produce complex responses such as playing with blocks. We have to be careful, however, in our thinking of brain areas as strictly independent agents associated with specific functions. As emphasized throughout this chapter, the organization of the brain's elements is probably even more critical for optimal brain performance. As Brian Burrell asked in his interesting book *Postcards from the Brain Museum*, what *exactly* is being localized when we speak of localization of function? Even with the most sophisticated of brain scans and technologically advanced methods, many brain terms are still uncomfortably ambiguous.[7]

In Search of the "On" Button: Brain Sparks and Liquid Assets

The brain switch, ironically, was stumbled upon indirectly by an impressive demonstration of dancing frog legs by Italian physiologist Luigi Galvani in the latter part of the eighteenth century. When he applied an electrical spark to a dissected frog leg, the muscles would twitch in an eerie dancing-like fashion. Galvani then pronounced that the spark had triggered the body's natural electricity, which normally occupies the nerves, the enclosed tributaries of the brain.[8] Consequently, the idea emerged that the nervous system resembled a battery in the head with cable-like nerves extending throughout the body.

Frog demonstrations were exciting, but what about human brains and nerves? Did electrical sparks fuel our behavior as well? It wasn't long before Galvani shifted to demonstrations of "reviving" dead bodies with electrical sparks. To accomplish this feat, Galvani's nephew, Giovanni Aldine, collected fresh human heads from guillotines and found that he could trigger grimaces, eye movements, and eye openings by passing current through the brain's tissue.[9] The term *galvanism* was introduced to acknowledge Galvani's contributions to understanding the electrical nature of nerves. Soon the European scientific community was abuzz with excitement and controversy over ideas about electrical currents controlling behavior and even giving life to dead or inanimate human forms.

The English writers Lord Byron, Percy Shelley, and his young bride, Mary Shelley, were among those captivated by these medical developments. In their discussions, they linked galvanism with the Greek mythological figure Prometheus, whose bold defiance of the gods led to tragic and grotesque consequences. This cultural context inspired, among other writings, Mary Shelley's novel *Franken-stein; or, The Modern Prometheus*, published in 1818. In the preface she wrote that her conversations about philosophy, the nature of life, and galvanism influenced the novel. Her main character, Victor Frankenstein, describes how the creature he created first came to life:

> It was on a dreary night of November, that I beheld the accomplishment of my toils. With an anxiety that almost amounted to agony, I collected the instruments of life around me, that I might infuse the spark of being into the lifeless thing that lay at my feet. It was already one in the morning; the rain pattered dismally against the panes, and my candle was nearly burnt out, when, by the glimmer of the half-extinguished light, I saw the dull yellow eye of the creature open; it breathed hard, and a convulsive motion agitated its limbs.[10]

So, there you go, the story of Frankenstein was created first and foremost by inquisitive scholars wondering what turned on brains. This historical story of how curiosity about neural function helped generate gothic horror literature indicates just how much our "neural functioning" knowledge base has expanded over the past couple of centuries. When Mary Shelley wrote *Frankenstein*, few differences existed between fiction and scientific treatises. Today, although many unanswered questions remain, scientists are gradually unraveling the secret language of the nervous system. For those who have remained students of the discipline, this progress has diminished the mysticism of the body's controlling forces. Progress on this front, however, was slow and, at times, distractions interrupted the journey.

Keeping with the topic of frogs in the brain discovery process, in the early part of the twentieth century German physiologist Otto Loewi extended research conducted by English physiologist Henry Dale, who thought something more than sparks was behind the fine-tuned brain functions.[11] Working in the drug research industry, he began testing certain chemicals on the nervous system and is credited for identifying that a certain chemical, acetylcholine, at the time thought to be associated only with plants, interacted with the nervous system in interesting ways. His interests focused on the nervous system outside the brain. The brain and spinal cord are often referred to as the central nervous system, and the extensions of the nervous system in the forms of nerves make up the peripheral nervous system.[12] Dale's friend, German physiologist Otto Loewi, confirmed his suspicions that chemicals rather than electrical sparks contributed to the highly selective functions of the nervous system. Interestingly, a dream played a major role in this endeavor.

Loewi reported that he had a significant dream about confirming the importance of this plant chemical in the animal nervous system but, after awakening, couldn't remember the details. Then, as the story goes, after having the same dream a second time he decided not to take a chance on forgetting it again and went to the lab while the details were fresh in his memory. He suspended two frog hearts in a physiological solution, one with an attached nerve known as the vagus nerve and one without the attached nerve. When Loewi physically stimulated the vagus nerve the heart slowed the pace of its beating. This could have been caused by an elusive spark, but Loewi pushed on. He collected some of the fluid around the heart and bathed the second heart in it and, voila!—the second heart also slowed its rate of beating. The liquid around the heart seemed to be the key. At the time, Loewi referred to this liquid as vagusstoff since it seemed to be related to the vagus nerve that extends from the brain to the abdominal area, but later work concluded that it was indeed the acetylcholine that Dale had hypothesized playing an important role in the peripheral nervous system. It seemed that plants and animals shared some of their chemical roots.

Although some electrical stimulation exists between nerve cells, we have since learned that most of the communication is due to the release of specific chemicals. At that time another chemical, adrenaline, was known for activating the heart rate and other functions associated with a functional arm of the peripheral nervous system known as the sympathetic nervous system, which comes on the scene when we detect a threat or something meaningful in our environment. The vagusstoff known as acetylcholine, associated with the parasympathetic nervous system, calmed that threatened nervous system down. In 1936 Dale and Loewi shared the coveted Nobel

Prize for their work nudging the neural paradigm shift from sparks to chemicals.[13] Today, approximately 100 chemicals (known as neurotransmitters) that have specific neural functions have been identified. Although all of the neurotransmitters can't be addressed in this book, we'll discuss a few favorites—some I'm sure you've heard of because of the prevalence of our approved direct-to-consumer advertising by the pharmaceutical companies—old friends such as serotonin, dopamine, and oxytocin.

With the visualization of the neuron and information about the importance of related chemicals on board, researchers were getting closer to figuring out exactly what turned on a brain. The answer pointed back to the days of the electrical spark, but there was a twist. After technology was generated in World War I to amplify wireless signals, this technique was applied to neurophysiology. English neurophysiologist Edgar Adrian applied this technology to thin neuronal strands, known as axons, that extended from the cell body and determined that there were voltage differences between the inside and the outside of neurons. A tiny microelectrode was placed in the outside of the cell membrane and compared to voltage recorded by a microelectrode placed in the inside of the cell membrane. The inside was found to be about 70 millivolts more negative than the outside. This observation was later referred to as the resting membrane potential, and its discovery suggested that, even at rest, the nervous system is a bit perturbed and ready for action. But as information is detected by the neuron, a shift in the positioning of electrically charged ions occurs, changing the membrane potential. English physiologists Hodgkin and Huxley used a neuron from a giant squid to map these changes. An essential part of the initiation of a neuron impulse appeared to be movement of these tiny ions, namely positively charged sodium and potassium ions, across the membrane—but that was just the first step in neural communication. The second important step involved the previously described neurochemicals.[14] If an incoming message from either the surrounding environment or somewhere else in the brain was strong enough to move these ions to a predetermined threshold, an impulse of electrical activation propelled down the neuron's extension until it arrived at its final destination at the end of the axon. After making its way down the axon, the activation stimulated the release of a cellular package of neuro-chemicals, which traveled across tiny little gaps known as synapses to potentially activate the next neuron in the circuit.

Are you still with me? Obviously, our burning desire to peer under the brain's hood has been a bit of a mixed blessing. Each step of the discovery journey has been simultaneously fascinating and intimidating, as a full understanding of the brain's complex workings appears to be farther and farther from our immediate grasp. Re-gardless, researchers have identified some of the brain's tricks for adapting to changing demands in the world around us, and one of the most impressive neural feats is discussed in the next section.

The Gift That Keeps on Giving: Neurogenesis

Although considerable energy has been devoted to determining the number of existing neurons in the brain, one of the most interesting aspects of the brain's design may be the neurons that aren't there—yet. In the early days of neuroscience research, it was thought that we were born with a stable number of neurons, and that initial set of neurons persisted throughout life. In the 1960s, however, research-ers discovered that new neurons continue to be produced in certain areas, known as neurogenic zones, throughout the brain.[15] Recent findings suggest that neurogenesis is more prevalent during child-hood in humans, but more research is necessary to fully understand the rate of neuron production across the lifespan.[16] We're still trying to identify the function of these new neurons, but they likely are involved with our ability to change and adapt to new environments. This idea is supported by findings that neurogenesis is enhanced when animals are housed in enriched and complex environments.[17]

According to German neuroscientist Gerd Kempermann, a key to the most insightful and fine-tuned brains is found in an animal's neurogenesis strategies. One of the neuron producing zones is an area of the brain known as the hippocampus, positioned just under the brain's outside cortical layer. The hippocampus is known for its role in learning and memory. A component of this structure, the dentate gyrus, is one of those zones that arrived late on the evolu-tionary scene, Kempermann points out. Whereas the hippocampus or hippocampus-like structures can be seen in a diverse array of animals including fish, reptiles, and birds, the more recently evolved dentate gyrus may give mammals a distinct advantage in the survival game by assessing new and relevant events in the environment. If you are investing in the stock market, you wouldn't look solely at last year's returns, you would search for the current status of the market and consider any prevalent trends and factors that are currently influencing return rates. That is, if you want to avoid investing in another financial bubble that will burst before paying off in the future, relevant current information needs to be integrated into the historical analysis of the stock performance. The streamlined neurogenesis in the dentate gyrus may provide this added survival service. Neurogenesis in the dentate gyrus can be thought of as a real-life neural stock brokerage firm, where the environmental waters are tested to determine if new neurons and connections are necessary to process changing conditions. Kempermann refers to this ability to determine where neural energy will be invested based on current contextual demands as "cognitive flexibility." Even though ants can navigate their way in monotonous desert habitats, they would be completely lost if relocated in a dense forest. Mammals with a dentate gyrus may be able to plug new information into the navigational system and survive such a drastic move.[18] The ability to alter neural and behavioral responses in changing environments is referred to as plasticity. This cognitive flexibility represents one of the most sophisticated behavioral responses programmed by the mammalian, especially human, brain.

Of course, there is a delicate balance between our neural circuits' ability to remain stable and, at the same time, modify existing circuits in the face of changing environmental characteristics. The hardwired behavioral programming of the ant greatly diminishes its ability to be flexible. On the other hand, if past experiences aren't translated into stable neural circuits, an animal is going to be reinventing the wheel constantly. This balance is referred to as the stability-plasticity dilemma and is likely just as relevant for the survival of businesses as for the survival of animals. As Kempermann states, "Networks that are too stable cannot acquire anything new, whereas networks that are too flexible cannot remember because they cannot lastingly store information."[19] Interestingly, the human hippocampus is approximately four times larger than that of our earliest primate ancestors after they have been theoretically enlarged to a comparable body weight. In addition to our endowed hippocampus, potentially enabling humans to move into virtually any habitat on the planet, additional unique characteristics of the human brain have been identified.

The Human Brain's Hidden Treasures

I have learned through the years that information about all mammalian brains is necessary to fully appreciate the uniqueness of the human brain.[20] In fact, on most levels, the human brain is amazingly similar to other mammalian brains. As previously indicated, with a few exceptions such as the absence of a language center in rat brains, humans share the same basic brain structures and neurochemicals as other mammalian species—and there is even considerable overlap with fish, reptiles, and birds. Based on the inventory of our brain structures and chemicals, the human brain is nothing to write home about. But, somehow, these structures are arranged in such a way to produce qualitative differences in our behavioral output. Although other species have evolved sophisticated forms of communication, humans are the only species generating such diverse communication styles as poetry and computer code. To my knowledge, we're also the only mammalian species contemplating the functions of their own brains and minds, planning for future generations that don't yet exist, and devoting resources to creating survival nonessentials such as abstract art. And, an observation appreciated by my college and university professor colleagues, humans are the only animals devoting a considerable amount of time and resources to obtain various documented "academic degrees" that may or may not enhance our evolutionary fitness. The name humans assigned to the mammalian order that we occupy—primates—after *primata*, meaning first rank, conveys that we have always thought we were something special.[21]

So, how did these "cognitive riches" manifest themselves in the human primate brain? How did we reach the pinnacle of the "first rank" mammalian species? The most obvious answer is the large size of the human brain—approximately three glorious pounds of neural tissue brimming with neural connections. But that can't be the critical factor because humans don't have the largest brains in the animal kingdom—we are easily beat in the brain weight category by elephants, dolphins, and whales. Although these species are respected for their cognitive riches, humans perceive that their abilities outrank those with larger brains.

What about *relative* brain size? Elephants, dolphins, and whales have really large bodies, so when brain weight is considered in the context of body weight, does the human brain stand out? Humans have a brain/body ratio of 1.86 percent, dolphins sport a ratio of 1.5 percent, and chimps' ratio is .88 percent. The parrot, considered to be one of the cognitive champs of birds, has an index of 1.72 percent—uncomfortably close to humans but since they're not mammals maybe their brains shouldn't be compared with mammals'. When the numbers are in, does the relative brain size ratio place humans on the top of the list of mammals and potentially explain the human cognitive riches? You already know from reading the previous chapter that there is an unexpected mammal that crushes the human brain/body ratio—the tiny shrew has an index of 10 percent.[22]

When brain scientists generated a new formula known as the encephalization quotient (EQ), which takes into consideration growth and maintenance factors influencing varying body sizes, the rankings seemed more expected. Under this new index, the mighty shrew has an EQ of 2.54, much lower than the human EQ of 6.54. Whale dolphins (*Lissodelphis borealis*) are close behind at 5.55, and, interestingly, baboons at 2.63 rank higher than the gorilla at 1.75 (lower than the shrew). Although the cognitive genius of baboons may just be untapped at this point, most primatologists have failed to uncover it. And, since this measure is sensitive to body weight, the EQ of obese humans drops in a manner that doesn't reflect changes in cognitive abilities. Then there's Einstein, the emperor of cognitive riches. His EQ was 5.76, much lower than the average adult human male EQ, probably due to the fact that Einstein's cortex was thinner than normal even though he had more densely packed neurons.[23] For these reasons, some researchers have suggested that, at least in primates, absolute brain size is a better predictor of cognitive ability (broadly defined as possessing diverse learning abilities such as detecting patterns, identifying concepts, exhibiting flexibility, and even using tools).[24]

So, the EQ is interesting but doesn't seem to be the final indicator of cognitive prowess. What if Einstein's neural dense cortex provided an important clue about sophisticated cognitive abilities? Is neuronal density a factor that could shed some light on contingency calculations and sophisticated behavior? One of the most innovative neuroscientists I have ever had the privilege of meeting, Brazilian neuroscientist Suzana Herculano-Houzel (currently at Vanderbilt University), has attacked this question with a vengeance. Suzana became interested in neuron numbers when she was developing a neuroscience education program following her graduate training. As she was preparing her materials, she was struck by the lack of original references for one of the most basic parameters of the human brain— the number of neurons it contained. Until just a few years ago, any reputable neuroscience textbook always clearly stated that the human brain had 100 billion neurons. This was a nice round number that no one questioned, not until Suzana started organizing those educational materials, that is. She questioned her mentor Roberto Lent at the University Federal of Rio de Janeiro, asking how we could be sure that there were 100 billion neurons. Being a thorough researcher, Suzana continued to search for the original study that generated that number. She couldn't find that critical reference; textbooks referenced older texts, and there seemed to be no origin of this information. It was as if this so-called fact that was espoused in the classrooms of the most prestigious of academic institutions could be more aptly described as an academic myth.

Roberto argued that the number had to be true because everyone knew there were 100 billion neurons. However, he quickly recognized this response was no more appropriate than a parent answering a persistent child's question with "Just because" or "That's just the way it is." As scientists, Roberto and Suzana knew that this question was far from settled.

Granted, there was good reason why no one had actually sat down and counted all of the brain's neurons. Once a brain is sufficiently stained and sectioned so the neurons are visible under a microscope, it would take a very long time to count 100 billion neurons one by one. If you could count one neuron a second, which would be a rapid pace to maintain, it would take nearly 32 years (working nonstop!) to quantify 1 billion cells. For 100 billion cells, we're talking about nearly 3,200 years. But maybe you could just count cells in a smaller representative sample of brain tissue and then generalize to the entire weight of the brain. That's a good idea, but the density varies in different brain areas so you would need to count a representative number in as many different brain areas as could be discerned. This strategy has likely been attempted to some degree but a discussion of it or its results has apparently never been officially published. And we haven't discussed the fact that it has been estimated that there are ten times more glial cells (a type of supportive cell in the nervous system) than neurons.[25] The years of counting brain cells are adding up!

Troubled with the need to provide accurate information in her educational program, Suzana came up with what she called a crazy idea and presented it to Roberto. Why not dissect each distinctive section of the brain, then, section by section: brainstem, cortex, hippocampus, etc.; one could homogenize or blend the targeted area into something of a brain smoothie. Then, the resulting neuronal liquid representing each area could be exposed to chemicals that stained the nucleus of each cell. Each cell has only one nucleus so this should work. She was able to double-stain the cells with a specific stain that reacted only with neuron nuclei as opposed to glial nuclei. Next, a certain amount, or aliquot, of the brain smoothie was extracted and placed on a slide to count . . . this procedure was repeated several times to obtain a representative number of neurons and glia for the specified amount of brain smoothie. Next, she just multiplied the specified sample volume to reach the full quantity of the liquid generated by the brain section (since the cells were equally distributed in the suspension). So, once the neuron count was subtracted from the total cell count, voila—they had estimates of both the neurons and the glia for the cortex, cerebellum, hippocampus, brainstem, etc. In stark contrast to the thousands of years it would take to count all the cells in the brain individually, an entire human brain could be quantified in a matter of days. And this was accomplished with a brain and a blender—is that innovation, or what?

I became aware of this amazing scientific achievement at a meeting of the International Behavioral Neuroscience Society meeting in Rio de Janeiro, Brazil. Roberto Lent presented this work as I furiously took notes for a textbook I was about to begin writing. The process of making a brain smoothie actually has the more technical name isotropic fractionation. This technique has determined that the human brain has 86 billion neurons, with about the same number of glia—very different numbers than had been printed in textbooks.[26] When compared to about 40 different mammalian species, the human brain holds the record for the most densely packed neurons in the cortex. For example, if a rat had a brain the same size as the human brain, it would have only 12 billion neurons. For the rat brain to have the same number of neurons as a human brain, the rat brain would need to weigh a whopping 77 pounds, more than eight times larger than the largest known brain on earth, that of the blue whale. This is because, following the rodent neuronal scaling rule, the size of the neurons increase as the brain size increases. This isn't the case with the primate scaling rules. In primates, the neuron size remains constant as brain sizes increase. But focusing just on primates, if a small squirrel monkey's brain was scaled up to the size of the human brain, the number of neurons would be comparable to that of humans. So, for primates, as suggested by Suzana in an article title, the human has a *remarkable but not extraordinary brain*. The interesting exception in the primates is the nonhuman great apes. The gorilla's body size is larger than a human's, but its brain is a modest one pound, with a lackluster 33 billion neurons.[27] Considering that the human brain utilizes about 20 percent of all the energy a human consumes, the great ape may have directed more of its energy toward maintaining body structure and functions than to fueling neural functions.

Animals would have difficulty eating enough food to maintain a brain the size of the human brain. Anthropologists have theorized about humans' success in supporting such a huge brain size and the failure of other apes to do so. Harvard anthropologist Richard Wrangham has suggested that the discovery of fire may have fueled the eventual large size of the human brain. With fire came the ability to cook food so that meat and tough vegetables could be softened for easier chewing and digestion (requiring less energy)—an advancement that paved the way for securing enough caloric energy to maintain the impressive human brain.[28] To my knowledge, humans are the only species who cook their food. This advancement likely led to the eventual diminished tooth and stomach sizes so that less energy was needed to be diverted to these areas. No longer needing to chew tough vegetables hours and hours a day, the mouth may have evolved toward a structure that became more conducive to spoken language. Language also likely fueled unprecedented brain advances. Thus, our brains and associated neurocognitive functions may have expanded when our stomachs constricted.

I contacted Roberto Lent after the conference in Rio and asked him about a few research ideas. Roberto introduced me to Suzana— and we have been collaborators ever since. She is helping me investigate a question about a specific mammal that captured my attention as a child and has persisted, morphing into a professional obsession. This animal is the North American raccoon—known for being clever, curious, and mischievous—cognitive and behavioral riches that I haven't been able to fully capture in my rodent models. Not unlike human pioneers, raccoons migrated to North America and have thrived; additionally, they have thrived wherever they have been introduced, such as Germany and Japan—much to the dismay of the human inhabitants of these areas. My rodent research emphasizes the importance of being able to manipulate environmental contingencies through experimental manipulations. Similar to the impressive ability of rats to use their paws to manipulate their surroundings, raccoons have brilliantly engineered forepaws that facilitate amazing feats, especially when the animals coordinate their use. Because raccoon paws are represented on the outer cortex of their brain just about as prominently as human hands are on the outer cortex our brains, I have always thought that raccoons could reveal meaningful secrets about how organisms interact with their environments in opportunistic, contingency-building ways. So, I pitched the advantages of looking at raccoon brains to Suzana, and she took the bait. Thus far, our research has certainly reinforced my suspicion that their brains would be worth investigating. Of all the mammals that Suzana has profiled, the raccoon scales closest to primates. Based on our current information, the raccoon brain is quite comparable to an owl monkey's brain. Scaled up to the size of a human brain, raccoons would have the same number of neurons. Now you understand why the raccoons frequently outsmart humans when it comes to breaking into garbage cans and attics. On a theoretical neuronal scaling level, we may have truly met our match in raccoons.[29]

In comparing raccoons to other carnivores, it currently looks like the cortical density of neurons is more impressive in the raccoon versus the golden retriever or the lion, but there is more research to be conducted in this area. My point of bringing up these preliminary data, other than the fact that I love to discuss raccoons whenever possible, is to indicate that species that have evolved adaptations for manipulating the environment and building contingency inventories may have an advantage in the survival game. Even so, raccoon brains seem to pale in comparison to the neural treasures of the human brain. In the case of raccoons, their proclivity to manipulate their environments often gets them into trouble . . . life-threatening trouble. It's as if the raccoons proceed through life with no contingency filters about potential dangers or threats—the ultimate optimists that never consider the negative contingencies. This is probably why raccoons in the wild often die prematurely, even before they turn three years old, when they can easily live to almost twenty if they stay out of trouble. Thus, as the brain mechanisms for reinforcing the contingency circuit are considered in the next chapter, it is important to be mindful of the brain's gas pedal and brakes when making decisions about interacting with the environment. The raccoons remind us that one-way contingencies are inadequate. All potential outcomes, both risks and benefits, should be included in the calculations.

To turn back to humans, in addition to the density of neurons other variables have been considered as being influential in the production of our remarkable brains. A considerable amount of attention has been focused on the outer cortex of the brain, the most recently evolved area. Whereas I was initially taught that a majority of neurons were housed in this brain area, we now know (thanks to the Brazilian team's isotropic fractionator methods) that the most prized brain real estate is the area involved in coordinating movement (among other functions), the cerebellum. In fact, we now know that about 19 percent of the neurons in the human brain are in the celebrated cerebral cortex, whereas a whopping 79 percent are in the cerebellum . . . with the remaining scarce numbers of neurons scattered throughout other brain areas.[30] These proportional differences aren't exactly the same but are similar in the rodent. Apparently, the brain has invested a lot of neural energy in our ability to effectively and safely move around in the environment. Effective maneuvers are, of course, a product of both the cerebellum (coordinated movement) and the cortex (contingency calculating and decision-making)—a fact that is reinforced by the neuronal distribution patterns.

The size of the human cortex doesn't distinguish itself in comparison to other mammals; we don't really stand apart in either the absolute size or the foldings of the cortex. We do have a slight advantage when cortex is expressed in proportion to total brain mass. The human cortex represents about 75 percent of the human brain, compared to a range of 71 to 73 percent in chimps, and 74 percent in horses.[31] A more specific area of the cortex, known as the prefrontal cortex, is distinguished in the human, occupying 29 percent of the brain, compared to 17 percent and 12 percent for chimps and rhesus monkeys, respectively. A key reason for this larger size in humans appears to be more white matter than is typically observed with the number of neurons in this area.[32]

A cortical area known as the insula has received recent attention for its diverse functions including emotional awareness, self-recognition, empathy, and decision-making under uncertain conditions. In order to pull off these jobs, this brain area interacts with multiple areas monitoring incoming sensations, outgoing responses, and all the intermediate processes between. This brain area is certainly a contender for enabling mammals to make optimal decisions and subsequent responses in changing environmental conditions, tasks necessary for effective contingency calculations. Recent research suggests that certain components of the insular cortex are the most expansive in humans in comparison with our closest living relative, the chimpanzee.[33]

In addition to a potential advantage in the human prefrontal cortex in terms of expansiveness, the connections between the two hemispheres, or halves, of the brain may be a factor. The principal connection between the two is a structure known as the corpus callosum, which in humans contains just shy of 200 million neurons. If you have a business partner, the way you integrate your activities is critical to productivity and effectiveness. If you and your partner both carry out the same functions, you're operating only at the level of a single person, or maybe worse. However, if you're able to integrate and coordinate efforts by assigning specific functions to each of you, then you'll achieve twice the productivity level. Although there is redundancy between your brain's hemispheres, some functions have been assigned to a specific hemisphere, such as language to the left hemisphere and facial recognition to the right hemisphere (generally speaking). In other functions such as vision, the hemispheres share their information to provide us with a seamless view of an expansive visual field.[34] There is some evidence that as brains got larger and it took longer for the two hemispheres to communicate, enhanced specialization occurred within the hemispheres to facilitate split-second decisions.[35]

The assignment of specific functions to specific hemispheres is known as brain lateralization; for example, as previously mentioned, language is lateralized to the left hemisphere. Lateralization of certain functions may provide the benefits of two brains in some cases. This is certainly seen in dolphins, which, as they sleep, relegate one hemisphere to sleep at a time; that way the other hemisphere can remain vigilant throughout the duration of the animal's slumber, enabling them to continue breathing and safely navigating their environment.[36]

Interestingly, it has been hypothesized that Da Vinci's genius was a product of both a lateralized brain plus a more prominent corpus callosum, enabling him to integrate information held in each hemisphere in unique ways. Of course, Da Vinci predated functional brain images so we really don't know the specific characteristics of his brain, but he was left-handed and was speculated to have exhibited homosexual tendencies, two phenotypes that have been associated with varying lateralization. Thus, hemisphere specialization and integration may have contributed to Da Vinci's creative abilities and unprecedented views of animal and social equality. He also included images of hands in his artwork at a time when it was traditional to have just the chest and face in portraits—arguing that the expressive nature of the hands was the gateway to the windows of the mind. Thus, although these ideas related to Da Vinci's brain may not be adequately confirmed, it is very likely that the unique lateralization and interhemispheric communication in humans influence cognitive riches and behavioral flexibility.[37]

As you can discern from this brief tour of the human brain, many candidates for the neural underpinnings of cognitive "riches" have been proposed—too many for an exhaustive discussion here. However, there is one more candidate that has caught my attention lately, a unique type of neuron known as the von Economo neuron. These neurons are also known as spindle neurons due to their elongated structure. They are also quite large compared to other neurons, and they may facilitate the speed of communication among neurons with their rather streamlined processes that may be able to quickly receive and relay information from a substantial "patch" of cortical tissue. Even with all the brain components in place, the speed of information transfer is also a factor that is influenced by many variables— one of which may be these specialized neurons. Further, these neurons are located in the insular cortex, as well as in areas that regulate emotions, and have been implicated in some rather sophisticated responses that appear to be uniquely human such as embarrassment, guilt, deception, and resentment.[38] They have also been targeted as potential causes of psychiatric illnesses such as autism.[39] However, we now know that these neurons are certainly not specific to primates, and the evidence is still too preliminary to make broad claims about their role in human cognitive functions and psychiatric health. Still, I will certainly continue to follow these interesting cells, as the distribution patterns rather than their presence may be the most influential aspect of the von Economos. If these cells facilitate the speed of neural processing, this may increase the speed at which various contingencies are calculated for competing responses, leading to success in social competition challenges. Recently, I collaborated with Kent State University's Mary Ann Rhaganti and Mount Sinai School of Medicine's Patrick Hof to explore the presence of von Economo neurons in raccoon brains (Figure 6). These cells are present in the insular cortex in healthy numbers. Although we're not yet sure what this means, we're continuing our investigations of these animals in their natural habitats to learn more about their authentic response-outcome strategies.

The Human Brain—A Neural Soufflé, Not a Neural Casserole

So, after surviving a chapter filled with neuroanatomy and neurophysiology, you have witnessed the current state of confusion about what makes the human brain stand out. More than anything, the

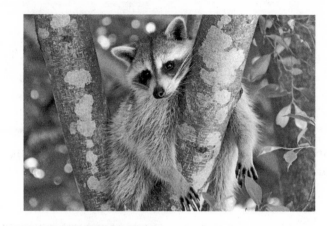

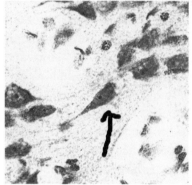

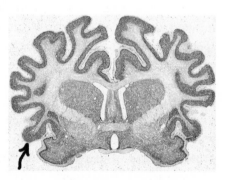

Figure 6. Raccoon von Economo Neurons. *We have been amazed by the complexity and flexibility of raccoon behavior—even switching from being active at night (nocturnal) to being active during the day (diurnal) in a population we studied in Miami. One of the animals we observed in this population is seen at top. We were thrilled to see von Economo neurons (indicated by arrow in middle photo) in the insular cortex (indicated by arrow in bottom photo), although the function of these elongated neurons remains a mystery. (Photos courtesy of Tim Landis and Molly Kent in the Lambert Neuroscience Laboratory, University of Richmond)*

human brain blends in with all the other mammalian brains, yet it is different in some ways that are often difficult to articulate. This makes me think of a poppy seed chicken casserole recipe. You may have made this dish yourself. My brother seemed to inherit the cooking gene in my family, and he loves to prepare the most complex and exotic dishes he can find for his friends and family. Although I enjoy cooking when I can find the time, my culinary boldness is much more limited. Knowing this, my brother sent me the chicken casserole recipe when I was newly married and included a note saying that "even you can cook this." He went on to make some statement about it not being possible to mess it up. And he was right—I just needed to mix the basic ingredients in any order with a pretty wide range of quantities. Boiled chicken, cream of chicken soup, sour cream, and salt and pepper mixed with crackers and poppy seeds and drizzled with a little butter on top, then baked at 350 degrees for about a half-hour, and voila! Yummy chicken casserole every time. My kids always loved it. Other casseroles follow this same pattern: add whatever at pretty much any time, just mix it all in, and out comes a tasty treat.

Then there's the soufflé. I'm not going to pretend that I have ever attempted to cook a soufflé. It just always seemed so intimidating. The ingredients—eggs, butter, and sugar—are basic enough but there seems to be a mystical element about rising and falling that appears almost impossible to master. It may not be truly impossible, but it's clear that timing, ingredient amounts, handling, and sensitive cooking conditions are all critical factors. Brains in general, especially the human brain, with all the functional bells and whistles, certainly align more with a soufflé than with a casserole. Unlike the user-friendly casseroles, when it comes to soufflés there is no forgetting an ingredient and throwing it in later. For human brains, there are also critical windows for exposure to certain life ingredients, such as loving parents, visually enriching scenery, and physically challenging surroundings, that can't be forgotten and then added later. Certain developmental events merge to elevate the human's cognitive riches to a level beyond expectation given the same ingredients found in other brains—neurons, glial cells, etc. Just as the tiny bubbles of hot air contained within the perfectly blended delicate structure provide the lift to soufflés, the structure of the cortex, speed of processing, and appropriate environmental surroundings seem to be blended in the perfect evolutionary recipe for the uniquely human cognitive riches.[40] Similar to a soufflé, the delicate cortical structure of the brain ensures that it is always vulnerable to "falling" in the form of damaged tissue and impaired functions. In a sense, soufflés and human brains are never "finished"; they are constantly changing in response to varying environmental conditions. In the next chapter, the importance of harnessing complex neural circuits to calculate the most optimal contingencies will be considered.

CHAPTER FOUR

Building the Brain's
Contingency Circuit

WHEN I INITIALLY READ Spencer Johnson's 1998 best-selling business fable *Who Moved My Cheese?*, I was intrigued but had no way of knowing that I would be assessing similar "life lessons" with mice, rats, and students in my own lab over a decade later.[1] For those of you who missed this classic, the characters consist of a pair of mice, Sniff and Scurry, and a pair of miniature humans, Hem and Haw. You can probably guess the pair with the least decisive and adaptive response to uncertainty. As the story goes, these two pairs live in the same maze but go their separate ways each day to find their favorite food, cheese. And find cheese they did, in a part of the maze called Cheese Station C. Both groups were excited about this rich source of cheese but responded a bit differently to their good fortune. Whereas Sniff and Scurry continued to explore the maze and notice slight alterations in the amount of cheese each day, Hem and Haw went directly to the cheese station, not feeling a need to continue to gain information about the remaining areas in their environment. In fact, their inflated confidence about the permanent status of the cheese station blinded them to the changing environment around them. Consequently, when the cheese supply was diminished, it didn't surprise Sniff and Scurry, who had seen it coming. Hem and Haw, however, were in shock.

The everyday behavior of the two groups obviously influenced their response to the uncertainty that accompanied the eventual realization that the cheese had been removed from its predicted location. Because Sniff and Scurry had explored the environment each day, they felt confident about setting off to find cheese in other parts of the maze, which they did. On the other hand, Hem and Haw kept going back to the same empty cheese station, lacking the confidence to venture out in the maze to find new cheese. Johnson emphasized several bits of wisdom throughout this business fable, reminding corporate leaders that change (and uncertainty) will always happen— and the best businesses will monitor the inevitable change and, consequently, will be poised to respond in adaptive ways.

Regardless of how appropriate it is for CEOs to monitor changes in their respective businesses, the plot of this parable is a point of central interest in this chapter. How do we respond when our world changes, and how do we know how to respond most appropriately to this uncertainty? In technical terms, this "change" is known as a prediction error—the cheese is no longer where it was predicted to be, hence the error. Since the world is full of uncertainty, it should come as no surprise that brains have a few tricks up their neural sleeves to respond to these changing conditions. When our life, or even a good menu entrée, is on the line, we need to employ these tricks to recalibrate contingencies in our favor.

Just Decide Already: Neuroeconomics Revisited

I introduced some of the fundamentals of neuroeconomics in Chapter 2, but I saved additional information for this chapter—thinking it would be more easily digested after learning more about the brain in the previous chapter. There is certainly much to learn about contingency calculations from the burgeoning new area of neuroscience. As previously discussed, neuroeconomics has provided considerable information about how we make decisions between two or more competing choices. For example, how do we decide what entrée to order when faced with a lunch menu containing 15 different yummy options? It's typically difficult to make a decision in this situation because there are just too many darn choices. Who needs 15 entrée choices for lunch? Did our ancestors encounter such difficult decisions? According to neuroeconomics pioneer Paul Glimcher, an abundance of choices sometimes dilutes our ability to make a final selection by evaluating the value of each individual choice. Neural activity spills over from one area of the topographical cortical map to another, leading to that blank stare on your friend's face as he considers all the menu options. So, before you blurt out, *Just decide already!*, it may help to understand that the restaurant has seriously compromised your friend's decision-making circuits by including such an extensive list of options.[2]

According to neuroeconomics findings, when you select an orange over an apple, certain brain areas are activated because you value the orange more than the apple—at least in that moment when forced to decide. If you recall the Coke vs. Pepsi study described in Chapter 2, the posterior parietal area of the brain's outer layer, or cortex, was implicated in that decision challenge task. Further research requiring monkeys to make difficult choices in ambiguous problem sets indicates the role of a more specific area, the lateral intraparietal (LIP) cortex, within the parietal cortex in making decisions in an uncertain situation. Hence, this area plays the role of *Behavior Director* as it zooms in on the most relevant stimuli and responses.[3]

The processing of probabilities and values in neuroeconomics tasks is referred to as the utility computation.[4] Glimcher's research prompting human subjects to decide between various consumer goods such as books and DVDs confirmed that, in addition to the LIP area, two additional brain areas were implicated. The medial prefrontal cortex (also implicated in the Coke vs. Pepsi study) and the area around the brain's reward center, the ventral tegmental area, are important in establishing value of certain choice options and, consequently, facilitated the evaluation of these consumer items.[5] Another component of the brain's emotional system, the amygdala, classically known for its involvement in fear, also influences our decisions by communicating with the medial prefrontal cortex.[6] Hence, the multiple cortical players in the decision-making game are modulated by subcortical emotional areas, especially those related to reward and fear. Decision-making, however, may get a little trickier when you select the salad over the burger and fries. In this situation, another area of your brain's relatively recently evolved cortex, the dorsolateral prefrontal cortex, is activated to try to inhibit your impulse to grab the burger and fries because you are trying really hard to value low calorie meals when you're on a diet.[7] The key cortical areas in decision-making challenges are depicted in Figure 7. The integrated processing of these areas to make an adaptive decision in ambiguous situations represents top-down processing at its best. Even though these decision-making exercises require processing in multiple cortical and subcortical areas in our brains, in the grander scheme of real-world decisions and behavioral output these laboratory exercises fall in the category of rather simple choices.

A precursor to the field of neuroeconomics was the Nobel prize–winning decision-making research conducted by Dan Kahneman and Amos Tversky, who worked together at Stanford University. Kahneman wrote about the fast and slow thinking introduced in Chapter 2. The classic research conducted by Kahneman and Tversky identified consistent errors in our thinking strategies when we are forced to make decisions presented in a multiple choice test format. For example, suppose you're told that in a certain population of interest 70 percent of the people are teachers and 30 percent are lawyers. When we're given a vague description of a young professional and then asked to guess the person's career, knowing that 70 percent of the sample consists of teachers doesn't really influence our guess. Because we have no obvious tip that the person is a lawyer, it makes more sense to just guess that the person is a teacher since such a large percentage of the population is made up of this profession. Nope, that's not the way most of us play it. We think we have some special insight and see a characteristic that aligns more with lawyers and select that choice option, ignoring the important prior information influencing probability outcome.[8]

In his book *Misbehaving* University of Chicago behavioral economist and recent Nobel Prize–winner Richard Thaler noted an interesting decision-making error his students made—this time in relation to their actual scores on a midterm exam in one of his classes. After giving a challenging test designed to differentiate the students who "got it" from those who didn't understand the material, the students were in an uproar when they learned that the average score was 72 percent. That average score sounds fair to me, but Thaler

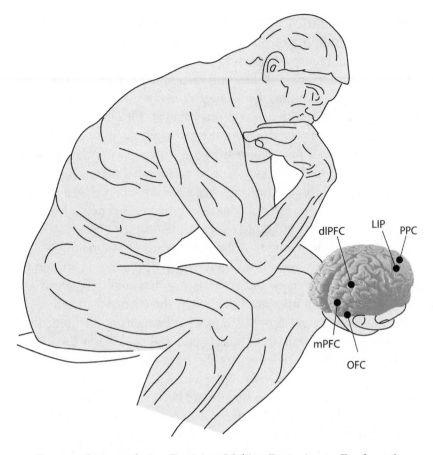

Figure 7. Contemplating Decision-Making Brain Areas. *Far from the specificity of brain functions proposed by early brain endeavors such as phrenology, most responses require the integration of multiple brain areas. For example, decision-making requires the contribution and integration of many brain areas positioned across the cortex. As described in this chapter, the technical names for these areas are: medial prefrontal cortex (mPFC), orbitofrontal cortex (OFC), dorsolateral prefrontal cortex (dlPFC), lateral intraparietal cortex (LIP), and posterior parietal cortex (PPC). (Image by Bill Nelson)*

thought he would try to satisfy the students without compromising the integrity of his exams. He explained that a score of 80 would actually be transformed into a grade of A and scores above a 65 would be in the B range. Even after this generous offer of higher letter grades, the students were still upset that the average numerical grade

was 72. Then he tried a little experiment on the next exam by making the total number of points add up to 137 and then giving the
students their raw score instead of the score representing the percent correct. This way, if they still responded correctly to only 70
percent of the questions, the average raw score was a more positive
sounding 96 points (that is, 96 out of 137). Of course, the letter
grade distributions for the second exam were no different than in
the first exam, but for some reason the students were thrilled with
this outcome. On the surface, this score sounded better, just as the
decision that a fictional character was a lawyer rather than a teacher
sounded better, regardless of what accurate contingency calculating
revealed. This was yet another form of consumer misbehavior informed by Thaler's earlier collaborations with Kahneman.[9]

Although the wayward problem-solving practices identified by
Kahneman and Tversky and the exciting data emerging from the
field of neuroeconomics are fascinating, the events that lead up to
these decision points, as opposed to what happens in the immediate
moment, are the emphasis of this chapter and book. How do our life
paths result in different values for different choice options that lead
us to value an orange over an apple? Further, there are so many important decisions in our lives that extend beyond these forced choices,
choices classified as complex decisions, that aren't clearly prompted
by a single symbol or object. At what point do our contingency calculators determine that our current job isn't really going anywhere
and it's time to think about a career change?[10] These types of decisions are very different than determining if someone is more likely
a lawyer or a teacher in a given group of people. It's the backstory
leading up to decision points that influence subsequent contingency
calculations, regardless of whether someone is solving a forced immediate problem of telling the Starbucks barista a specific order or
making a more open-ended decision to purchase an engagement ring
and present it to a significant other.

Although an individual's experimental backstory isn't always emphasized in neuroeconomics-related research, the notion has been
around for quite a while. Early in the twentieth century Edward
Tolman, an experimental psychologist who spent most of his career
at University of California, Berkeley, introduced the term *latent
learning* to the field of psychology. His research with rats and mazes

suggested that rats didn't need to be rewarded to learn information about their environments; on the contrary, they developed cognitive maps of their worlds just by exploring them. For example, when rats that were allowed to randomly explore a maze without being rewarded were compared to rats that had received rewards each time they entered the goal box in the same maze, they performed similarly once the rewarded trials in the maze commenced. Once the rats caught on to the fact that the goal box now contained the desired reward, their prior exploration history of the maze paid off. Similar to the story of Sniffy and Scurry, rats in Tolman's lab demonstrated learning in a maze after just spending time exploring and accumulating knowledge about the maze—without the rewards that the behaviorist pioneers declared were imperative for learning to occur.[11] Regardless, this idea of an experiential backstory in learning research was placed on the back burner for years until the behavioral and cognitive scientists felt more comfortable integrating their ideas.

Similar to the Talking Heads classic rock song "How Did I Get Here?," neuroscientists are currently exploring ideas of how specific pathways lead to our minute-to-minute responsive brains. Comparable to Tolman's exploring rats, and to the smart mice of *Who Moved My Cheese?* fame, certain neural buttons are pushed throughout our lives that guide our responses in specific scenarios. If specific neural buttons are repeatedly pushed, then neural networks, our brain's go-to neural "playlist," emerge. Neural networks consist of coordinated neural responses to various stimuli in the world around us—sculpting our personalities, habits, and dreams for the future. Unlike the types of decision-making scenarios that can be assessed in the laboratory, our lives also consist of the tough questions that require layers of life experiences to make the most informed decisions. These life experiences, our earned contingency capital, transform our brains' neural networks, influencing both our decisions and our actions as specific contingencies are calculated.

In our changing world, my life experiences are very different from your life experiences, and these accumulated experiences influence the values that are established in our respective brains' neural networks. What is crystal clear is that the phrase "same as it ever was" in the Talking Heads song mentioned above doesn't accurately describe our brain at any given time. Our neural hardware and associated functions change with every passing second—brains that are the *same as they ever were* would lack the ability to adapt to changing environments that would ultimately compromise survival. In order to investigate how past experiences influence our established values and subsequent decisions and responses (that is, using our scientific jargon, response-outcome contingencies), I had to turn to my long-time business partners, the rats, for clues about how informed contingency calculations lead us to the most strategic decisions and actions throughout our lives. No surprise, they didn't disappoint.

Who Moved My Froot Loop?

Throughout the past century, researchers have designed clever devices and tasks to test the learning ability of various animals. Mazes dominated the early days of animal learning. In a fascinating history of mazes written for the popular magazine *Slate*, journalist Daniel Engber reports the rather somber story of the demise of the rodent maze. Even so, when they were initially introduced, they were quite glorious. The earliest maze was designed by Willard Small at Clark University. Patterned after the elaborate Hampton Court hedge mazes, this early maze was huge, about the size of most rodent laboratory testing rooms today (six feet by eight feet), and included an open area in the middle with six cul-de-sacs for the rats to explore. In these early days, Small was interested in how the rats explored and learned about the maze. Although other species were tested in the maze, the rat became the standard laboratory animal and was associated with mazes from that point forward. Pioneer behaviorist John B. Watson used the rodent maze for his dissertation research at the University of Chicago. He compromised various senses such as vision and audition in the rats to determine if these deficits diminished the rats' ability to navigate the maze. He found that they could learn the maze without depending on these senses.[12]

There have been many creative versions of the early rodent mazes. Today, the Morris Water Maze is used to allow rats to swim to a hidden platform in a specific quadrant of the circular arena. And a plus-sign structure elevated on stilts, with two covered and two open arms and known as the elevated-plus maze, was designed to assess a rat's anxiety in approaching the open arms. As different spatial mazes were popping up on the laboratory scene, in the 1920s the highly mechanized and quite unnatural operant chamber was introduced by B. F. Skinner. Compared with observing how quickly a rat could learn to navigate a maze, lever pressing seemed much more efficient for assessing Skinner's interests in reinforcement learning. For a premier behaviorist, Skinner certainly streamlined the rat's behavior in the tasks he designed—the minimalist behaviorist.

The spirit of those early rat mazes and rodent learning tests lives on in my laboratory with the Dry Land Maze that I adapted from a spatial maze created by Ray Kesner at the University of Utah.[13] I am less interested in the rat's ability to navigate spatial challenges and more interested in assessing prediction errors and responses to uncertainty, what I consider to be the "big questions" in the world of behavior. Full disclosure—my own spatial ability is sorely lacking, so I guess it's no surprise that I'm not excited about linking spatial ability with more generalized intellectual capacity. Even so, navigating spatial terrains is very important for the survival of rats, so it is indeed an appropriate strategy when assessing learning in rodents.

Perhaps a tour through the Dry Land Maze protocol is in order. Similar to the early mazes, this circular apparatus is rather large—about six feet in diameter. The floor of the maze is sprinkled with the rats' normal laboratory bedding material (that is, dried corn cob pieces), and the walls are about a foot high so the animals can't jump out (or at least they're not supposed to jump out). Around the periphery of the maze are eight small plastic soda caps that are drilled in the floor so they will remain in exactly the same place throughout testing. On the first day of training, the small pieces of Froot Loops are placed in each of the food wells and the rats are given 10 minutes to familiarize themselves with the apparatus, or to just check the place out.

Even though the rats used in these studies have had experience eating Froot Loops, their initial anxiety produced from being in a completely new environment typically trumps their hunger. Still, even if they don't eat any of the rewards on that first day, the point is that they explored the arena and hopefully saw the food wells and treats. On the next day of training, alternate wells are baited with the sweet cereal so that the rats are learning that every well isn't always baited in the maze. On the third and last day of habituation, only two of the wells baited on the previous day are baited. The next day is critical for this test, as it's the rats' first introduction to the maze having only ONE of the originally baited wells actually baited with a Froot Loop. Hopefully, by this time, we have systematically taught the animal that the Froot Loop is in a single well. From this day forward, during the three test days, the rats experience three 3-minute trials in which they are positioned in the maze at different start points for each trial. During these trials my student researchers record how fast the rats retrieve the Froot Loop reward, as well as additional behaviors such as exploring the other wells, grooming, or trying to escape from the maze. As you may predict, by the third day these rats "have got this" and typically have no problem orienting themselves as they head toward the payoff well after being dropped in the arena like special operations soldiers.

All of this training and testing is merely the backstory for what I'm really interested in investigating. After all the test trials have been conducted, the probe test is employed by placing the rat in the apparatus to which it is now accustomed, but this time the Froot Loop isn't where it's supposed to be. In fact, for the first time in the rats' short maze careers, there is NO Froot Loop in the entire appa-ratus. Of course, the rats don't actually say it, but you can almost hear them thinking, "Who moved my Froot Loop?" Now we have created a prediction error similar to what was encountered by Hem and Haw and Sniff and Scurry. Then the question becomes, will they utilize the strategies of Hem and Haw—the passive, indecisive little humans—or Sniff and Scurry—the information-gathering, resource-ful mice?

I never get tired of observing rats in this situation. What's a rat to do? In the Morris Water Maze, when the platform is removed for a similar test, it is thought that the intelligent response is to swim around in the same quadrant where the platform was originally lo-cated. As if to convey . . . it was here yesterday . . . it's supposed to be here . . . where is that darn platform? Indeed, this persistent searching in the same area confirms that the rat remembers where the platform used to be . . . so that strategy seems adaptive if you're interested only in memory. But we're interested in more complex decision-making and contingency processing, so we just watch the rats to see what they tell us. The rats that have the healthier stress responses and exhibit more adaptive behavior in other assessments use several strategies to try to solve the problem. Sure, they go to the previously-baited well just as Hem and Haw did, but once they thoroughly explore the area and confirm that the reward is no longer there, they utilize another strategy—torn from the playbook of Sniff and Scurry. One of the additional strategies we observe is the rats' exploration of other wells that were previously baited in the training process. Although this may be considered an error by some researchers, in my opinion it makes perfect sense, since at one point earlier in the training process all the wells contained Froot Loops. Other rats rear up on their hind feet as if they're closely examining the arena for any clues about where the Froot Loop may be. Much like Sniff and Scurry searching for the lost cheese station, it appears that the smartest rats are those that utilize the greatest number of strategies when faced with a prediction error in this task. I can almost see the contingency wheels turning—especially if I have provided a contingency boot camp prior to their exposure to this Froot Loop maze.

The "contingency boot camp" we developed to build contingency circuits in rats was briefly introduced and described in Chapter 1 as effort-driven rewards and is quite simple. In contrast to classic psychology research known as learned helplessness, in which animals learn there is no connection between efforts and rewards, similar to a depressed individual who finds it difficult to get out of bed since all the person's effort seems to lead to no positive consequences, I was interested in enhancing the connections between effort and rewards in order to reinforce a connection between specific responses and outcomes. So I sent my rats to the fields, the laboratory fields in this case, to harvest Froot Loops. Each day, rats are placed in a four-foot square arena that contains small mounds of their familiar bedding material with coveted Froot Loops buried in them. After a few weeks, rats learn to look for the mounds and then dig for their sweet cereal treats. After about six weeks of approximately six-minute trials each day, it becomes clear that these rats, known as the contingent rats, understand their task—they look for mounds and dig up Froot Loops. The true test of all of this contingency building comes when the rats are exposed to a very different problem-solving task following their contingency boot camp training. Again, we em-

ploy a low-tech task for this assessment consisting of a standard plastic cat ball toy containing a little bell. This new object is somewhat
anxiety provoking—especially with that odd sounding bell. The
pièce de résistance is that the ball contains a desirable Froot Loop
that can't be removed—even though we hope that the rat thinks it's
worth the effort to try.

When we do these studies we have another group of rats that
are exposed to a different version of the contingency-building boot
camp—the version where we don't want them to build contingency
circuits. When these rats are placed in the digging arena, they are
simply given their Froot Loop rewards without having to work for
them. It's obvious why this noncontingent group is known as the
trust fund group in comparison to the contingent worker group.
When faced with the problem-solving cat ball task, the contingent/
worker rats spend more time than the non-contingent/trust fund
rats trying to retrieve the Froot Loops from the weird cat ball.[14] Instead of learned helplessness, we're modeling *learned persistence*.

But what impact does the contingency training have on the rats
in the Dry Land Maze Probe test when someone moves their Froot
Loop? Well, compared to the trust fund rats, the worker contingent
rats employ more problem-solving strategies by spending more time
at the previously baited well but also more often rearing up in the
maze to gather additional information, as if the rats are hitting the
"recalibrate" button in their brains. We also record behaviors such
as grooming, and the trust fund rats exhibit more disrupted bouts of
grooming; that is, they start their highly structured grooming bouts
but seem to get confused and have to start over . . . or just skip a few
strokes here and there.[15] Additionally, the worker rats had healthier
levels of stress hormones. In our lab, we extract evidence of these
hormones in their poop—a biological sample the rats seem all too
happy to offer to their investigators. We look at the typical stress
hormone, corticosterone, in addition to a hormone correlated with
resilience, DHEA (technically, Dehydroepiandrosterone). When we
evaluate DHEA/corticosterone ratios, the contingent workers have
higher values, suggesting that they are producing ample levels of
DHEA to combat the toxicity of the stress hormones.

According to the worker and trust fund rats, contingency training in one task appears to extend to other tasks. If this finding is

generalizable to humans, it implies that interacting with the environment and gaining a sense of mastery and self-efficacy (for just a few minutes each day) appear to provide a buffer against the endless bouts of uncertainty we experience throughout our lives. How does the brain orchestrate all these changing conditions and probabilities to generate the most optimal responses? Scientists have placed their bets on a gambling task to learn more about this process of building sufficient contingency muscle to get us through the prediction errors of life.

Building Cognitive Capital

If one of the most important functions of the brain is to generate realistic contingencies to guide our behavior, how exactly does that happen? Now that scientists know the general working parts of the brain and have some insights about their functions, we're more poised than ever before to get to the bottom of this mystery. Moving beyond the simple choices emphasized in the classic decision-making research (à la Kahneman and Tversky) and neuroeconomics, a more complex task is needed to simulate real-world uncertainty. Such a task should enable subjects to make choices about responses that may pay off in the future, and responses that are too risky. If that sounds like gambling, then we're on the same page! The classic task for this complex behavior is known as the Iowa Gambling Task, and it assesses responses to uncertainty by presenting subjects or patients with two decks of cards. The consequences for selecting cards from each individual deck are unknown at the beginning of the task, but the participants quickly learn that some cards result in payoffs and some in financial penalties. In the beginning, all a person can do is gather information by selecting cards from each of the two decks— and taking mental notes along the way. Kim Sterelny, a biological philosopher at Australian National University, refers to the information gathered in such phases as a version of accumulating *cognitive capital* to guide future decisions. In his view, our predisposed neural circuits require personal interactions with changing environmental conditions in order to build optimal cognitive tools, an experiential repository of sorts, to help us navigate novelty when it is invariably introduced into our lives. Faced with ever-changing environments, our predisposed neural responses that we inherited from our genetic capital fall short of informing us about the best responses in the barrage of new contingency challenges we face day to day.[16]

So, cognitive capital that is essential for navigating the Iowa Gambling Task is gained through experiencing the cards and their consequences in real time. After a while, some contingency patterns begin to emerge. One deck (Deck A) is associated with bigger pay-offs and bigger penalties, whereas the other deck (Deck B) is associated with smaller payoffs and smaller penalties. To an observer taking careful notes, it is clear that the smaller payoff pile ultimately yields the bigger payoff, but that requires resisting the temptation to go for the larger, more immediate payoffs in Deck A. The interesting aspect of this task is how long it takes the human participants to come to conclusions about the differential payoffs of the decks. Neuro-psychologists have observed that individuals with damage to their prefrontal cortex area take longer to realize the contingency pat-terns, if they do at all.[17] In this task they are likely to keep selecting cards from the high payoff/high penalty deck. And, in the real world, these individuals may persist with low (or no) payoff strategies in their social or professional lives by sticking with a dead-end job or an abusive relationship, mistakes that keep them from realizing their desired goals in life. Outside of clinical studies, the Iowa Gambling Task has also become a popular task that has informed us about spe-cific areas of the brain contributing to successful performance.

Before considering the brain areas regulating behavior in such a contingency-challenging task, it's important to point out another fascinating aspect of this task—an aspect that should make us cau-tious about using human self-report data. In the Iowa Gambling Task, healthy subjects most often start to respond appropriately by select-ing more cards from the small payoff/small penalty deck even though, when asked about their responses, they aren't clearly aware why they are responding in such a manner. Interestingly, when subjects are asked why they are selecting more cards from the "smart" deck, they can't really articulate beyond saying that they have a "gut feeling" or a "hunch" about the deck.

This reporting error is fascinating for two reasons. First, it con-firms that the research participants are generating contingency out-come data that are ultimately guiding their behavior, in some instances *before* they are aware of why they are responding in a certain way. Such findings remind us to be cautious when asking individuals to provide accurate reports of their behavior.[18] This reporting error is also seen in research in which subjects are asked to estimate the slant of a hill—they verbally report that it's much steeper than it actually is. For example, subjects often estimate that a hill has a thirty-degree slant when it actually has just a seven-degree slant. Yikes! We obviously aren't very good at verbally describing this incline. This isn't a big deal, as it is probably related to the brain's ability to focus attention on the hill in front of us. However, when we try to walk up said hill our muscles appear to know the exact movement to match the incline. Again, our neural processing and related behavioral output are literally a few steps ahead of our cognitive awareness. My colleague Cedar Riener, working with his former research supervisor Dennis Proffitt at the University of Virginia, found that self-report of the steepness of inclines is further biased if subjects are in a depressed mood . . . that is, they report steeper slants when depressed.[19] When you're feeling bad, that mountain really does look too steep to climb.

These biased perceptions are likely related to available energy reserves that are ultimately adaptive but confirm that we can't always trust our laboratory subjects—or our own self-awareness. In other words, our brains are ultimately processing knowledge much more accurately than we can verbally acknowledge the situation. We are also champs at making up stories to resolve inconsistencies between responses and outcomes. If a student doesn't perform well on a test, he may blame the types of questions on the exam when a more realistic explanation is that he didn't spend enough time studying. As described in *The Lab Rat Chronicles*, I sometimes prefer to work with nonhuman animals because they don't have a cover story the way that humans, with their complex brains, often do, generating both fact and fiction, mostly fiction![20] In addition to not-always-trustworthy human self-report data, the delayed realization of the contingency patterns in the Iowa Gambling Task confirm that there is a complex neurobiology directing our hunches and gut feelings. Hunches are far from random, fleeting feelings; they are the early signs of accumulating experiences and cognitive capital that are pointing our responses in certain directions.

Interestingly, researchers have developed a rat model of the Iowa Gambling Task known appropriately as the Rat Gambling Task. Untrainable to draw from a deck of cards, they are given the opportunity to stick their noses in openings that result in varying payoffs of food pellets, sweet sucrose solution, or penalties in the form of time-outs in which they can't respond for another payoff. In these rat casino scenarios, more fine-tuned analyses of brain areas involved in successfully discerning the smart contingencies leading to more payoffs can be determined. For example, Francoise Dellu-Hagedorn at the University of Bordeaux has systematically aligned specific areas of the prefrontal cortex with problem-solving in the Rat Gambling Task. In addition to various areas of the prefrontal cortex, the involvement of the cingulate cortex and related areas (involved in mediating between emotions and cognition) plays a role in regulating the contingency processing in this task.[21] More specifically, the speed at which the animal arrives at the correct contingencies associated with specific nose-poking portals is regulated by the anterior cingulate, which may be very important in enabling the brain to acquire adequate cognitive capital to identify strategic contingency payoffs.

Whereas the anterior cingulate may be setting the pace for building cognitive capital and making decisions based on that capital, the orbitofrontal cortex (OFC), a portion of the prefrontal cortex located behind the eyes (and also depicted in Figure 7) is becoming increasingly known as a "contingency critic" in the brain. A different rat model in which certain odors predict the presentation of a sucrose solution (payoff) or of bitter-tasting quinine solution (penalty) is used to explore brain areas activated when contingency calculations are challenged. Once associations between odors and solutions are formed, Geoffrey Schoenbaum and colleagues, working at the University of Maryland, mix up the associations, requiring the rats to engage in cognitive flexibility to keep up with the constantly changing predicting odors. Healthy rats can rapidly recode the changing odor-outcome situations, but the rats with damage to the OFC have problems changing their behavior in pace with the changing conditions. These researchers concluded that the OFC is important for signaling expected outcomes, such as one odor no longer predicting the sweet rewarding solution. Thus, the OFC may be the ultimate contingency regulating brain area. But it certainly doesn't work alone. In line with life observations that "everyone's a critic," there are many brain area critics that ensure we are indeed detecting these important prediction errors when they arise. Schoenbaum and colleagues also refer to these prediction errors as teaching signals, suggesting that the brain recruits input from more basic areas such as the reward centers to mark the importance of these errors.[22]

It's easy to appreciate the role of errors as teaching signals when you think of learning to drive. It's difficult to imagine how any amount of virtual training could replace the old-fashioned real world experience of building contingency capital by actual behind-the-wheel training. Young drivers need to drive a real car on a real road to acquire the appropriate amount of experience to become a competent driver. Making mistakes such as drifting off the road, cutting off drivers when making lane changes, and not changing lanes in time to exit a highway all provide expectancy discrepancies and prediction errors that prompt our brains to recalibrate for those driving surprises (i.e., near misses). Although these are considered simple response-outcome contingencies, driving serves as an informative model for understanding how we rely on errors to recalibrate response-outcome contingencies. As described in Chapter 1, when injured patients are relearning to walk, it's important for them to make mistakes and correct those specific mistakes as opposed to being told what they need to do to improve. Before progress can be made in physical therapy or in other areas of life, it's important to own the error and recalculate accordingly.

Optogenetics: Spotlighting Contingency Circuits

Even after reading respected peer-reviewed journal articles on the rather new brain technique known as optogenetics, I have to remind myself that this technique isn't science fiction. In a nutshell, light-sensitive proteins known as opsin proteins have been found to alter cellular functions in certain microorganisms. When natural light hits these microorganisms, tiny channels on the surface of the neurons open or close depending on the specific opsin protein and the nature of the light, ultimately prompting neural responses. This was all very interesting in the world of simple organisms, but would these light-sensitive opsins have an influence on mammalian brains? That question seems like quite a stretch, but that is exactly what optogenetics is all about. These opsin proteins are harvested from microorganism hosts and infused in a specific brain area in a mouse, with optic fibers positioned just above the brain area so that, after the opsins have matured, pulses of light can be delivered through a cap placed on the animal's head to the opsin-infused brain area.[23]

Does this light technique have an impact on the mammalian brain and associated behavior? Indeed it does. Early research with optogenetics resulted in dramatic demonstrations of rats sleeping before the laser was turned on and, after it was turned on, awaking from their slumber.[24] Depending on the area infused with opsins, specific behaviors can be choreographed under the direction of neuroscientists. Just like cartoons with a light bulb positioned over a character's head to depict the generation of a thought, turning the lights on inside the rodent brain generates neural impulses. Thus, with the recent discovery of optogenetics, these cartoons with light bulb bubbles take on a new meaning.

I enjoyed reading about this new neuroscience technique but never envisioned incorporating it into my own research. This was a bit more sophisticated than the investigatory tools we typically use in my undergraduate research lab. However, after some consideration and conversations with colleagues, it appeared that this technique could offer a more mechanistic explanation for some of our research findings. Although this optogenetics is no doubt being explored for potential therapeutic uses in humans, I had something different in mind.

What if we could test the effectiveness of contingency training in the effort-based reward Froot Loop digging task (nice old-fashioned behavioral therapy) by pitting that experience against real-time brain activation or suppression via optogenetic techniques? Based on our past work, I had evidence that the behavioral training was modifying brain activity as had been observed with optogenetics. Could the contingency-behavioral training and its associated neural circuitry hold its own against cellular channels of animal brains being opened and closed with fast pulsating lights? This was very different from my more naturalistic research programs, but I was getting excited about using this technology to determine if brain circuits built

by the experience of "work" resulted in comparable activation compared to the laser lights penetrating specific areas of the brain. I was
fortunate that Garret Stuber, one of the research stars in this area,
and his enthusiastic postdoctoral fellow, Jenna McHenry, agreed to
collaborate on this project.[25] They welcomed two of my brave undergraduate students, Emily Kirk and Brooke Thompson, to their
lab at the University of North Carolina at Chapel Hill to train the
mice in the effort-driven reward task. I didn't mean to engage in
"rodent profiling," but I was a little nervous that mice couldn't handle this intensive training program—I had always placed my trust in
the more cognitively complex rats. Time would tell . . .

Although the data generated from this endeavor are preliminary, it turned out that this brain technique certainly added a valuable layer of explanation to my investigation of the effectiveness of
rodent behavioral training models. To maximize efficiency, we decided to expose mice that had already had opsin proteins implanted
in a brain area associated with the stress response, an area known
as the paraventricular nucleus of the thalamus. This is a centrally
located structure located below the cortex. To be overly simplistic,
if this area is inhibited with specific laser administration, it should
make the animal more relaxed. Following either the infusion of opsins in this brain area or the delivery of opsin blanks for a control
condition, the mice were trained for five long weeks in the effort-
based reward task. Each day these mice would "go to work" for 10
minutes, searching for mounds of bedding and digging up Froot
Loops. The trust fund mice that served as the controls for the training group just had to show up and receive their sweet rewards.

At the end of training, the mice were exposed to the emotionally
challenging problem-solving task consisting of the scary new stimulus (cat ball) filled with rewarding Froot Loops. This was similar to
the problem-solving persistence task we used for the rats. Would the
mice approach or avoid this challenge in the new unfamiliar context? I drove from my home in Virginia to the Stuber Lab in North
Carolina to observe these critical trials that my undergraduate students were conducting. After five weeks of training, all of the data
would be generated on this one day in the lab when the animals were
tested in the learned persistence task.

After the mice were connected to the optic fibers that would deliver pulsating light to the affected opsin area, my students and I watched each mouse's response to the challenge by following them on a remote video feed. Even before formally analyzing our data, I could already see that some animals were spending more time perched on top of that cat ball that had been securely positioned in the center of the arena. Were the contingent worker animals persisting longer to get to their rewards? Or, did the opsin treatment modify their anxiety responses, allowing them to feel more relaxed about obtaining those rewards? I couldn't stand the suspense! Although this was an exploratory study, the trends we observed were very interesting. Compared to noncontingent/trust fund and sham surgery animals, both opsin inhibition and contingency training resulted in the animals appearing less stressed. For example, both "therapies" resulted in the animals approaching the challenging task faster, but the contingent-trained group spent more time on top of the cat ball as if they were trying to figure out a way to retrieve the Froot Loop. On the contrary, the opsin-treated animals spent more time rearing up on their hind legs, perhaps to recalibrate or gather new relevant information. On one level, it seemed that it was pretty much a draw between the two therapies, but the contingency training resulted in more "on-task" behavior, so maybe it had the potential of having a higher efficacy rate. The true tipping point, however, is the fact that the contingency training required no invasive procedure and, further, has no known negative or long-term side effects. This observation corroborates human findings that behavioral cognitive therapy—a noninvasive, nonpharmacological therapeutic approach for humans—is more effective than many other treatment strategies, a topic that will be further discussed in Chapter 8.[26]

The Ultimate Decision Points Theater

In April of 2013, George Bush's Presidential Library and Museum opened in Dallas, Texas—complete with what the facility calls a "Decision Points Theater."[27] Because I had begun to focus my rodent research on decision-making and associated neural responses, I wanted to learn more about Bush's version of informed decision-making.

Of course, President Bush received a good bit of criticism about his own decision-making ability, especially for his decision to invade Iraq following the traumatic terrorist attacks in 2001. Many citizens who supported this decision, even those who shared his belief about the presence of weapons of mass destruction, later changed their minds as the war progressed and clear victories seemed out of reach. Because this book is about behavior influenced by neural responses, not politics, I'll skip any supportive or critical political narrative and focus on the fundamental decision-making lessons disseminated in this intriguing interactive exhibit.

Visitors who enter the Decision Points Theater are greeted by a virtual guide, who invites the audience to select one of the famous "decision challenges" that faced Bush during his presidency. Among the events are the Iraq invasion and Hurricane Katrina. Again, since Bush was criticized for how he responded to both, I wasn't sure where they were going with this exhibit. Which decision points would be emphasized?

Once the audience selects a decision challenge, four minutes of comments from various experts on the topic are flashed across the screen—words of advice from politicians, military officers, law enforcement, government administrators, etc. That's great—the exhibit participants are building cognitive capital! The audience is asked if they believe the brief statements along the way and then, at the end of the advice blitz, they are asked to select what they conclude to be the best response among three options, including the one selected by Bush, the self-proclaimed "Decider."

I suppose the idea is that the audience will make their decision based strictly on the information presented in the exhibit, which presumably presents the information that Bush had in order to make his decision. However, most of the audience members likely are familiar with the actual events and the consequences of Bush's decisions. For this decision challenge to work objectively, audience members either would have had to live in a bubble protecting them from world news for decades, or they would have to be able to wipe their memory slate clean upon entering the theater—both highly unlikely scenarios. Similar to the song lyric I mentioned earlier, in this exhibit the status of decision-making for each issue is erroneously *the same as it ever was*. At the end of the challenge a virtual version of Bush appears on-screen and explains why he made his decision, and his is apparently viewed as the "correct" decision. The exhibit is not scientific because it assumes that none of the audience members have updated their opinions and perceptions since the time of the original events and therefore won't have the benefit of hindsight. Also, the advice is presented so quickly, with no background or debriefing for each piece of wisdom, so it's difficult to generate relevant values for the response options as is required for effective decision-making. At this point the contingency-building cingulate cortex and the outcome-discrepancy-detecting OFC are most likely throwing up their symbolic neuronal hands in despair. Even though this "blank slate" strategy is being endorsed in this political demonstration, a healthy brain, void of reality-distorting brain bubbles, simply can't suspend its awareness and limit its decision-making in this way.

Based on this confusing information about presidential decision-making, I'm returning to my rats for insights about how the brain's recently evolved cortex represents the ultimate and authentic decision theater. Certain sections of this cortical theater inhibit responses, others predict the outcome of our decisions, and still others monitor internal and external factors to make critical decisions about responding one way over another. In the most ideal decision-making scenarios, we are constantly updating this information that is necessary for our brains to make the most informed decisions—far from being *the same as it ever was*. The Decision Points Theater may or may not have been revised, but, based on what I observed, I think I'll stick with the more naturally evolved decision points theater (that is, our neural networks) . . . and hope that we can preserve the integrity of this theater in the midst of our technologically advanced society.

With so many working parts, it's no surprise that things can go wrong with this optimal decision-making process. When the brain loses its ability to make informed, real-time decisions, a person's well-being is compromised—at its very worst, these factors may lead to the most tragic of responses and result in our demise. The best decisions and contingency calculations are the result of the acquisition of authentic cognitive capital. When this capital isn't realistic or is distorted in any way, the brain loses its ability to make accurate predictions, resulting in lousy decisions. In the next chapter, we'll discuss several examples of mismatches between real and perceived cognitive capital.

CHAPTER FIVE

When Life Distorts the
Contingency Filters

ALTHOUGH THE IMPORTANCE OF realistic contingency calculators is emphasized in this book, in full disclosure, there is
one area of parenting where I completely blew the accurate contingency calculator rule. A few years ago, I wrote
an essay for the *New York Times* entitled "Santa on the Brain" in which
I publicly confessed to being guilty of generating and propagating a
multilayered, long-term contingency distortion for my two unassuming daughters. After happily sustaining the myth of Santa for several
years, one day I received a call from my husband telling me that an
older child in the neighborhood had persuaded the girls to look
in the attic for presents—where they saw everything that Santa was
supposed to bring that year. I absolutely panicked at the thought of
robbing my two young daughters of their beliefs in Santa and, from
some unknown neural origin, a story started spewing from my lips.
"But the contract," I anxiously told my daughters, Lara and Skylar,
"Santa made me sign a contract that you wouldn't find the presents
until Christmas morning." They looked at me with their confused
little faces and my deception-oriented neural circuits kept cranking
out this story that surprised even me as I was saying it. I went on to
tell the girls that Santa was having back problems and his doctor and
Mrs. Claus had demanded that he take care of himself and ship the

bulk of the presents before Christmas so it would be easier on his back. "The problem is," I continued, "now that you have seen the presents, I am contractually obligated to send them back." "No, no, Mommy! You don't need to do that, we really didn't see anything." I put on my best contemplation face to look like I was seriously evaluating the choices and confirmed that if they hadn't seen too much that maybe Santa would understand if we just kept the presents.[1]

Why would a serious-minded neuroscientist, and passionate author of this book emphasizing the importance of NOT distorting reality, fight so hard to distort reality on so many levels? As I described in the *NYT* essay, prior to developing the skeptical mindsets my college-age daughters currently have, the story of Santa represented a sense of imagination, whimsy, anticipation, and even magic that seemed to be valuable for a developing child's mind—especially at a juncture when it seems possible that reindeer just may be able to fly. Once all the neural connections have developed, it gets harder to go to such an imaginative emotional place, and as their mom I wanted to create a few positive emotional cubbyholes for my daughters to revisit throughout their adulthood. I wanted them to relive that warm, familiar emotional response during each future holiday season as they experienced the conditioned cues marking the presence of the season. The familiar smells of fir trees and holiday desserts, in addition to seeing holiday decorations and hearing those old familiar holiday songs—all of these sensory experiences would represent access portals to these holiday memories. In my mind, this is a form of emotional time travel back to the safety and boundless anticipation of childhood—a gift I was adamant about giving to my daughters. Fifty years from now, I can't predict what my daughters may be facing during the holiday season, but it gives me some comfort to think that I may have created little pockets of predictable emotional retreats for them, even during a time when they may find themselves surrounded by unpredictable conditions and stress. This was the gift that my holiday-loving mother gave to me, allowing me to revisit those almost-magical childhood emotions each time I encounter those familiar holiday cues—even twenty years following her death.

There are likely several examples of distorted contingency filters that may be advantageous, or at least not harmful, to our emotional and cognitive lives—a few examples (e.g., play and creativity) are discussed in Chapter 10. However, one has to proceed with caution when the actual interactions between responses and subsequent outcomes are blurred. Distorting reality may be okay for the short duration of watching a movie or visiting a theme park, but for day-to-day living, being in tune with reality is extremely important for maintaining a functional brain. Outside of the Santa reality detour, I worked hard to maintain a sense of authentic, not distorted, reality for my daughters. In this chapter, we'll discuss the impact of many life variables that impair our ability to build cognitive, emotional, and social capital reserves necessary to generate the most accurate and authentic contingency calculations. Among these distortion candidates, we'll consider the impact of celebrity, privilege, poverty, suicidal thoughts, endless arbitrary awards, and religion. To round out the chapter we will end where we started, with a potential beneficial distortion, in this case an optimistic attitude.

The Man in the Mirror

Mirrors are valuable in that they provide a somewhat representative image of ourselves—that is, a healthy dose of reality. Even in the Brothers Grimm fairy tale "Snow White and the Seven Dwarfs," the magic mirror responded to the evil Queen's question of identifying the fairest in the land with the truthful answer that it was Snow White. Outside of fairy tales, the value of such truthful reflections can't be underestimated. Mirrors allow us to see if that spinach salad is stuck in our teeth before making an important presentation, or if the coffee stain on our shirt is visible enough that we need to change before heading to work. In these cases, our reflection in the mirror provides important information necessary for us to respond accordingly to correct or improve the situation.

Life mirrors are a little more complicated. How do we know if that conference talk was effective or if our chatty, upbeat personality works with the new co-workers? The list goes on . . . we need feedback about our cooking, parenting, driving, social skills, study habits, financial investment strategies, and sense of fashion . . . just to name a few lifestyle choices that benefit from a healthy dose of monitoring. Where do we obtain this valuable feedback? Where are the best life mirrors?

Based on the important ties between our responses and outcomes, the outcomes themselves represent the best reflections of the effectiveness of our responses—that is, if the outcomes are accurately presented to us and we can accurately interpret them without any distorting filters. For example, even if your friends are trying to be supportive, telling you that your new diet must be paying off because you look like you have lost weight even though your bathroom scale is telling you otherwise, that particular social feedback life mirror falls short of providing accurate information to assess the effectiveness of the diet. Thus, it's not such a bad thing if everyone around you is a critic, at least an honest critic. In the real world, where we need to be at our best, yes-men or -women serve no purpose. In fact, such dishonesty can lead to our demise in the same way that being dependent on drugs that give us the false and fleeting perception of pleasure and happiness can destroy our lives.

It's ironic that, although one of the epic entertainers in recent history, Michael Jackson, had a hit song, "Man in the Mirror," that stressed the importance of using a reflection in a mirror to prompt change, his own distorted life mirrors likely led to his personal undoing. In his real life, Jackson didn't heed the important message of this song and, sadly, ended up surrounding himself with unrealistic and distorted mirrors as his celebrity grew. In addition to his physical appearance, which seemed distorted after so many plastic surgeries, his behavioral responses appeared equally distorted, so much so that they likely contributed to his early death. But how so?

Although the specifics of Michael Jackson's life and health status aren't documented in the academic journals that I typically rely on, there are plenty of accounts in reputable news and entertainment sources conveying that his reality became increasingly warped as his fame increased. He built a fantasy-like theme park home he called "Neverland," after J. M. Barrie's fictional *Peter Pan*. Adding to the Disney-like amusement park theme of Neverland was a personal zoo with animals such as giraffes, apes, and an elephant—animals that don't belong at a private home. He had a chimp named Bubbles that he dressed like a small child and kept close to him. Jackson invited children to Neverland in many different capacities ranging from charitable events to personal visits. The personal visits from children, especially when they involved sleepovers, ultimately contributed to accusations of child molestation.

The life bubble that Michael Jackson created for himself grew more intense and dangerous as his life mirrors provided less and less realistic and authentic feedback about his lifestyle choices. Thus, his misguided behavior lacked the ability to self-correct itself and, like an unchecked tumor, grew until it ultimately overcame him. A *Rolling Stone* article written after his death questioned Jackson's distorted views: "Sometimes you had to wonder whether Jackson had any real idea how his actions struck the world . . ."[2]

The ultimate undoing came because Jackson's unrealistic lifestyle bubble extended to his basic physiological and health functions, resulting in his untimely death. In 2011, the British Broadcasting Corporation published a list of drugs found in his body at autopsy. This long list of chemical assists in the form of pills tells a compelling story of just how much control Jackson had lost of his most basic physiological and emotional functions. The media certainly covered Jackson's use of the sedative propofol, a drug typically administered in the hospital as an anesthetic, that he started using as a sleep aid in his home. Using such a strong drug to enhance sleep in one's home was unprecedented. Its chronic use had unknown effects in Jackson's nervous system and subsequently diminished his ability to sleep without this pharmacological agent. In addition to sleep problems, Jackson likely had severe issues with anxiety considering that evidence of at least three anti-anxiety drugs (diazepam, lorazepam, and midazolam) was found in his body. Perhaps to provide some arousal to compensate for all of the sedative and anti-anxiety drugs, ephedrine, a stimulant, was also on board, in addition to the local anesthetic lidocaine.[3] This pharmacological inventory suggests that Jackson had provided an artificial chemical environment for his brain . . . to an extent that it didn't seem able to survive with or without the medications. He incorporated a pharmacological regime that reduced anxiety and pain during his waking hours and promoted an unnatural form of sleep when he needed to escape his distorted daytime reality. With his drug-impaired brain unable to monitor any semblance of reality, it became increasingly difficult for Jackson to continue to function in a healthy way. Compared to a healthy brain managing its chemical inventory naturally with self-generated neu-rochemicals in response to life's events, Jackson's incorporation of such a complex mixture of pharmacological assists likely had a pro-found impact on his physiological functions. Psychoactive drugs probably represent the fastest paths to reality-distorting brain bub-bles, typically of the most dangerous form. Consequently, Jackson's case was a brain tragedy in every sense of the word.

Privilege and Poverty

Michael Jackson's tragic story of interrupted realistic contingency calculators confirms that, although most of us think that financial security will solve all of our problems, financial "prosperity" often leads to the production of new challenges. On the other end of the financial spectrum, poverty can also distort life's contingency filters in the most powerful way—by distorting the brain's landscape.

A recent study followed nearly 1,100 children and analyzed how socioeconomic status (SES) affected neural and cognitive function. In this type of research, SES is generally considered to be a product of income, education, and occupation but is often reduced to simple income for easier calculations. For behavioral neuroscientists like myself, however, SES is about modified interactions with the envi-ronment that ultimately influence neural functions and outcomes. In this study, researchers Kimberly Noble at Columbia University and Elizabeth Sowell at UCLA focused on the use of MRI scans to look for any neural footprints left by extreme variations of SES.[4] This type of brain exploration is interesting but tricky, as many fac-tors are involved, and sometimes it's not clear whether a thicker or a larger part of the brain is good or bad. You may think, for example, that a thick cortex is advantageous, but it may mean less surface area, which is also an important factor for brain processing. Adding to the confusion, cortical surface area continues to increase through the early teens and then slowly shrinks through middle adulthood. Children with higher intelligence scores have thinner cortices with more surface area. As an aside, for those of you in your early forties who have had a scan and were told that you had a relatively thick cortex, don't panic—intelligence is positively correlated with corti-cal thickness as we approach the middle-adulthood years.[5]

So what did these researchers find? Family annual incomes for participants in the study ranged from $5,000 to $300,000, and those with higher incomes exhibited increased brain cortical area. Children from families with an annual income not exceeding $25,000 had 6 percent less cortical area than children from families earning at least $150,000. Interestingly, at this higher SES level, the advantages of higher SES increments leveled off. Additionally, parental education, which is often intertwined with SES, was positively correlated with cortical surface area; children of parents with a college degree had approximately 3 percent more cortical surface area than children of parents with a high school education. Regarding the brain's func-tional output, higher SES was associated with enhancements in four cognitive abilities that were assessed, including inhibitory control, working memory, vocabulary, and reading. It was also noteworthy that neither race nor ethnicity had an influence on the results.[6]

These results were supported in a similar study conducted by Seth Pollack, a neuroscientist at the University of Wisconsin–Madison, and his colleagues. In this study, poor academic performance in chil-dren living below the federal poverty level was also tied to matura-tional delays in the cerebral cortex. In this case, developmental delays in the frontal lobes, which are involved in executive functions, and the temporal lobes, which are involved in the processing of emotional information, were observed.[7]

As previously described, neuroeconomics focuses on how the brain makes choices throughout our life, hopefully based on acquired cognitive capital and informed experiences that point to the choice leading to the best outcome. Although there are exceptions, low SES may be associated with substandard prenatal care, poor nutri-tion, impoverished living conditions, increased stress, exposure to environmental toxins, and less-stimulating lifestyles.[8] Increased stress and restricted resources don't provide an adequate climate for ex-ploration that builds contingency repertoires for informed problem-solving throughout a child's life. Thus, low economic status appears to have a significant negative impact on the brain's ability to build appropriate contingency capital for optimal decision-making.

The long-term effects of poverty are clearly seen when considering the likelihood of a child from a family with low SES graduating from college. Almost two decades ago, the U.S. Department of Education embarked on a longitudinal study following current eighth-grade students through the next 12 years—that is, throughout their high school, college, and early employment years. The results are shocking. When the students' eighth-grade math test scores were divided into low, middle, and high score ranges, the students scoring in the lowest achievement category but in the highest income category were just as likely to graduate as those scoring in the highest achievement category in the lowest income category. Looking at it another way, if you were a high achiever in the highest income category, you were 250 percent more likely to graduate from college in comparison to a student with the same ability but in the lowest SES category.[9]

Regardless of the specific mechanisms through which poverty conditions compromise brain functions, their potentially toxic impact is quite clear. These concerns highlight the importance of intervening and providing additional support when children face these conditions. Possession of similar academic abilities in no way creates a level academic playing field when children are on opposite ends of the SES spectrum. Kenneth Oldfield, a professor of public administration at the University of Illinois, shared his story of being a first-generation low-SES college student in an emotional essay entitled "Humble and Hopeful." In it he discusses the risk facing first-generation college students due to a deprivation of "cultural capital" that the students never obtained during their childhood and adolescence. In college, a good bit of cognitive, social, and cultural capital is necessary to navigate the financial, social, advising, and lifestyle mazes that accompany college life.[10] Obviously, these issues need to be taken seriously so that a disproportionately large group of high-achieving students from middle- and low-SES categories doesn't fall between the academic cracks. If given appropriate information, students can enhance their knowledge of necessary resources—that is, cognitive capital—in order to make the best decisions throughout their college experience.

Of course, living a privileged life in the highest SES category doesn't necessarily protect a person from the neural compromises and behavioral mishaps accompanying distorted contingency filters and insufficient cognitive capital. As seen in the case of Michael Jackson, access to a personal drugstore appeared to have exposed his brain to a toxic chemical environment, ultimately shutting it down. A privileged life characterized by an abundance of resources without clear authentic contingencies linking responses and outcomes may also compromise future decisions and responses.

The media extensively covered a recent case in which an "affluenza" defense was used by lawyers for 16-year-old Ethan Couch after he killed four bystanders and injured 11 people while driving under the influence of alcohol and other drugs. The term *affluenza* was first used by psychotherapist Jessie O'Neill, granddaughter of a past president of General Motors, in her 1996 book entitled *The Golden Ghetto: The Psychology of Affluenza*.[11] In this context, the term referred to the potential damaging effects of growing up or living in an affluent world.

In the controversial legal defense for Couch, however, the term was used to describe the abnormal condition of growing up in an affluent household with no opportunity to learn that certain behaviors have specific outcomes. This condition isn't considered a mental disorder or formal condition by the psychological/mental health industry, but it raises an interesting question about the contingency deficits that likely result when children are not allowed to experience the rightful outcomes of their responses. During the investigation, Couch's mother reported that she had no memory of ever disciplining her son. Further, he was apparently given everything his heart desired regardless of his behavior (a human version of my trust fund rats!)—including his own 4,000-square-foot house, complete with a pool, along with plenty of money that gave him access to alcohol and drugs. Pioneering behaviorists J. B. Watson and B. F. Skinner wouldn't have been surprised by Couch's situation, considering that the authentic outcomes of responses were distorted and filtered by parental interventions.

Persuaded by this controversial defense, the judge gave Couch no jail time. Instead, he was sentenced to 10 years of probation and sent to a private rehabilitation center. The judge in this case was criticized for denying this teen the opportunity to treat his affluenza by exposing him to a dose of *contingency-building therapy* in the non-affluent environment of a prison. To no one's surprise, the judge's version of rehabilitation therapy failed to change Couch's response patterns, as he was arrested two years later for violating his probation and fleeing to Mexico with the assistance of his anti-contingency-building mother.[12]

With SES extremes leading to potential contingency-building deficits that threaten an individual's ability to survive and thrive in today's world, there is no denying that poverty creates the deepest and longest lasting wounds in the brain's ability to process information and make the best decisions throughout one's life. Regardless of SES category, parenting is a complex process that can be easily compromised if authentic connections between responses and outcomes limit a child's ability to accumulate knowledge about important life resources. Just as it is difficult to let go of a toddler's hands as he or she takes those critical first steps, or to take the training wheels off a child's bike a few years later, it is difficult to let our children free-fall into the negative consequences that they will inevitably encounter if they are successfully parented. The parents who just can't let go are given labels such as helicopter parents—hovering over their children while they micromanage their lives. More recently, the label snow plow parents has been introduced describing parents who clear their children's life paths from the usual obstacles encountered by other teens. I realize that it is extremely difficult to let our children build their own contingency inventories, but mentally healthy children need to encounter these experiences, complete with positive and negative consequences, to avoid creating the brain bubbles that compromise their ability to thrive. More information about the best parenting strategies for building important contingency capital inventories in our children is discussed in Chapter 7.

And the Award Goes to . . .

What could contribute more to a child's confidence and competence than presenting him or her with various awards acknowledging impressive performances in the classroom, sports field, or dance floor? If just exerting effort was enough to be recognized as a winner, this would be an effective way to build authentic response-outcome behavioral inventories, but we all know this isn't the case. Our obsession with awards may very well be the biggest brain-building scam ever introduced—a true crime against humanity and naturally pre-disposed contingency-building brains.

I can't imagine a rat working for a shiny medal to hang around its neck or an inscribed plaque to decorate its cage. As appealing as having the title of "Laboratory Rat of the Year" or "Most Creative Path through a Maze," the rats just aren't motivated by such distinctions. Instead, laboratory rodents want the real deal—food, safety, social contact, even some gentle stroking from an experimenter (Figure 8). In fact, award ceremonies are distinctly human, as I know no other animal that will work for trophies or certificates. Other animals learn to associate verbal expressions with the subsequent presentation of tangible rewards such as food, but medals, ribbons, and accolades are specific to human motivation. Awards are designed to distinguish one individual from a group of individuals, a goal that doesn't register for most nonhuman animals.

I have worked my entire career in higher education. During this time, I have become painfully aware of how obsessed the academic community is with awards. For as long as I can remember, we have had an "awards day" each spring semester, during which the entire college comes together for an honors convocation, recognizing so many students, faculty, and staff for *distinguished* achievements that they're practically running across the stage so that the ceremony won't spill over into the evening hours. There are exceptions, how-ever, to the fast-paced academic recognition awards. A few of the most-distinguished awards are accompanied by an especially gen-erous deluge of remarks praising the recipients' accomplishments. These beautifully written comments give us all warm fuzzies as we applaud those among us whose extraordinary accomplishments have stood out over the past year.

Don't get me wrong—it's great to receive an award. When I have been fortunate enough to receive one, I have relished every minute. Our brains appear to soak up this acknowledgement like cocaine. As the engraved plaque and ceremonial handshake are dis-pensed, an emotional high floods our neural circuits. Even so, the reality of how much I actually deserved an award typically sets in after just a few minutes. With so many impressive professors on my cam-pus and beyond, it quickly becomes quite obvious that my efforts aren't distinctive. I am fully aware that the kind administrator pre-

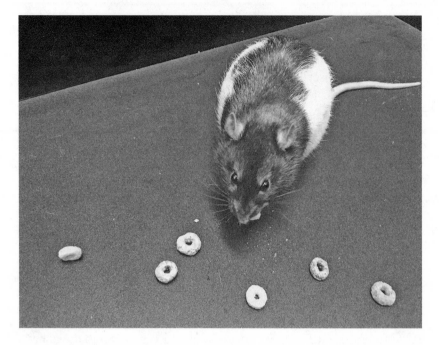

Figure 8. Rats Work for Primary Rewards. *For the most part, rats in my laboratory can be trained to do just about anything for an appetizing Froot Loop. As described previously (Chapters 1 and 4), these sweet treats are the rewards used in the effort-based reward contingency-training studies designed to build emotional resilience. In other studies and demonstrations, we have trained rats to run through hurdles, climb ropes, even drive a little rat race car, all for an anticipated Froot Loop. Although some animals may work for a secondary reward such as a token they can trade in for food or other primary award, humans seem to be unique in that they will work for medals and certificates that aren't clearly associated with traditionally viewed primary resources. In the case of humans, peer recognition associated with awards rises to the level of food, shelter, and other important resources. (Photo courtesy of Lambert Neuroscience Laboratory, University of Richmond)*

senting the award could have cherry-picked nice observations about other professors and presented equally impressive accolades. Consequently, after graciously accepting such an award I make an effort to recalibrate quickly with a healthy reality check to avoid adopting a distorted view of my actual accomplishments.

One of the few social scientists conducting research on awards, University of Zurich's Bruno Frey writes that the motivation for social distinction seems to be a hardwired characteristic of human nature.[13] Relevant to this chapter is the influence of these awards on subsequent realistic action-outcome associations. That is, do such "achievement awards" enhance or distort our contingency filters? Aside from academic institutions, other distinguished accomplishments are acknowledged in the forms of awards . . . the Academy Awards, the Nobel Prize, Pulitzer prizes. Whereas many sports awards are determined based on objective quantitative scores such as the fastest time in a race, the most points scored on the basketball court, or the height cleared in a pole vault attempt, many of the most recognized awards in our society are rather subjective. Thus, sports awards based on such objective measures provide more authentic feedback about performance than do other awards.

The Nobel Prize, created by Alfred Nobel in 1895, is designed to honor the scientists who "have, during the preceding year, conferred the greatest benefits on mankind."[14] Wow . . . how do you quantify that? Is there a test or some assessment tool for determining the greatest benefits on mankind? The fact that most of these awards are given to individuals based on a scientist's overall career achievement suggests that it's impossible to look at a single year and make such a conclusion. Even examining a person's lifetime achievement is problematic. How do you decide if a discovery that leads to environmental conservation is as important as a finding leading to a potential cure for a specific disease? There are plenty of quantitative ways to measure a scientist's success including number of publications, amount of grant money received, or number of other accumulated awards, but the contribution of these variables to the greatest benefits on mankind isn't always obvious.

Related to authentic response-outcome associations and authentic perceptions of reality that are necessary for adaptive contingency calculations, the point of this section is that it may be smart to take the more subjective awards with a grain of salt. It's probably best for Nobel Prize winners to understand that they may or may not have actually produced the most important scientific contribution on the planet. If we actually believe that we deserve all these awards that we're trading with one another, it's likely that our contingency filters may be distorted in maladaptive ways. In fact, recipients of the Fields Medal, a comparable award to the Nobel given every four years to mathematicians under age 40, actually experience a decrease in their scholarly productivity when compared to equally productive mathematicians who did not win the award. There are several potential reasons for this decline in productivity, such as the observation that recipients of the Fields Medal tend to expand their interests beyond the specific area that led them to the top prize.[15] Similar decreases in productivity have been observed with Nobel recipients.[16] Whether or not these declines are a product of a distorted contingency filter, or are even a negative outcome, is debatable. However, as observed with the Fields Medal, it's interesting from a behavioral perspective that winning the top prize in one disciplinary area makes researchers more likely to apply their interest to other areas where they don't have expertise. This confidence to work outside one's area of training may certainly contribute to a decline in traditional measures of professional productivity. Thus, although most everyone appreciates receiving an award, if the "honor" distorts reality, it may result in compromised contingencies.

Overriding Reality-Based Contingency Calculations with Religion's Blessings and Curses

I have been fortunate to experience religion from several different vantage points throughout my life. Growing up as a conservative Southern Baptist in Alabama, I had a front row pew to this version of religious teachings, preachings, and various rituals and practices several times each week. As I entered the world of higher education I became less conservative and enjoyed expanding my view of religion to one that tolerated neurobiological and behavioral perspectives.

Rather than making any judgments about the appropriateness of religion in our lives, I'm more interested here in reporting how religiosity may affect our life views to determine any impact on our contingency calculations and subsequent decisions and responses. Of course, I have to focus on humans for this investigative endeavor as, similar to the humancentric fixation on awards, no other species has been observed to exhibit religious beliefs and behaviors.

Neuroscience research indicates that one reason religion is so prevalent across different cultures and feels so natural for those who practice it is that the familiar neural networks involved in important social and cognitive functions are the same circuits involved in maintaining religious beliefs. This is why religious experiences feel like "real" experiences—they activate the same brain areas as nonreligious experiences. Consequently, we interpret them as we do any other experience. Not surprisingly, the brain is much more engaged when experiencing religion on a more personal level through imagery or prayer than it is from a more academic level. Thus, although many aspects of religion are controversial, religious *beliefs* do exist and can be studied in the neuroscience laboratory.[17] Subjects asked to think about their religious beliefs exhibit more activation in brain areas associated with emotions, self-representation, and cognitive conflict in fMRI brain scans than do subjects asked to recall nonreligious memories.[18]

The process of building "religious capital" is very different from the process required to build cognitive capital necessary for calculating authentic contingencies in the reality-based world—the same world that individuals enter after leaving their churches, synagogues, monasteries, or mosques. Further, these processes may be at odds in a person simultaneously living in both secular and religious worlds. For example, a person who is diagnosed with breast cancer builds cognitive capital by reading about successful treatments and speaking to appropriate medical authorities about treatment options leading to the highest probability of curing the cancer or entering the longest period of remission. In contrast, religious capital is gained through prayer and other abstract means such as interpreting scriptures. Sometimes these approaches complement each other; other times they may not. Advice from the medical establishment may suggest that no treatment is available for a successful recovery, whereas religious guidance may suggest that a full recovery is imminent. As you will learn later in the chapter, our brains are a bit biased toward more positive outcomes so the belief that one is protected, regardless of conflicting information, will typically override the more traditional and often gloomy real-world belief. In this situation, the real-world contingencies are often rejected in favor of the spiritually based contingencies.

There was perhaps no bigger example of the confusion of natural and supernatural contingencies than the Salem witchcraft trials of the seventeenth century. When the authoritative members of this Massachusetts community observed women experiencing hallucinations and other distorted thoughts, their Puritan beliefs pointed them to supernatural, rather than physical and natural, causes of the bizarre behavior. Because these responses were rather novel, little cognitive capital was available to draw from to provide plausible explanations. Other odd yet familiar behaviors such as vomiting were known to be caused by eating certain foods or by other forms of illness; however, these new behaviors were more difficult to explain.

Because uncertainty is often viewed as aversive, the notion that men and women exhibiting the questionable responses were influenced by supernatural causes such as demonic possession was readily adopted. If people are possessed by demonic spirits, the town leaders told themselves, they could be made to engage in these bizarre behaviors, hence the demonic-possession/bizarre-behavior association. By September of 1692, 20 women and men were accused of being witches and were subsequently executed; of these, 19 were sent to the gallows and 1 was pressed to death. Although others were condemned the next year, the executions abruptly ended.

If the religious leaders had changed their focus from supernatural to natural causes during that summer, the outcomes for the accused would have been very different. It wouldn't be until centuries later, in 1976, that a more logical and plausible analysis of the causes of these symptoms would be introduced in a paper published in the journal *Science* and entitled "Ergotism: The Satan Loosed in Salem?" Of the countless scientific papers I have read throughout my career, I found this paper to be among the most brilliant and eloquent. Its quality is all the more impressive considering that the author, Linnda Caporael, was an undergraduate student when she conducted innovative research leading her to the novel convergence of evidence supporting the ergotism hypothesis.[19] She reported that during her senior year she needed one more general education course to graduate and added a history course just to fulfil the requirement. That course led her to the fascinating topic of the bizarre behaviors in Salem. She was a mere graduate student when the paper was ultimately published as a single author paper.

When told that she had to write a paper for that course, Caporael chose Ann Putnam, a witness at the Salem witchcraft trials, as her topic, since she had just seen Arthur Miller's play *The Crucible* and wanted to explore the thesis that women could be just as wicked as men. While reading the court documents of the trials she was intrigued by the descriptions of unknown "distempers" that initially afflicted a group of about eight girls. Caporael recalled her previous reading about ergot poisoning, similar to LSD in its effects on mental and behavioral responses, in Europe, and her contingency wheels started turning. What was the probability that the disordered speech, gestures, and postures described in these seventeenth-century court documents were the result of ergot poisoning? Ergot is a parasitic fungus that grows on many types of grains, especially rye, which was used for bread making in Salem at the time of the trials. It was known to produce ergotism, a condition associated with tingling, vertigo, crawling skin sensations, distorted sensations, hallucinations, and convulsive-like muscular contortions. Caporael investigated whether the accused were likely to have been exposed to rye and ergot through preparing or eating bread. She also confirmed that the warm, damp weather conditions in 1692 were conducive to survival of the ergot fungus. The following year, when the weather conditions were less hospitable for the fungus, the symptom outbreaks seemed to have subsided. This was all circumstantial evidence based on archival data, but Linnda Caporael was one impressive scientific sleuth in that undergraduate history class.

John Hale, a Salem minister involved in the witchcraft trials, wrote about the extreme measures taken that deadly summer and the darkness of those times. He regretfully confessed that "we walked in the clouds and could not see our way."[20] In this case, the contingency calculators of the ministers and magistrates of Salem appeared to be distorted by their Puritan beliefs. Even though a plausible explanation wouldn't be proposed for a few centuries, a much needed reality check casting doubt on the witchcraft hypothesis would have quickly redirected the treatment of these individuals. Thus, when we ignore the influence of natural stimuli on various life outcomes, we increase our chances of distorting response-outcome associations and generating contingencies that not only lack any benefits but can be damaging in some way.

Fatal Distortions Leading to Suicide

Our brains enable us to calculate future outcomes so we can navigate through the journey of life. The future and its prospects drive our responses as we desire certain outcomes over others. Although neuroscientists have confirmed that the brain is fueled by the movement of various ions and neurochemicals at critical times, at another level hope appears to be the ultimate fuel that keeps us going through the ups and downs of daily life. In the 1999 movie *Jakob the Liar* Robin Williams's character Jakob Heym, who was trapped in Nazi-occupied Poland, made the profound statement, "Hunger for hope may be worse than hunger for food." Without hope, humans have very little to live for.

When one's life lacks hope for a desirable future, sometimes the final contingency decision of ending one's life may be considered. Suicide is currently a significant public health problem, with approximately 1 million people around the world taking their life each year. In the United States, suicide is the fourteenth leading cause of death.[21] It is thought that, in about 90 percent of cases, a psychiatric illness is involved. Most often, depression is the psychiatric illness associated with suicide, with about two-thirds of suicide victims having this diagnosis.[22] Among adolescents, suicide is the third leading cause of death, behind unintentional accidents and homicides; on college campuses suicide has surpassed alcohol-related incidents as the leading cause of death.[23] Suicide attempts have also increased among veterans, especially those who served in the army.[24] Sadly, many years after his role as the powerful and inspirational fictional Jakob Heym, Robin Williams, who may have suffered from dementia and who had spoken about past mood fluctuations and addiction challenges, committed suicide.[25] Even though more research is currently being conducted on this important topic than ever before, the causal factors related to this final response-outcome calculation of suicide still elude us.

When the sad case of University of Pennsylvania student Madison Holleran's suicide was covered by many media outlets in 2014, I did a double-take. Suicide?[26] This beautiful young woman was a high-achieving student and a track star, and she appeared to have a loving and supportive family. Her pictures looked like those of a person bursting with hope for the future. How did her decision-making calculators ever arrive at this final decision?

While reading about Madison's suicide, I was struck by a few comments she had made about her classes after her first semester. She told her family that she was anxious about a few of her grades; it didn't matter what she did to improve her performance, she couldn't earn the A's that she was accustomed to earning. In her opinion, she wasn't getting feedback that allowed her to alter her responses to obtain the outcomes she desired; consequently, she kept getting the same undesirable grades. Her father later conveyed that she ended up receiving a good grade in a course once the grades were evaluated on a curve at the end of the semester, but Madison didn't feel that she had earned it. On top of the many other sources of anxiety that accompany a freshman's first semester, this disconnect between her effort and grades added to the anxiety mix. After remaining the same for most of the semester, her grades suddenly and for no identifiable reason were higher. The perception of a lack of control in classes is likely an increased risk factor at universities such as the University of Pennsylvania, where the academics are so competitive. At the time of Madison's death, her school had reported six suicides in a 15-month period.[27] Added to the vulnerability of being a freshman is the perception that everyone else's life looks picture-perfect on social media. Thus, although her life looked perfect on the outside, internally Madison's sense of control over the positive outcomes in her life may have seemed to slip away, altering her contingency calculations as the old rules that worked so well in her precollege life didn't seem to work anymore.

Although there were most certainly many factors involved in Madison's decision to end her life, her anxiety related to academics, athletics, and social acceptance serves as a strong reminder that professors and staff in colleges and universities need to be vigilant about reinforcing authentic and realistic response-outcome contingencies to maintain our students' healthy brains and contingency calculators. My students will confirm that I'm not suggesting diluting academic rigor in any way . . . just doing my best as a professor to deliver valuable, timely feedback so that motivated students have the best chance to recalibrate their efforts and master the material in time to earn the grade they desire. Further, it's important for parents and professors to acknowledge the distorted nature of social media. Everyone has insecurities, awful days, and doubts about the future, but these are rarely evident on social media—where we're more likely to see image after image of smiling, beautiful people regularly reporting about their triumphs throughout life. In this new world of "generic perfection," in which everyone is perceived to be AWESOME at everything she or he accomplishes, it would be refreshing on occasion to see a few posts showcasing a pretty horrible grade, an image of a bad hair day, erupting forehead zits, a bathroom scale indicating those extra five pounds put on through the holidays, or a terribly messy room that a person just can't bring him- or herself to clean. These images are closer to the realities experienced by most individuals. If authentic information is critical for our decision-making neural circuits, it's important to let go of this elusive perfection once and for all and teach our children and students just how much can be learned from both our successes as well as our inevitable failures in life.

Beyond case studies, what does the research tell us about reducing the risk of suicide, and does it align in any way with reducing one's distortions of reality? How does one conduct research on the inner workings of suicidal brains? There are two general categories of research strategies in this area—research conducted on autopsied brains of suicide victims, and assessment of brains and mental functions of at-risk individuals reporting suicidal thoughts.

We'll start with the autopsied brains and remind ourselves that these data are correlational, and may or may not lead us to actual causes of suicide; nonetheless, it's a place to start. One of the most prevalent findings is a difference in the receptors that are activated by the neurotransmitter serotonin. One study found that receptor binding for a particular version of serotonin receptors known as serotonin 1A receptors was higher than expected in the suicide cases, especially in the problem-solving area of the prefrontal cortex discussed throughout this book.[28] However, decreased binding of another serotonin receptor, the serotonin 2A receptor, has also been found in the prefrontal cortex.[29] Another neurochemical implicated in suicide is GABA (gamma-aminobutyric acid), one of the most prevalent chemicals in the brain, known for its function in inhibiting actions. Robert Poulter, a researcher at the University of Western Ontario, and his colleagues have found abnormal or reorganized distributions of a specific GABA-A receptor in the frontal cortex area in the brains of suicide victims compared to those who died of other causes.[30] Considering that GABA often serves as the brakes of the brain's functioning, these GABA effects may be related to a disruption in the inhibition of the suicidal attempt.

Focusing on brains at risk for suicide has also revealed interesting results, but no absolute answers. Lena Brundin at Michigan State University has reported alterations in another neurotransmitter, this time the most prevalent excitatory neurotransmitter, glutamate. Patients who had attempted suicide had higher biological markers of glutamate activity in their cerebrospinal fluid than did patients who had not attempted suicide. This biological marker of glutamate— that is, quinolic acid—is also activated during inflammation, suggesting that neuroinflammation may be another risk factor for suicide.[31]

In addition to brain markers, thought patterns of suicidal patients are also being investigated. Matt Nock, working at Harvard University, uses what's called the Implicit Association Test, which requires patients to quickly associate various terms linked to life or death with either themselves or others. Compared to nonsuicidal patients, individuals with a history of suicidal thoughts are faster to associate the death terms to themselves than to other people. Interestingly, individuals with this tendency have up to a sixfold increase in the likelihood they will attempt suicide in the next six months.[32] In such cases, the contingency filters are tipping toward death outcomes. Although this doesn't point to a specific cause of suicide, such a test may be used as a determination of risk or, alternatively, a marker for the success of various treatment interventions for suicide.

Nock and his colleagues have considered many psychological factors that have been associated with suicide-related behaviors. Past research suggests that suicide is related to having a strong feeling of being a burden to others, a low sense of belongingness, a high tolerance for pain, and intense feelings of defeat and entrapment (not being able to escape from stressful, defeating, or humiliating circumstances). Suicide is often associated with a negative life event either in the past, such as child abuse, or some traumatic event occurring closer to the suicide attempt. Being inflexible and unable to shift one's attention toward other factors or events in one's life are also viewed as risk factors, as is compromised problem-solving abilities.[33] Cognitive styles such as being more pessimistic or exhibiting signs of hopelessness have also been associated with increased suicide risk.[34]

The convergence of all of this evidence suggests that the many factors related to increased suicide susceptibility may distort the contingency calculators in significant ways, rendering an individual unable to see anything other than the pronounced negative outcomes associated with one's life at that very moment. The ability to think of alternative outcomes beyond the thoughts fixed in the person's mind—or even to direct one's thinking away from the negative circumstances momentarily—seems impossible. The life perspective filters seem to get all out of focus. In her suicide letter Madison Holleran wrote, "I thought how unpleasant it is to be locked out, and I thought how it is worse perhaps to be locked in. For you mom . . . the necklaces . . . For you, Nana & Papa . . . Ginger snaps (always reminds me of you) . . . For you, Ingrid . . . the Happiness Project. And Dad . . . the Godiva chocolate truffles. I love you all . . . I'm sorry. I love you."[35] From her note it appears that Madison was trapped in her thoughts, unable to envision alternative solutions and outcomes.

When I view brain tissue under the microscope, my perception changes drastically as I progress from a high magnification lens to a lower magnification lens. When I view the tissue under the high magnification lens—for example the 100x lens—I can focus only on a few cells at a time, with very little informative context to let me know exactly where I am in the brain. It's only when I back off of the magnification, using the microscope's nosepiece to shift from 100x to 40x, to 20x, to 10x, or lower do the more familiar and informative brain territories come into view. As I see these structures—the hippocampus, amygdala, anterior cingulate cortex, basal ganglia—everything starts to come into perspective and I have a better idea of how the cells and activated circuits I had been so focused on fit into the larger brain context.

It appears that an individual with suicidal thoughts gets stuck or, using Madison's terminology, *locked in*, at the high magnification mode, and so are unable to see beyond the moment and calculate context-appropriate contingencies. As devastating as a failed relationship, a bad grade, or a lost job appear to be at the moment, these experiences typically pass and have minimal impact on a person's long-term success or happiness. Neurobiological and psychological factors, ranging from alterations of neurochemicals in problem-solving areas of the brain to impaired cognitive strategies leading to inflexibility due to heightened senses of defeat and entrapment, make it difficult for someone to refocus from this personal high magnification reflection to more varied perspectives. Of course, sometimes a person finds oneself in a situation with little chance of improvement, such as terminal illness, and the prospect of living with ongoing pain and fear may bring increased suicidal thoughts. In such a situation, the brain's "nosepiece," which allows the individual to see his or her situation from different perspectives and time points, isn't impaired—unfortunately, it is working quite accurately.

As a professor, my job is to encourage students to meet high academic standards, emphasizing the importance of pushing themselves to attain their goals and develop a strong sense of achievement. Even so, research pointing to the emotional vulnerabilities of college students reminds me to also continue to help these students use their neurobiological and psychological nosepieces to view a bad grade from multiple perspectives, moving on to try to improve the situation and consider actual, rather than distorted, impacts on the bigger picture of their lives. This balancing act is sometimes difficult but it is imperative for the emotional health of students. The more I can emphasize failure and disappointment as *transient* emotional outcomes necessary for eventual success, the less likely the contingency filters are going to be distorted, or stuck, in these young adults. It is here that the lines blur between being a professor and being a parent. The same guidance and advice holds for both of these important roles.

Optimism: Healthy Distortions of Contingency Filters?

At the beginning of this chapter I confessed that I had actively sought to distort my daughters' contingency filters on occasion, hoping that this would enhance the occasional emergence of joy in their future lives. Not to be outdone, it appears that nature has similarly tinkered with reality in ways that may give us a slight reprieve in tough times. How has nature accomplished such a feat? Through a phenomenon we know as optimism—you know, seeing that glass half-full instead of half-empty. It turns out that this is a pretty big deal for perpetuating our neural functions. Research indicates that a healthy dose of optimism leads to a greater probability of graduating from college, an enhanced ability to determine when to exert more effort, and an increased emphasis on goals.[36] Thus, optimism appears to emphasize potential positive outcomes and keeps us working toward our goals. Of course, costs typically accompany such benefits. A vivid example of a negative consequence of this optimism bias is seen in the 2008 crash of the U.S. housing market and, as an extension, the broader financial market.[37] As described by Michael Lewis in *The Big Short*, the banking and real estate industries exhibited an extreme positive bias, ignoring information suggesting that there was indeed a housing bubble.[38] As it turns out, brain bubbles precede housing bubbles.

Tali Sharot and her colleagues have investigated optimistic bias in her neuroscience laboratory at University College in London. The subjects in her studies were asked to guess the probability of certain events occurring in their lives, such as a cheating spouse, developing kidney stones, experiencing financial bankruptcy, dying before turning 70—fun stuff like that. In general, subjects tended to underestimate their probability. Even when they were presented with the actual probabilities so they could accurately update their prediction errors, that didn't always happen. When their brains were scanned, activity in frontal cortical areas involved in problem-solving and the cerebellum (involved in response coordination and other varied functions such as learning processes) accompanied a subject's estimation errors when that person persisted in downplaying the actual probability of the negative event.[39]

The most optimistic among us are very adept at ignoring updated information when it diminishes the positivity of the outcome. You may think . . . *the odds are 250,000,000 to 1 that I will win the lottery, but what the heck, you never know.* Of course, there is a happy medium between blatant denial and wallowing in despair when it comes to our various interpretations of reality.[40] The 2008 financial crisis is a vivid reminder of the notion that something appearing too good to be true probably is too good to be true even though we may be a little slow in realizing this truth.

With increasing evidence of the importance of optimism for

healthy responses, neuroscientists have started to investigate this cognitive ingredient in rats. Yes, you read those words correctly: optimistic rats. It's not likely that optimism popped onto the evolutionary scene only with the arrival of humans. Such important cognitive styles were likely expressed in many other animals prior to affecting humans. Is it possible for rats to be optimistic? After working with them for three decades my inclination is to say yes, but of course we need some systematic evidence to support my informal claims.

Rafal Rygula has tackled this problem in his laboratory at the Polish Academy of Sciences, with a clever research design enabling him to profile rats as optimistic or pessimistic. Using old-fashioned behavioral techniques, he exposes his rats to two tones—one 2,000 Hz tone that is associated with a positive outcome, such as sugar-flavored water if the rat presses a lever on the left side of the cage, and a 9,000 Hz tone associated with a punishment, such as a shock if the rat fails to press the lever on the right side of the cage. Of course, loudness of the tone is consistent between the groups. Once the rats exhibit proficiency in this training, the true test is presented. To determine cognitive bias, a 5,000 Hz ambiguous cue is presented to the rats. Do you see where this is going? If a rat is optimistic, it interprets this ambiguous cue as positive, hitting the left lever for the sweet reward. Alternatively, the pessimists among these Polish rats interpret this ambiguity as being the worst outcome and hit the bar on the right side of the cage associated with avoiding punishment. Following this cognitive bias screening and the assignment of rats to their proper cognitive bias groups, they are exposed to another learning task in which they have to exert more energy in the form of more lever presses to obtain the desired outcome. The optimistic rats worked harder than the pessimistic rats to obtain the reward, whereas both groups worked similarly to avoid the negative shock stimulus. Thus, confirming findings in the human studies, this experiment indicates that increased levels of optimism are predictive of increased rates of working and exploring.

As an extension of this optimistic rat work, Rygula investigated an optimistic intervention program of sorts. He did this by gently tickling the rats, scratching their bellies in a playful, unpredictable fashion. When rats are tickled they produce a vocalization (hence the laughter designation) that is similar to the vocalizations they emit during other positive encounters such as sex, eating, and positive social interactions. Rygula tickled the rats prior to exposing them to the cognitive bias screening described above and found that the rats were more likely to be profiled as optimistic if they were just coming off a tickling spree.[41] Although few parents consider how the belly laughs resulting from tickle fights with their kids may bias their contingency calculations, a good tickle binge may increase the chances of finicky kids actually agreeing to try the new squash casserole for dinner.

I'll end this chapter with another positive story about rats and optimistic views—one that may or may not represent reality. I recently received an interview request from a television reporter in New York City about a viral video known as the "pizza rat" video. Go ahead, google it if you haven't already seen it—it's quite impressive. On the surface, it looks like this rat has a lot of optimism as it maneuvers a slice of pizza larger than itself down a steep set of stairs in a New York City subway station. If a rat could evaluate such a situation and then make the choice to engage in this behavior so that it could enjoy a private feast on this food prize, I would say that is one optimistic rat. Not to burst your contingency bubble on this story, but the reporter revealed that it was likely this rat wasn't as optimistic as it appeared. His sources suggested that the rat video was a hoax. It seemed that the pizza rat had allegedly been trained to perform this trick so the rodent behavior could appear to be captured spontaneously on a bystander's cell phone—a video release, mind you, that ultimately led to handsome amounts of licensing fees. Then came the merchandise—pizza rat Halloween costumes, hoodies, and advertisements for video views. The reporter wondered if I had any insight into how difficult it would be to train a rat to do this. I'm not sure what concerned me more—that the pizza rat may have been a hoax or that I was the go-to "expert" to defend a subway rat's potentially sketchy behavior.

My answer? Of course a rat could be trained to perform this simplistic trick. The trainer, however, would have to be mindful of the environment. Since rats tend to avoid new environments, they should be trained in similar surroundings to those in which the actual "trick" will be performed. Regardless of whether the pizza rat was real or a hoax, the video likely went viral because it resonated with our own cognitive bias toward optimism. The idea that New York City rats could be optimistic and gritty as they navigate the city appears strangely familiar and comforting to humans. Similar to Frank Sinatra's song "High Hopes," describing a little ant that thought it could move a rubber tree plant, brains are prewired for high hopes through activation of higher cortical brain areas that sometimes work by suppressing reality.

We're treading on thin ice, however, with these reality distortions and should be careful about maintaining a healthy contingency balance. Even though it's fine to stray from reality every now and then, it's time to focus once again on generating optimal, accurate contingency calculations and their subsequent positive outcomes. We won't stay on this pure-reality track for the rest of the book, however; in the final chapter we'll consider additional healthy versions of reality-distorting brain bubbles.

CHAPTER SIX

Fine-Tuning the Contingency Calculators

Well-Grounded Lessons from Rats, Comedians, and Triple-Crown Horse Owners

ALTHOUGH THE TERM *well-grounded* is virtually absent in the neuroscience research literature, it deserves serious consideration. According to Merriam-Webster, well-grounded refers to receiving "good training" in a subject or activity. It is generally thought that well-grounded individuals are the most prepared to get the job done. In my opinion, a neurobiological exploration of how well-grounded brains accurately process past response-outcome experiences in order to pump out real-time contingency calculations for healthy responses is as valuable as investigating how healthy hearts efficiently pump blood. The authenticity and relevance of our experiences are as critical as the natural composition of our blood—synthetic, diluted, or artificial blood falls short of fueling the body with healthy energy reserves.

Even if we figure out how to have a fine-tuned, well-grounded brain, we have to beware of emerging brain bubbles that can wreak havoc on our contingency circuits. As confidence is gained with practiced contingency outcomes, our vigilance may become relaxed as we gain more and more trust in our perceived abilities, ignoring relevant feedback from the surrounding world. All of a sudden, our perceptions of ourselves and our environment are no longer authentic, and these distorted perceptions compromise the hard-earned contingency-building inroads to our brains. We have now entered the realm of the *contingency conundrum* in which our impressive ability to learn from our environment and past experiences ultimately leads to a heightened confidence and accompanying diminished capacity to engage in experiential learning.

According to neuroscientist Jennifer Beer, director of the Self-Regulation Laboratory at the University of Texas at Austin (but also referred to as the cleverly titled Laboratory of Intoxicating Science!), arrogance may be the most debilitating self-generated condition that exists for our neural networks. Arrogance can be viewed as straying from authentic contingency outcomes as one's inflated confidence begins to influence the calculations. When she scanned the brains of her subjects while asking them questions about their positive and negative characteristics (used as the measure of arrogance), she found that the most arrogant subjects had less brain activity in the orbitofrontal cortex (OFC). In fact, the effect was quite dramatic, with evidence of reduced connectivity with other important areas of the brain such as additional sections in the frontal cortex, as well as temporal and occipital lobes, in comparison with the more accurate self-assessment forecasters. As you'll recall from chapter 4, rats with lesions to the OFC had difficulty making adjustments to changing conditions in their environmental surroundings, limiting their capacity to establish accurate predictions about future outcomes. Thus, arrogance literally short-circuits an area of our brain involved in some of the most important aspects of decision-making—making it next to impossible for arrogant individuals to remain grounded in appropriate contingency calculations. It's important to point out that the decreased role of the OFC in positive self-assessment flips to an increased role when having to defend a threat to one's self-esteem, a more complex cognitive endeavor. Go ahead, think of the most arrogant individuals you have encountered in your life . . . Jennifer Beer's findings may explain a lot.[1]

Regardless of whether a person is suffering from the arrogance bias or a less-dangerous bout of optimism bias (discussed in the previous chapter), the neural contingency areas are somewhat altered. With the diminished capacity to drink up pure doses of reality, the likelihood of making the most informed decisions starts to diminish. Consequently, the focus of this chapter is the importance of keeping our neural circuits grounded to run interference between our external and internal worlds as well as our past, current, and anticipated experiences—all to finely tune our ability to calculate the most informed response-outcome contingencies necessary for optimal performance. These grounded circuits serve as a vaccination against arrogance, optimism bias, or any other threat to our brain's perception of reality.[2]

Jay Leno Revs Up His Brain with Several Ground Checks

"You know, Jay, Jerry, Dave, and Tim—they're all car guys," Mike Lacey, owner of the Comedy and Magic Club outside of Los Angeles, told me. As we spoke, my brain quickly searched for more identifying information . . . Jay *Leno*, Jerry *Seinfeld*, Dave *Letterman*, and Tim *Allen* . . . a veritable who's who of successful comedians.[3]

Why was I so interested in the mechanical interests of these comedy superstars? Could the more grounded contingencies accompanying strategic engine repairs facilitate the more ambiguous comedy contingencies in these performers? Were they grounding their neural circuits by routinely adjusting mechanical circuits? Jay Leno's tinkering with the 100-plus cars in his personal collection could easily be viewed as a contingency-building boot camp, similar to the effort-driven reward training of my Froot-Loop-digging rats. As the hands work in complex ways, one gains expertise as a successful mechanic and enjoys brain-reward hits of various neurochemicals and neural networks along the way. Indeed, hearing an engine purr or seeing a dilapidated old car restored so that it looks like it just came off the assembly line likely gets the brain's reward circuits revved as well. In a world filled with uncertainty, knowing that replacing spark plugs, valves, and pistons can restore malfunctioning cars provides a foundation for fine-tuning contingency circuits to maintain mental health. There may not be a clear connection between working on cars and delivering a perfect monologue, but Jay Leno's contingency-building repertoire aimed toward fine-tuning cars may also fine-tune activity among the brain's reward, incentive, motor, and decision-making areas.

Even though Jay doesn't use the exact phrase, his recollections suggest that he has incorporated a healthy contingency-calculation regime most of his life. After realizing how much passion he had early in his childhood for making people laugh, he became a student of human behavior to understand more about this fascinating laughing response. In his book *Leading with Your Chin*, Jay recalls watching his father practice jokes for his insurance conventions and learning the importance of understanding and reading an audience in order to get the best laughs.[4] His father told him that the phrase "run like hell" was fine with his insurance buddies, but "run like blazes" was better for more religious groups. Jay took this lesson to heart as he started to train to be a comedian, performing his act anywhere before an audience. He was building an impressive stockpile of comedic response-outcomes scenarios.

Before Jay landed his coveted job as the host of NBC's *The Tonight Show*, the range of venues he had previously performed in was quite diverse, including strip clubs, prisons, convalescent homes, Kiwanis club bars, taverns—the list goes on. Jay seemed to realize that the stakes were high if he wanted to be a successful comedian—he had to be able to evaluate which jokes were keepers and which jokes should be tossed. He had to evaluate various important factors regarding the composition of the audience—such as age, gender, occupation, socioeconomic status, and level of intoxication—when attempting to generate laughs. He could learn these valuable methods of fine-tuning his laughter contingencies only through these diverse grassroots comedy experiences.

Jay's commitment to being well-grounded with his humor education served him well on the most important night of his career. During Jay Leno's formative years, the ultimate measure of success for a comedian was an invitation to perform on *The Tonight Show* when Johnny Carson was host. After being passed over several times and told to work on enhancing his joke inventory, Jay was finally asked to perform on March 2, 1977. He was told that he would know immediately if Johnny approved, because he would be invited to join him at his desk for conversation at the conclusion of his performance. If Johnny was less than impressed, the director would shoo him off the stage to contemplate what had gone wrong. No pressure there!

After years of a comedian observing and receiving feedback from audiences, it's difficult to imagine your chances of success coming down to just a few minutes standing in front of a crowd of strangers on national television. His lone goal was to quickly arrive at an understanding of the audience's collective cognitive conscious enough to lead them down a path to laughter. Although comedians often have a rehearsed monologue, the best are ready for the unexpected— comedic prediction errors. On this night, it turned out that all of Jay's sweat equity performing for any and all audiences paid off. During that critical performance, the unimaginable happened midway through his act when an audience member started heckling him. Heckling was worse than an audience that remained silent and did not laugh—an unimaginable outcome for Jay. He quickly processed what was happening and strayed from his rehearsed material to turn that potentially unnerving experience into joke material—in real time. This is comedy contingency calculating conducted at superhero speed. He cleverly told the audience that the heckler was the kind of guy who talked to his TV each evening—saying something like, "Hey, Kojak, there's the bad guy behind you," with Kojak responding by expressing his gratitude and waving to the at-home viewer (Kojak was a police detective played by Telly Savalas in a popular TV series at the time). When he finished his act and was acknowledging the applause, Johnny invited him over to talk after what seemed like an eternity.

After Jay's *Tonight Show* appearance his career took off, and he eventually became *Tonight Show* host himself when Johnny retired, serving in that position for 22 years. Even when he reached that pinnacle, Jay never stopped fine-tuning his comedian contingency circuits, and he regularly continued to perform stand-up away from his show. He could often be seen at the small Comedy and Magic Club in Hermosa Beach, California, where he could test the waters with new jokes and make probabilistic decisions about their potential outcome if used in his *Tonight Show* opening monologue. Far from the arrogance studied in Jennifer Beer's lab, Jay continued to work as a student of comedy—and he still does. By continuing to be grounded in real-world comedy, he maintained the ability to read his audiences and strategically deliver the jokes that generated the desired laughs.

Interestingly, Jay's practice of combing through newspapers for potential comedy material led to a joke about my own rodent research. This happened as a result of work my colleague Craig Kinsley and I presented at the 1999 Society for Neuroscience meeting in Los Angeles, where we discussed our work describing how rats with maternal experience outperformed virgin rats in various learning tasks. I still can't believe that this research about our rats and their impressive brains ended up on the front page of the *Los Angeles Times* the next day. In his monologue that evening, Jay described the findings of scientists in Richmond, Virginia, who reported that pregnancy makes a woman smarter. However, he continued, after becoming pregnant, it was then too late to realize what a jerk the baby's father was. Of course, Jay's delivery was better than mine, but it was a lot of fun hearing about our mama rats on *The Tonight Show*, even though virtually no part of the joke reflected what we actually found. We worked with rats as opposed to humans, assessed the rat moms after their pregnancy instead of during the pregnancy, and used various forms of mazes to assess the navigational skills of the moms as opposed to evaluating the intelligence of fathers, but those details didn't get in the way of a little neuroscience humor.

Comedians receive better feedback from sober audiences, and because Mike Lacey wanted his Comedy and Magic Club to support the professional development of comedians, he implemented a two-drink *maximum*—as opposed to the more traditional two drink *minimum*. Even though he would make more money if patrons drank themselves into oblivion, this wouldn't be helpful to comedians' ability to gather feedback and realistically evaluate their material.

So, kudos to Jay Leno for maintaining passion and resilience in his work assisted by his outside interest in his car collection, all the while keeping himself grounded in his comedic career by consistently seeking real-world feedback. As previously described, celebrity can be a dangerous distorter of reality and instigator of brain bubbles but Jay has certainly figured out how to pull ahead of this risk and stay in life's authentic contingency-building lane. In the next section, the importance of learning from our contingency mistakes will be discussed as we consider ways to improve our probabilities for success in the future.

The Value of Failed Contingencies

When David Ring, an arm and hand surgeon at Massachusetts General Hospital, sat down one day to review his patient files following a long shift, he had a horrifying realization. According to one file, a patient needed a surgical procedure on her left ring finger (yes, David *Ring* was performing surgery on a patient's ring finger!) to stop it from becoming stuck when the patient moved it in certain ways. He panicked when he realized that this wasn't the surgery he had actually completed on this patient, as he instead wrongly performed a carpal-tunnel-release surgery. In a subsequent interview, he reported, "Just imagine the worst thing that's ever happened to you and that's how it feels."[5]

As we all know, like any of our best-laid plans, established procedures can fall apart. Although David Ring thought he had followed the proper surgical protocol, it had obviously been compromised. And these wrong-site surgeries aren't as rare as we might think. From March 2009 to June 2010, 137 such surgeries were reported in the United States. In our culture of mistakes being associated with blame and shame, Ring's response to his mistake was quite remarkable. He immediately reported the mistake to the hospital and patient, admitting his error and offering to perform the corrective surgery at no charge. Although the prospect of lawsuits was looming, everyone was very forthcoming regardless about the unfortunate mistake.

As uncomfortable as it is to learn that one's intense training, knowledge, and expertise had not served as protection against such a mistake, these circumstances present a wonderful opportunity for our brains to upgrade any faulty expectations or ineffective strategies as conditions change throughout our lives. David Ring saw this as a valuable opening to learn more about what led to this mistake, so instead of just putting this embarrassing situation behind him he brought it to the forefront. He investigated each element of that day to learn more about how he conducted the wrong surgery on his patient. This incident was especially surprising considering the existing safety procedures such as a "time-out" session prior to each surgery, during which nurses and doctors confirm the identity of the patient, the surgery site, and the correct surgical procedure. With so many checkpoints, how could anything go wrong?

It turns out that the day in question could be described as a perfect storm for this type of mistake. On this particular day the surgeon had a long shift of surgeries planned. Adding to the stress was the outcome of another patient, who had an emotional and painful reaction to her carpel-tunnel surgery. Ring reported that he felt a lot of anxiety as he listened to her describe her pain. After this interaction, and toward the end of the long day of surgeries, the patient who received the wrong surgery was prepped according to protocol, with her wrist accurately marked. But then there were delays and complications in Ring's schedule. Due to a shortage of surgical venues, the patient was moved to a new operating room, a change that was accompanied by a change of staff. During this delay Ring was called once again to tend to the emotional pleas of the stressed patient, and he recalled telling himself that the next carpel-tunnel surgery he performed would be the best one ever so the patient wouldn't experience these painful postsurgical effects. He then went to perform surgery on the patient with a trigger finger. The patient in question spoke Spanish only, and, lacking an interpreter, Ring spoke to the patient in Spanish to explain what to expect during the surgery. During this time the new nursing team prepped the patient again, unaware she had already been prepped in the original operating room. But in the process the team inadvertently washed away the marked surgical site. Further, the team misconstrued the Spanish-language exchange between surgeon and patient and concluded it was the required time-out, in which all the important details of the procedure being conducted are reviewed. Consequently, as a result of his anxious, fatigued, and distracted mental state in combination with all the miscues, the surgeon proceeded to conduct the wrong surgery.

Ring immediately reported his error to his administrators and told the patient exactly what had happened, expressing his apologies. Further, exhibiting an extraordinary degree of courage, he published the details of his blunder as a case study in the *New England Journal of Medicine*. He wanted to highlight these circumstances so others would be vigilant; he also hoped to start conversations about additional protective measures to ensure that the correct procedures were conducted in surgical settings, reducing the likelihood of repeating this unfortunate outcome. Although he feared a negative response pointing to incompetence, he received quite the opposite reaction from his peers. His colleagues were impressed by his courage and were collectively grateful for his analysis of this important case study.[6] Ring used this experience to fine-tune his actions in future similar situations. His honest response to this error was further acknowledged by his colleagues in 2013 when he was appointed as chief of the Hand and Upper Extremity Service at Massachusetts General Hospital Department of Orthopedic Surgery.

Although it's not my intention to focus on the mistakes of medical doctors, Read Montague's neuroimaging research, using medical doctors as research participants, provides brain evidence of why it is important to focus on both failures and successes throughout our lifetime. In one study, Montague and his colleagues recruited 35 experienced physicians and performed functional magnetic resonance imaging (fMRI) while they learned about two hypothetical medication treatment modes through virtual patient interactions. As the physicians were engaged in this trial-and-error learning process, making both inaccurate and accurate responses, Montague was peering in on their brains by analyzing their fMRI scans. After training, the physicians were separated into high performers and low performers based on the accuracy of their responses. The group of high performers exhibited equal rates of brain activation in both the successes in the virtual training session (the virtual patient responded well to the medication) and the failures (desired response was not obtained from the medication). Alternatively, the low performers exhibited the biggest brain response in the successful responses, but not so much during the failures, a response that, in the real world, would lead to suboptimal treatment of their patients. The brain scans revealed that the high-performing physician brains responded with heightened activity in the dorsolateral prefrontal cortex and adjacent parietal cortex in response to the failed trials, whereas the low performers exhibited heightened activity in these areas in response to the successful trials. Also interesting was the activation of the brain area known for both reward and anticipation, the nucleus accumbens, when the low-performing physician subjects were presented a trial. It's as if they anticipated being successful before really processing the details of the case, engaging in what the authors of the study referred to as success-chasing.[7] Thus, it appears that the brain anticipates more successes than failures, so we have to make an exerted effort to push through the pain and focus on our failures enough to learn from them. Focusing on failures is essential for fine-tuning our contingency-calculating brains.

Montague's research helps us understand the processes that the brain utilizes in order to make sense of the world. When we encounter a new situation, which factors do we tag as important for subsequent desired outcomes? Sometimes the selection of supposed predictive and relevant factors seems far from a grounded reality. As I was writing this chapter, a news story reported that a group of observers in formal coats and top hats had gathered at Gobbler's Knob in Pennsylvania to await the emergence of a groundhog affectionately called Punxsutawney Phil. After the observers knocked on the door to his tree stump of a home, Phil emerged and was picked up and placed on top of his stump so that it could be determined if he could see his shadow. There was great applause when it was determined that he could not see his shadow, evidence pointing to an early spring. This contingency forecast has been practiced in the United States since 1886, likely a spin-off of a European ritual focusing on February 2 as the midway point between the winter solstice and the spring equinox. Determining the future weather forecast was important for settling various debts and anticipating payoffs from future crops.[8] It is important to acknowledge that, regardless of their name, using groundhogs in this manner is not an effective way to enhance accurately derived, well-grounded contingency calculations!

This groundhog contingency example, coupled with Read Montague's research, reminds us just how much brain activity is likely diminished during many of our brain's faulty determination of future forecasts. Even though there is scant evidence that a large rodent seeing its shadow predicts an early spring, we have embraced this tradition—with some individuals perhaps actually believing it. However, although most of us would acknowledge the flaws associated with groundhog-generated weather predictions, many of our beliefs about predictive factors leading to desired outcomes are perceived as less obviously flawed even though they are just as faulty in their predictions. We need to employ every tactic available in our neural arsenals to avoid welcoming future Punxsutawney Phils into our decision-making neurocircuitry. For most of us who don't rely on crops for our incomes, weather forecasts play a minor role in the big scheme of our lives. So, perhaps it's okay to let our guard down on that light topic. However, most of us take solace in acknowledging that we would *never* let our contingency guard down when making informed forecasts about the important things in life—selecting our life partners, adopting parenting strategies for our children, choosing political leaders—nah, that would never happen! On the contrary, no part of our life appears to be totally immune to a compromised contingency calculation, regardless of its short-term or long-term impact. The next section discusses a neurochemical that is often implicated in our persisting contingency-calculating forecast screwups.

A Dash of Dopamine

Whereas the brain's preference for evaluating only positive outcomes over failures can get us into trouble, the neurochemical dopamine may provide the fuel to drive us through the most important contingency-building experiences of life. And, it turns out that the true identity of this neurochemical has been updated recently, thanks primarily to the impressive investigative prowess of John Salamone at the University of Connecticut.[9]

Although students in every psychology and neuroscience course are introduced to dopamine as the neurochemical substrate of reward, that association is less than accurate. Just as Watson and Crick wrote that the structure of DNA they had identified had "novel features which are of considerable biological interest," the claim that dopamine is exclusively involved in reward or pleasure is quite an understatement.[10] Beyond early research suggesting that the interference of the brain's dopamine system and activity in the brain's nucleus accumbens interrupted a rat's likelihood of obtaining rewards, this claim has become much more qualified and complex throughout the past half-century.

In a more updated list of dopamine functions, Salamone and his colleagues broaden the core function to facilitating motivation, a rather vague prospect. Generally, it is thought that dopamine influences one's assessment of the probability of obtaining a desired rewarding stimulus or outcome. And, considering the power of effort-driven rewards in my laboratory rats, it's not surprising to learn that motivation and movement are intricately intertwined, even derived from the same word—*movere*, meaning "to move." After decades of processing research in the relevant scientific literature, Salamone offers a new professional profile for dopamine, one that involves many aspects of motivation including the following: behavioral activation, exertion of effort directed toward acquiring our goals, flexible behavior, and monitoring of energy expenditure. Translated to behavior, dopamine seems to be more involved in the anticipation of the reward than the actual experience of the reward. Of course, no neurochemical works in isolation, and there are many relevant neurochemicals influencing our day-to-day actions. Dopamine interacts with other neurochemicals such as the inhibitory neurotransmitter GABA (gamma-Aminobutyric acid) in the brain area extending from the middle of the brain to the lower part of the frontal lobe known as the mesolimbic area.[11] Additionally, small pockets within this area—known as "hedonic hotspots," which work independent of dopamine and utilize opioids and marijuana-type receptors—have been identified.[12] Even so, dopamine is indeed a contender in this important area of directing us toward the highest payoffs in life. Whereas a healthy dopamine system will keep us working hard and making an extra effort to achieve our goals, a compromised dopamine system will keep us picking the low-hanging fruit, always opting for the easy way out even if the outcome isn't as desirable as the more effort-demanding approach. In short, healthy dopamine systems *invigorate* our behavioral responses to tolerate challenging work and delays and respond in flexible ways to achieve our goals. What incredibly important stuff! In the big scheme of all things important for our well-being and survival, this neurochemical ranks near the top in real-world importance. Considering that money doesn't grow on trees and, for most of us, we aren't handed everything on a silver platter, it's dopamine that decreases the *psychological distance* between our current selves and the rewards we want to acquire in the future.[13]

Thus, in a sense, dopamine may be the neurochemical bridge that leads to our dreams and desires, or at least to our current goals.

Without it, we're perfectly happy accepting the status quo. For example, take two students who want a career in the medical field. A dash of dopamine could indeed be the difference between one student's decision to pursue extensive education all the way through medical school, and the other student's choice to become an EMT (emergency medical technician) and bypass the many additional years of school. Both are important and respected careers, but the preparatory effort required for each profession is quite different. In addition to invigorating our responses, dopamine likely keeps the contingency-calculating areas of our brain sufficiently primed for acknowledging the most desired response-outcome contingencies.

Colin De Young, a neuroscientist at the University of Minnesota, has proposed that dopamine is a driver of exploration. This fundamental ingredient for building behavioral repertoires leads to effective means of gaining experiential capital for determining optimal contingency calculations as we navigate our way through life.[14] This system is likely involved early in childhood development as witnessed by a toddler's propensity to put everything in his or her mouth, touch everything in sight, and experiment with various vocalizations and movement strategies. Brains have to experience these things to determine future response/outcome contingencies. Dogs give sloppy kisses, the fireplace screen is hot, Mommy laughs when she hears silly noises, fast steps lead to falls and boo-boos . . . these are the initial ingredients of the most complex behavioral recipes, all driven initially by dopamine-induced explorations.

Peter "Pete" Pidcoe, a professor of physical therapy at Virginia Commonwealth University, has recently provided a wonderful exploration-enhancing treatment option for children with movement disabilities associated with neuromuscular disorders such as cerebral palsy. If our brains thrive on reducing the psychological distance between ourselves and our goals, which for an infant is typically just to touch something in its visual field, imagine how debilitating it is when that psychological distance can NEVER be diminished through self-initiated movement and discovery. Parents carry children around to show them objects in the environment that they think are interesting for these infants, but that's no substitute for the lack of self-initiation in the discovery process. So, Pete combined his engineering and physical therapy expertise to produce the Self-Initiated Prone

Progressive Crawler (SIPPC), which is essentially an elaborate skate-board; an infant can be strapped in and taught to move, or crawl, similar to an infant crawling on its hands and knees, to inspect the irresistible elements in the immediate environment. With this de-vice, an infant likely experiences healthier brain activation patterns necessary for laying the groundwork for critical neural circuits. Ad-ditionally, this experience builds the child's sense of self-agency, or sense of mastery, over controlling its movements, enhancing its sense of control over aspects of its environmental interactions. Thus, the SIPPC builds both bodies and brains as infants scoot around in a fashion similar to that of their infant peers without neuromuscular challenges.[15]

Not only is self-initiated discovery imperative for building expe-riential capital during early development, it is also critical through-out our lives, especially when neuromuscular systems are challenged by a stroke. John Krakauer, a neurologist and neuroscientist at Johns Hopkins University, has been concerned by the lack of self-discovery in the rehabilitation process. After experiencing the trauma of a stroke and subsequent lingering paralysis, many patients are faced with seem-ingly unending repetitions of boring movements in their rehabilita-tion sessions, with no apparent immediate function or outcome. Fur-ther, due mostly to insurance restrictions, this movement therapy is dispensed in such low doses that it is not likely to have an impact. If dopamine-driven discovery and invigoration are indeed important for neural growth necessary for rehabilitation, similar to infants, then these boring movement repetitions aren't sufficient to spark the new brain growth required for recovery.

Discouraged by the outcomes of traditional rehabilitation ther-apy for stroke patients, Krakauer recruited a rather unconventional research team to address these deficiencies. He hired artists, animators, engineers, and computer programmers to staff his Brain, Learning, Animation, Movement (BLAM) Laboratory. Krakauer's plan was to throw a dash of dopamine into the rehabilitation process by adding motivation and reward—attempting to make the process fun! He wanted to capture the childlike curiosity that drove the development of the patients' brains when they were infants and toddlers.

Krakauer's team developed a high-quality rehabilitation video game starring a dolphin named Bandit. Patients learn to control a type of joystick to guide Bandit through the water—finding food and friends, and warding off the occasional shark. As patients move their joystick in this virtual reality context, their bodies merge with the animation, forming a motoric connection with their perceived environment. Further, decisions are made at a rapid pace in this exercise, building and solidifying new neural circuits. In order to increase the odds of rehabilitation success, the dose of interactive time with Bandit was a generous two hours per day.[16]

So, has Bandit and the Johns Hopkins team been successful? The actual data are still being collected and evaluated, so it's too early to tell. Still, kudos to this team for thinking outside the box in an attempt to fuel the brain's ability to regain experiential capital and optimize contingency circuits.

Crossing the Contingency Line with Secretariat

Not far from Randolph-Macon College, where I worked for 28 years (before recently moving to the University of Richmond), is a beautiful homestead in Doswell, Virginia, known as The Meadow. Although it is the site of the Virginia State Fair today, this homestead became famous in the early 1970s due to the celebrity of two of its residents, horse racing's Triple Crown winner Secretariat and his equally impressive owner, Helen "Penny" Chenery. In 1973, this duo's accomplishments graced the covers of *Newsweek*, *Time*, and *Sports Illustrated*. Secretariat and Penny's story illustrates the level of achievement that is possible when the work of several well-grounded individuals, human and equine in this case, converge.

Penny Chenery always had the "horse bug," as she called it, a passion for horses that was patterned after that of her father, Chris Chenery. She lived in Colorado with her husband and four children when she received a call that her mother had passed away. At that point, Penny decided that her father needed help with his thoroughbred racing business in Virginia. He had renovated the old family home at The Meadow and had spent decades learning the strategic ropes of the thoroughbred horse business, and with his advancing age it was getting increasingly difficult for him to manage this expansive enterprise. Penny's brother and sister were in favor of dissolving the business, but Penny computed a more positive contingency forecast. She saw an opportunity and decided that she could help preserve her dad's dream and perhaps even capture the elusive Kentucky Derby prize, a long-held but as yet unrealized dream of Chris Chenery.

Penny stepped into the family business at The Meadow, and began acquiring the appropriate experiential capital to navigate the multiple layers of decisions leading to the highest probability of a Derby win, maybe even the Triple Crown title. Penny immersed herself in the trade journals and sought the advice of experts, many of whom had been her father's longtime loyal friends. As a woman, she was certainly an outlier in race-horse owner circles. But with the combination of the MBA degree that she had already earned from Columbia University, her educational training in horse racing, and her overall passion for horses, Penny had the necessary discipline to gain an informed confidence in a relatively short period of time. Unlike Jay Leno, who had years and years to hone his craft, Penny needed to hit the ground running (alongside the horses) to maintain the success that her father's diligence had established. Fortunately for Penny, she had mentors who gave her freedom to make decisions for herself as opposed to encouraging her to follow their advice. This autonomy was probably critical in enhancing her vigilance for assessing contingency calculations, accelerating her rise to a respected player in this male-dominated field. Timing was everything, since two horses that needed her attention would quickly appear on the scene. According to Kate Chenery Tweedy, Penny's daughter, this new role was invigorating for her mom, who seemed to embrace it with both enthusiasm and passion. She was a woman on a mission. Perhaps dopamine was fueling this new invigorating, experience-driven role, paving the way for relevant learning and successful outcomes.[17]

Although it is not always easy to step into a family business and maintain its success (as will be discussed in Chapter 9), Penny's strategy for listening to and learning from the most informed and respected sources paid off. In fact, she didn't merely *maintain* her father's business: in just three short years she catapulted it into a realm of success that exceeded expectations—with a Triple Crown winner. Her achievement was literally the stuff of movies, with Diane Ladd playing the role of Penny in the 2010 Disney movie portraying her story. In 2013, Penny received an Honorary Degree of Letters from Randolph-Macon College for her fast-paced achievements. I was fortunate to be in attendance on this momentous occasion. After hearing Penny's insightful comments about her experiences at the nearby Meadow four decades earlier, I asked if she had ever felt intimidated as a woman in the old boys' horse racing network. Without missing a beat, she quipped, "No I didn't feel intimidated, they could have their old boys' network as far as I was concerned, because I had the damn horse!"

The truth is, considering the size of The Meadow's impressive stables and inventory of horses, Penny had a lot of horses. Her success came down to picking the right damn horse or horses to invest in each year. Through a combination of her recent experiences and the observations of her trainer, Lucian Laurin, Penny gained the valuable skill of detecting winners from the foals. Similar to humans, horses require training and relevant feedback to excel on the track, and the earlier this focused training begins, the better the odds of reaching its maximum potential. By listening to her trainer and staff, and appropriately applying her recently acquired experiential and cognitive capital, an early focus was placed on two horses, Riva Ridge and Secretariat. Just before Secretariat made his exciting debut, Riva Ridge was the first horse from The Meadow to win the Kentucky Derby. Although her father didn't live to see Secretariat win the Triple Crown, he lived long enough to hear the news that Riva Ridge had won the Derby in 1972. He was unable to speak at the time but he expressed his acknowledgment of the cherished news through tears that streamed down his cheeks. Just one year later, Penny's success would continue, with Secretariat winning the Kentucky Derby, the Belmont Stakes, and the Preakness Stakes—the coveted Triple Crown![18]

Although many may be tempted to attribute such achievements to luck, the theme of this book is that success is most often the product of well-grounded, finely tuned contingency building. But even if achievement is earned via appropriate experiential training, success can slip in and distort those well-grounded and hard-earned neural circuits. After all the hard work to produce the champion Riva Ridge, Penny made the insightful comment that "a good horse arouses ambition and compromises the lessons gained from hard work." Penny's informed insights about lessons learned from training Riva were timely, and a necessary recalibration put her team back on track in preparation for Secretariat. There was no place for overconfidence in this field; every horse presented a new and different experience. Riva was a sickly, nervous young horse that seemed to be running away from the herd in a state fueled by fear in his races, and Secretariat was a strong foal that developed into a dominant leader of the pack. The differences between these two horses emphasizes how important it is to notice the unique nuances and individual predispositions of each new contender.

As a scientist, I don't explain events in our world as magical or mystical, but I admit that the way Penny earned her experiential capital chops, added to the physical agility and cognitive prowess of Secretariat, produced something that seemed a bit like magic. Unlike magic, however, both Secretariat and Penny's achievements were the result of becoming well grounded through appropriate training.

Sadly, not long after Penny reviewed the manuscript for this book, she passed away after living an engaging and challenging life. As I interviewed her, however, four decades after her adventures with Secretariat, Penny was investing in her own brain and health in impressive ways. Before visiting her in Boulder, Colorado, I spoke to her on her 94th birthday and, when asked how she would celebrate her big day, she conveyed that she was playing poker with friends—for REAL money. This is just one of Penny's weekly activities that kept her neural circuits engaged—in addition to yoga, massages, exercise, art, discussions of current events—the list seemed endless. Her weekly schedule looked like the perfect template for maintaining healthy brains. Working around her active schedule for a visit, I witnessed her continued mental discipline as I had the opportunity to speak with her about her experiences with Riva Ridge and Secretariat. As she followed my questions with interest she became frustrated if the direction of the question wasn't clear or on target with the discussion. It was impressive to witness how deftly she was analyzing our conversation on multiple levels, and I could appreciate how, nearly a half-century earlier, her mental strategies enabled her not only to pick winners but to become a winner herself in a very challenging field.

Let's Make a Contingency Deal . . . with Statistics

Even the most adept individuals possessing the most effective strategies for building the cognitive capital necessary for making the most informed decisions reach their limit in some response-outcome scenarios. Consider the seemingly simplistic classic television game show *Let's Make a Deal*, originally hosted by Monty Hall. This show required the contestants to make "deals" by trading known prizes for unknown prizes, some of which were indeed prizes—perhaps a trip to an island—while others were valueless items referred to as *zonks*, such as a live goat or a broken washing machine. In 1990 Marilyn vos Savant, who wrote a weekly *Parade Magazine* column featuring intellectually challenging questions and dilemmas, issued a probability challenge using a hypothetical extension of the *Let's Make a Deal* format.[19] As vos Savant noted, there are absolutely no cues directed toward the door with the highest probability of hiding the prize. So the contestant just picks a door, any door—let's say door #1. Next the contestant is shown what's behind one of the remaining doors—and it is always an undesirable prize (such as the goat). At this point, an opportunity to switch to the remaining unopened door is presented to the contestant. With this information, the contestant must make a final decision to stick with door #1 or switch to the third door. What would you do? Most individuals see the chance of selecting the prize as 50/50 since there are two doors and it has to be behind one of them. Thus, it wouldn't matter if you stuck with your original choice or switched to the new door. In this case, no cognitive capital gained from game shows or opening doors in some other life scenario would appear to offer help with this decision, known as the "Monty Hall problem" . . . except if you had taken some form of a statistics or decision analytics course at some point.

Cognitive scientist Gary Klein has shared a solution to this Monty Hall problem. A key is a person's cognitive flexibility in having the ability to leave the 50/50 odds notion behind. Yes, this cognitive flexibility likely requires the actions of dopamine. It turns out that everybody increases their chances of securing the prize if they switch to the remaining unopened door. If you're scratching your head and doubting this detour in decision analytics, consider this exercise. Let's say that the prize is behind door #1 and you had already selected door #1; if you switch to the unopened door, you lose the prize. But wait a minute, that's just one scenario. For the second possible outcome, let's move the prize to door #2. Remember that you selected door #1. After being shown the joke prize behind door #3, you switch to door #2 and, bam, you win the prize. Stay with me, as we have one more condition to test with your choice of door #1. If the prize is behind door #3 and you are shown the undesirable prize behind door #2, and you switch to door #3, you win the prize. Now, do the math. If you selected door #1 and stayed with this choice, you would win 33 percent of the time, but if you switched, your odds of winning the prize increase to 66 percent. This is similar to the host offering you the door you selected or both of the other doors (which is the case since one is revealed and you can select the other one); presented in this way, you would go with the two-door over the one-door option. This will still result in losing 33 percent of the time even if you apply this information, but if you have the chance to become a serial player of this game, you could really increase your desirable prize outcomes using the switch technique.

This is a different type of cognitive capital—very counterintuitive, and it requires us to use our executive decision-making areas such as the dorsal cingulate cortex to override our tendency to believe that we have a 50/50 chance of winning the prize once the first goofy prize is revealed. In this case, having the ability to shed our prior conceptions as we learn new strategies enables us to fine-tune our decision-making abilities.[20] Just like the rats in my lab struggling with their prediction errors involving misplaced Froot Loops, we need to employ every strategy possible to update our ability to make more accurate predictions and avoid annoying prediction errors. Klein argues that the idea of just stockpiling experiences to generate the best decisions and responses sometimes requires a little house-cleaning and retrofitting, something he refers to as the *snakeskin strategy* of shedding old expectations and observations and updating when necessary.

In 2008, Nate Silver, a baseball statistician, applied his finely honed skills to the political arena and surprised everyone with his on-target predictions in the presidential election. Beyond the simple technique of sampling voters for the polls, Silver considers all relevant variables such as the age of the voters, the current mindset of voters, and recent events influencing the voters' opinions. He collates this relevant information with the best practices of sampling the population in order to generate the most accurate predictions. These predictions go beyond our intuitive abilities; we have to agree to disagree with our hunches and beliefs in these cases and look toward these sophisticated techniques. Thus, on top of us gaining relevant experience throughout our lives to fine-tune our knowledge and skill sets, statistics can sometimes give our decision-making abilities superhuman qualities. Today, in the midst of all of the news services polls in political races, Nate Silver serves as editor in chief of ESPN's FiveThirtyEight.com website, contributing relevant analyses to enrich the political analysis circus that accompanies each presidential election. Of course, it takes appropriate experience to know when to use or trust such statistical analyses. In informed hands, however, statistics-informed analytics can take experience-driven decision-making to a new level.[21]

Anne Milgram, former district attorney for New Jersey, saw a need for more formal decision analytics for the criminal justice system. Too much money was being spent on incarcerating too many individuals, and the recidivism rates were abominably high. Her plan was similar to the one depicted in the popular movie *Moneyball*, which was based on Michael Lewis's story of the baseball statistical whiz Billy Beane, who switched from relying on instinct to smart statistics about a player's playing history to generate a statistical predictor of success for the Major League Baseball team Oakland A's.[22] Milgram set out to "moneyball" the criminal justice system so that the judges would be better prepared for their contingency forecasts, arming them with a combination of experience-driven "instinct" and decision analytics. The results were impressive. Using massive data sets, Milgram's team created a risk assessment tool that facilitates a judge's prediction of whether a particular individual will commit another crime and, if so, the likelihood that it would be a violent crime. Less money was subsequently directed to house low-level crime inmates such as drug users so that more attention and resources could be directed toward more violent offenders. Anne Milgram's research confirmed that, without the benefit of statistics and analytics, the experiential and cognitive capital that the judges brought to the bench, even with the best of intentions, failed to increase the safety of residents of New Jersey. This isn't necessarily surprising; it appears that as decisions affect people beyond the individual, it is more difficult to rely on personal experiences. In these cases, statistics and decision analytics serve as a contingency prosthetic of sorts that generates the most informed and effective responses. In short, when the stakes are bigger than ourselves, the necessary decision analytic strategies will likely extend beyond our personal decision-making abilities.

Green Contingencies

If reading about all the hard work that goes into gaining the necessary experiential capital and decision analytics in order to fine-tune your contingency calculators is a bit overwhelming, you may want to consider closing this book and walking outside. That's right—walk through a park or a tree-lined street, or, if no such options exist, head for the closest potted plant in your office building. In contrast to the active strategies for fine-tuning our contingency calculations recommended throughout this chapter, simply spending time in naturalistic environments appears to be an effective technique for building some contingency muscle.

I became interested in how natural environments affect the behavior of laboratory rats several years ago when my students and I designed a variation of the classic enriched environment studies conducted in the 1960s. In the typical enriched environment study, groups of rats housed in environments with toys, activity wheels, and other enriching stimuli had richer neural connections than rats housed in more impoverished conditions. Thus, enriched environments seemed to be more engaging, leading to more neural activity. Decades later, research investigating the impact of enriched environments continues, with results continuing to reinforce the pervasive influence of complex environments. One recent study, for example, reported that the young adult offspring of rats that were exposed to an enriched environment during pregnancy (but then relegated to their more boring standard cages after giving birth) exhibited enhanced neuronal complexity—even after experiencing induced brain trauma early in life.[23] Thus, *prenatal* exposure to an enriched environment altered the behavior and brains of the offspring following birth and into adulthood—that's quite an intervention!

Although I have always been fascinated by the far-reaching impact of enriched environments, my students and I noticed that most of the studies in this area used artificial stimuli to provide stimulation. These artificial environments certainly produced interesting results, but was it the best type of environmental enrichment? Would an enriched environment with more natural stimuli—a hollow log instead of a plastic igloo for a hiding place, a stick instead of a plastic ladder for climbing, a rock instead of a marble—be more effective? As indicated in Figure 9, we referred to the natural and artificial enriched rats as "country" and "city" rats, respectively. A third condition housed the same number of animals but included no form of enrichment—this was the impoverished group. Marion Diamond, a neuroanatomist on the original "enriched environment" investigative team at UC Berkeley, and her colleagues conducted a similar type of study in which one group of rats was housed outside with natural elements. Although the few animals that were assessed appeared to have heavier brains, the results were never officially published.[24] So, this natural territory of research was also a new territory for research in behavioral neuroscience.

In addition to using a few traditional learning and emotional tasks in this new green line of research, we wanted to eavesdrop on the animals during the night hours, when they are active. We videotaped each cage for one hour so we could systematically compare the behavioral responses of each group—if they were grooming, interacting with the environment, resting, etc. Similar to the public service announcements asking, "It's midnight, do you know where your kids are?," although we knew where our rats were during the dark hours we were very curious about what they were actually doing. More like, "It's midnight, do you know what your kids are DOING?" After analyzing their spontaneous behavior we were surprised with the results. We anticipated that, after several weeks of living in these arranged assignments, the animals in the impoverished environment would spend more time interacting with one another since they didn't have objects for interacting. We were interested in any differences in engagement with objects between the natural and artificial enriched environments but weren't sure of the direction of the findings. Would it be more stimulating to live in the country or the city laboratory neighborhoods?

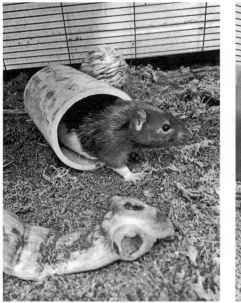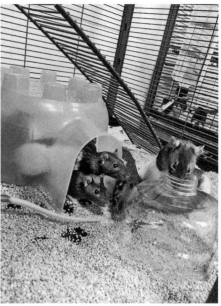

Figure 9. Country and City Rats. *In my laboratory we are exploring the effects of different types of enriched environments. The rat on the left is in a natural-enriched environment with dirt and sticks and a hollowed out log to hide in, while the rats on the right are housed in an artificially enriched environment with a plastic water bottle, manufactured bedding, and a plastic igloo for hiding. Although the "country" and "city" rats each demonstrate comparable learning abilities, the rats housed in more natural environments exhibit greater emotional resilience. (Photos courtesy of Lambert Neuroscience Laboratory, University of Richmond)*

It turned out that the natural enriched animals were the most engaged across the board. They interacted with more objects than did the artificial enriched environment animals and, surprisingly, interacted with each other more than the impoverished and artificial enriched groups did. The enhanced interactions with the environment observed in the natural group, perhaps increasing the groups' invigoration, scaled up the spontaneous contingency training and all of its associated benefits. We completed additional assessments and generally found that the cognitive skills were similar between the enriched groups, but the natural enriched animals exhibited enhanced emotional boldness. For example, in a threatening escape task, the natural enriched groups exhibited less activation of the fear-related nucleus known as the amygdala.[25] In a similar study, natural enriched animals exhibited the bold response of diving in a water tank as well as had healthier stress hormone profiles.[26] Enough said, time to move to the country!

Thus, if you are a laboratory rat, you may have healthier emotional responses if you are surrounded by a little dirt, rocks, and sticks. Test-taking, or cognitive, skills, however, may not be affected. But what if you're not a rat? If you're a human, can nature offer any cognitive or emotional advantages? David Strayer, a cognitive scientist at the University of Utah, and his colleagues have proposed the Attention Restoration Theory, suggesting that spending time in nature recalibrates the attentional systems of the prefrontal cortex. In one study, after spending approximately four days hiking in natural environments, the subjects performed 50 percent better on a test of creative thinking and problem-solving. Although the exact mechanisms still need to be investigated, the authors proposed that our normal everyday lives, complete with social media and never-ending distractions, compromise the ability of the prefrontal cortex to focus effectively on single problems. Nature, however, is proposed to replenish our neural activity, perhaps leading to more restful and focused introspection—an important ingredient for accurate contingency building.

So, if I asked you to generate a word that connects the following words: SAME/TENNIS/HEAD and you can't think of a word that connects them, you know where you need to go—grab your backpack and hit the trails. If you were able to generate "MATCH," your neural activity may be acceptable—carry on.[27] In a similar vein, a few years ago, when my colleague Massi Bardi and I took our comparative animal behavior class to the DuMond Primate Conservancy in Miami, Florida, we asked the students to sit in the beautiful rainforest exhibit for 30 minutes before collecting a saliva sample from each to assess their levels of the stress hormone cortisol. We compared the rainforest stress hormone levels to a sample taken a little earlier that morning at the base camp before class—a setting that didn't include the visual beauty and natural sounds of wildlife encountered in the rainforest exhibit. Interestingly, stress hormones were about 20 percent lower in the natural setting in this preliminary study. Too bad we can't bottle nature and dispense it in effective 30 minute doses!

Cold-Turkey Contingency Cuts

As we tune up our contingency calculators, our brain adjusts to being increasingly in tune with the world around us. These primed brains will serve us well—ensuring that authentic information is processed in a timely manner. But, caution is in order. Once a brain is in its contingency prime, it may experience a paralyzing blow if the contingency context changes. If we revisit the contingent-trained, Froot-Loop-digging rats who benefited from experiencing effort-driven rewards and strengthened contingency circuits, one study pointed to a slight hiccup.

In the laboratory we have explored the effects of various coping styles exhibited by rats. It turns out that rats generally profile as passive, active, or flexible in their responses to threatening situations. These responses can be thought of as temperaments and likely extend to humans—some individuals are consistently shy or inhibited when faced with a threat (passive copers), others come out swinging every time, complete with toxic elevations in blood pressure (active copers), whereas others' responses differ depending on the situation (flexible copers). You are probably already thinking that the flexible copers require more neural processing to determine contingency forecasts associated with various responses prior to generating the behavioral output.

Before going further, I'm guessing that you want to know how the rats' coping styles are profiled. I obviously can't rely on self-report assessment formats in rats. The origin of this idea started with pigs . . . in the Netherlands.[28] When researchers gently restrained young piglets on their backs, they noticed differences in the number of wiggles or struggles to free themselves, and this degree of reactivity persisted the next week. We adapted the "back test" to rats and added a third coping style to the more passive and active responses. When tested twice within a week, some animals weren't consistent; they switched from passive to active or vice versa. These animals were profiled as the flexible copers and, in multiple studies, exhibited markers of resilience. One resilient response, for example, is their adaptation to the threat of being placed in a swim tank. The first time rats are exposed to the water, they swim around looking for an escape route and, at some point, start to conserve energy by floating. Although some researchers have interpreted the float response as "conditioned despair" and a sign of giving up, perhaps even a symptom of depression, I have always had a different take on this behavior. Once an animal figures out that there is no escape route, it makes sense to conserve energy and float. If we expose the rats to three consecutive days of swim exposure, responses of the three coping groups are interesting. Whereas the active and passive copers gradually increase their duration of floating over the three days of swim stress, the flexibles exhibit more of a drastic increase on the second day, as if they figured out that there was no escape earlier in comparison with their more consistent responding counterparts. The flexibles switched their responding to match the context of the situation, real-time contingency tuning . . . pretty amazing stuff.

So, it gets interesting when we expose rats of different coping strategies to contingency Froot-Loop-digging training (effort-driven reward training) for five weeks prior to the swim task. I hypothesized that the contingency training would serve as a "behavioral therapy" for the actives and passives, bringing them closer to the coping capacity of the flexible copers. That didn't happen. The contingency training just made the flexibles super-copers, prompting them to have an even more drastic rise to increased floating on the second swim compared to the other groups. That finding was surprising but made sense in retrospect. We had tuned up the supertuned rats. If the flexible copers were already more tuned in to contingency building, then giving them training in this area just strengthened their ability to be accurate readers of their environment and enabled them to adapt accordingly in record time. There didn't seem to be a ceiling to this effect that would allow the less-effective coping groups to catch up. The biggest surprise came when we looked at the non-contingent, or the trust fund, group that received their Froot Loop rewards regardless of their efforts, masking any meaningful contingencies. The flexible copers in this group failed to adapt to the swim stress, exhibiting the same level of floating across the swim exposures. They were horrible at this task! The other groups were compromised as well, but the most drastic change was with the flexibles.

Again, in retrospect this makes sense as well—confirming that the rats were smarter than we were in this situation. If the flexible animals are prepared to read the environment and generate accurate connections between their responses and outcomes, when this successful strategy is suddenly squashed—cold turkey—in the trust fund situation, the effect is more drastic for these animals.[29]

If forced to categorize humans and their advanced decision-making abilities, I would put most of them in the flexible coping, contingency-sensitive category. I have argued that one factor contributing to the rising rates of depression in service-oriented, technology-driven societies is the removal of contingency training in our day-to-day lives. Instead of engaging in tasks that our ancestors did, such as cooking, cleaning, building, and gardening, requiring ongoing contingency calculations, we are more likely to sit around and push buttons for our resources to appear as soon as possible. Consequently, I fear that many of us are increasingly becoming the noncontingent trust fund group, with a diminishing ability to adapt to changes in our environment in effective ways. Regardless of whether we diminish our contingency-building activities suddenly or gradually, our sense of control and efficacy also diminishes, leading to emotional and cognitive challenges and, in the worst cases, psychiatric illnesses such as depression. The effects of placing flexible rats on a trust fund schedule are indeed very informative regarding our own mental health.

As explored in this chapter, contingency calculation abilities aren't carved in stone. Fortunately, they can be fine-tuned via a variety of methods that facilitate the availability of authentic feedback. Such methods range from including hands-on real-time activities, such as Jay Leno working on his cars, to enhancing awareness about our decision-making process by taking a statistics class, to priming and recalibrating our neural circuits for response-outcome contingencies by simply taking a walk in nature.

For most of our lives, we're accountable for our contingency-building opportunities, building a sense of self-efficacy and self-agency. Early in a child's life, however, contingency-building templates are influenced by parents and caregivers. The critical impact of parental responses on these essential contingency-building neural circuits is the topic of the next chapter.

CHAPTER SEVEN

Parenting

Time to Recalculate
Life's Contingencies

ALTHOUGH I HAD SEEN many maternal rats efficiently attending to their pups in my laboratory by the time I became
pregnant myself, I started to gain a new respect for the
seemingly effortless parental responses in these little rodents as my own delivery date approached. As I signed up for baby
classes at our local hospital and accumulated a stack of parenting
how-to books on my nightstand—including the popular *What to
Expect When You're Expecting*—my appreciation for the rat moms,
who just seemed to know what to do, grew immensely. Whereas I
had a wonderful husband to help with the parenting—and was sched-
uled to deliver in a hospital with elaborate equipment, a full professional staff, and the requisite buffet of drugs—my laboratory rat
moms were on their own. No classes, no books, no rat social support,
no baby rat showers, no rat mommy blogs, no hospital, no drugs—
nonetheless, most maternal rats successfully deliver 10–14 healthy
pups. I would leave the bulging pregnant rat in the lab on one day,
and the next day the new mom would be hovering over her tidied-up
nest and pups, almost looking tranquil as the little pink rat babies
huddled and suckled underneath her. She had it all under control.

By comparison, I felt woefully unprepared when held to the competency standards of nature's vast spectrum of prepared and resilient mothers.

And the rodent mom's impressive parenting skills don't stop there. Without other rats around to help (at least in their laboratory cages), and in the absence of any form of rodent day care for her clan of 12 or so pups, all of the caretaking is on her shoulders. Extended nursing periods ensue, with hungry offspring rigorously tugging at twelve nipples strategically located across her entire belly. These small animals quickly morph into larger, juvenile animals with teeth—all focused on this mama rat's nipple zone. In the midst of dispensing all of this nourishment, the pups aren't able to go to the bathroom on their own in the early days following birth—they require a little nudging in the form of the mother licking the anal-genital area to prompt them to eliminate their physiological waste. As seen in Figure 10, there are no wipes or diapers for these animals—it's protein out (of the pup), protein in (to the mother). It's not very scientific of me to say so, but EEEWWWWWW!

So now you understand my respect for these rodent mamas. In the lab during my first pregnancy I vividly remember watching the moms retrieve their pups, hover over them in their arched back position to provide equal access to her nipples during nursing sessions, and, when they weren't nursing, gently hold the pups upside down in their hand-like paws to lick their backsides. Wow, I was in awe. I hoped I would be as successful as these uber-mamma rodents were.

Both the mother and the neuroscientist in me wanted to learn more about these supercharged rodent mothers. Consequently, my long-time colleague from the University of Richmond, Craig Kinsley, who was embarking on his journey as a father at the time, and I took our parental curiosity to the lab and began a program of research that continues in my lab today, more than two decades later. Although our respective human children grew and thrived, suggesting some success on our respective personal parental fronts, our enthusiasm in the lab continued to grow as we learned more about the beautifully choreographed responses of these mama rats.

These impressive parental responses and the brain circuits that produce them may be viewed as the neuroarchitecture, or the brain's foundational groundwork, of sympathy, empathy, and various forms

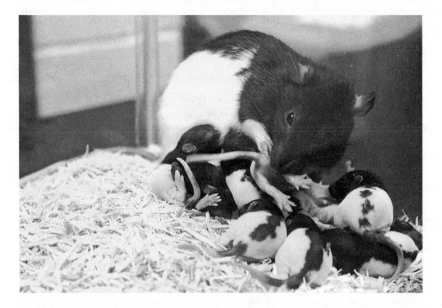

Figure 10. Rodent Supermoms. *This maternal rat has grouped her pups in a huddle and is keeping them clean and healthy by licking them, even around their hindquarters, to stimulate them to urinate and defecate. No diaper service for this rat mama! (Photo courtesy of Lambert Neuroscience Laboratory, University of Richmond)*

of social nurturing. Indeed, some of the traits that we perceive as distinguishing humans from other animals such as reptiles began millions of years before humans hit the evolutionary scene. These higher-order characteristics likely began when the first animal delivered offspring that depended on the parents for survival. With parenting behavior entering the brain scene, the evolutionary contingencies for survival were now drastically changing. Unlike the reptiles who would drop their eggs and go, leaving the baby reptiles to fend for themselves, this new version of animals hung around its offspring—building nests and providing nourishment through glands, mammary glands, on its body. How strange is that? The earliest of these nurturing prototypes likely lived in the shadows of the dinosaurs over a hundred million years ago. The prototypes, with names such as *Agilodocodon* and *Docofossor,* initially came in small packages of just a few inches in length, allowing them to go unnoticed and coexist with the massive reptiles.[1] Thus, the dawn of mammals, with all of their impressive adaptations and specializations, coincided with the dawn of nurturing and caring. That observation gives me a warm feeling every time I think about it—so glad to be on the mammalian side of the evolutionary family tree.

In this chapter we'll review the exciting ways a mother's brain changes as she transitions to motherhood. In fact, I can't think of an animal encountering a more drastic transition in contingency calculations than the massive impact reproductive experience has on a female brain and behavior. For example, the mother rat's former behavioral contingencies get an extreme makeover, as pups that were once viewed as aversive—relegated to the *avoid at all costs* category—become an object of desire and obsession. Of course, all mammalian species are successful parents; otherwise, species would go extinct. Hence, it is difficult to underestimate the importance of the changing contingencies accompanying parenthood in mammalian species. In addition to the rat moms that I have worked so closely with over the past three decades, we'll also review other parents, both mothers and fathers, including humans, to learn more about how neural and behavioral contingencies change to accommodate parental care for helpless offspring totally dependent on others for their survival. Along the way, we'll discuss the many changing contingencies that maximize returns on long-term parental investments in the form of healthy, functioning offspring. Unfortunately, parenting isn't a foolproof system; at times, the environment and other contextual factors compromise parental investments. Once problems are identified, appropriate interventions may be introduced to keep the parenting contingencies and eventual outcomes—in the form of high-functioning, healthy, and happy kids—on track.

Transformation of the Parental Brain: Lessons from the Rodents

As we began our research journey investigating the brain and behavior of the maternal rat brain, we initially focused on the areas of the brain involved in tweaking the contingency circuits so that instead of viewing the smelly, whining, hungry pups as somewhat disgusting, the mother would find them extremely appealing. The brain area known as the hypothalamus was the obvious first stop. The hypothalamus is the go-to brain area for all things motivation-related, as it influences our basic motivations such as hunger, thirst, sex, aggression, and stress responses. It's difficult to imagine that so many essential behaviors are regulated by something the size of an almond in human brains, but that seems to be the case. Of course, as is the case with most brain areas, the hypothalamus achieves its behavioral reach through connections with other brain areas so, it's important to emphasize that this brain area isn't working in isolation of other neural networks. Even so, this brain area is essential for many behaviors that are important for survival. Not surprisingly, maternal responses are also influenced by this small brain area. One of the "fathers" of maternal behavior, Michael Numan, began investigating the role of this brain area as part of his doctoral dissertation research at the University of Chicago nearly a half-century ago. In his groundbreaking work, Numan provided clear evidence that the hypothalamus was essential for maternal responses in rodents. If a small segment of this area, known as the medial preoptic area, was destroyed, the once doting maternal rats no longer paid any attention to the pups.[2]

We now know that, since the first mammals started scurrying around their dinosaur "earth-mates," the medial preoptic area of the hypothalamus has been the hub of maternal responses necessary to keep various species alive and functioning. Not unexpectedly, though, this brain hub receives help from other brain areas and is fueled with various reproductive hormones such as progesterone, prolactin, and oxytocin.[3] For example, the brain area traditionally associated with rewards, the previously discussed nucleus accumbens, is also a part of the rat's maternal circuit. When Craig Ferris, an inventive neuroscientist at Northeastern University, developed a rat-sized brain scanner he found that the maternal rats' nucleus accumbens lit up when pups were presented to them. And when presented with both pups and cocaine, the moms' brains showed more reward activation toward the pups.[4] This type of research confirms that a mom's offspring activate the brain's fundamental motivational and reward centers. Now we're starting to understand those helicopter moms among us.

Overall, in comparison to reptiles, mammalian brains clearly evolved to attend to the needs of others. However, Craig Kinsley and I, along with our students, were less interested in the broader

evolutionary adaptations and more interested in the individual transformation that happened each and every time a mammal delivered
offspring. The changes that occurred in the hypothalamus to help
orient the female to her offspring were essential for the offspring's
survival, but the successful maternal mammal had to do much more
than just tend to her offspring. In the real world, a mom has to feed
herself so she can maintain lactation for up to 14 additional animals,
regulate her emotional responses so that she doesn't waste unnecessary
energy on runaway stress responses or other unnecessary metaboli-
cally expensive responses, and keep a vigilant eye toward protecting
her offspring from predators. Thus, it appears that the maternal-
induced changes in the rat prepare her for "off the nest" behavior in
addition to the expected "on the nest" behavior adaptations. The
job description for being an effective mom was extensive, and we
wanted to know how the brain was providing a neural assist to help
the moms with these behaviors, the new maternal contingencies that
weren't typically considered to be maternal but were essential for
maternal success.

Because we were in psychology departments, it's no surprise
that we started with mazes. To protect their helpless pups, mother
rats need to be superefficient when they leave the nest to search for
food—a behavior known as *foraging* in the animal world (similar to
those energy-efficient shrews discussed in Chapter 2). As previously
mentioned, the rat moms need to expend as little energy as possible
and get back to the nest promptly. This isn't the time to take a stroll
through the food patch or go exploring in unknown dumpsters imagining what her nest would look like in that particular neighborhood.
The foraging response can be simulated and assessed with the various mazes described in Chapter 2. The Kinsley lab used the Radial
Arm Maze with eight arms radiating from a central area. The rats
learn to enter the arms to retrieve food rewards, with the most efficient learning to avoid arms that have no food. Thus, to perform
this task efficiently, the rats have to use a form of a working memory
to successfully complete this spatial foraging task. In my lab, we used
the Dry Land Maze that I described in Chapter 4, in which the rats
are required to remember the location of the single food well with
the Froot Loop among a group of eight previously baited wells.

A definite theme started to emerge in the use of both of these foraging tasks in our respective labs. The maternal rats, compared to their virgin counterparts that hadn't experienced any type of re-productive behavior, could get down to the business of working these foraging tasks very efficiently. In the Radial Arm Maze the mother rats made fewer errors, and in the Dry Land Maze the mother rats reached the baited wells the fastest. This didn't surprise us consid-ering how important it was for these single mother mammals to be efficient about getting their food and returning to the nest. Regard-less, it was impressive to see these maternal modifications reflected in these laboratory tasks.[5] When we made the foraging tasks even more relevant for rats by switching from Froot Loops to crickets for their snacks, the maternal rats remained superior to their virgin counterparts.[6]

But did these animals actually have to go through pregnancy and lactation to experience this foraging boost? We added a "foster mom" group to our maze studies and found that just being exposed to the pups enhanced the foraging skills of the female rats.[7] It's likely that the rats going through actual pregnancy and lactation may have been more specifically primed for their maternal modifications, but caretaking experience in itself (as seen in the foster moms) also ap-peared to be a significant factor driving the maternal brain and all of its contingency modifications. Interestingly, these offspring-driven contingency calculations continue to change throughout the paren-tal experience for these rats (for example, as told in one of my favor-ite rodent stories in my previous book, *The Lab Rat Chronicles*[8]). Rut-gers University neuroscientist Joan Morrell has repeatedly shown that rat moms with young pups prefer a chamber associated with pups over a chamber associated with cocaine. This preference changes, however, when the pups are a little older (about 16 days old), at which time the moms shift to preferring the cocaine-associated chamber over the pup-associated chamber.[9] Of course, these rat pups grow up much faster than our human kiddos, so much so that by the time they're weaned they're considered juvenile rats—so this contingency shift from parental nurturing to parental medicating preferences is happening about the time the rats are entering their preteen and teenage years. I'll leave it to the parents out there to confirm or deny that these effects observed in rodents may generalize to human par-ents during the teenage years.

After behavioral changes were established in the maternal rats, our next goal was to learn more about the brain areas regulating these additional tasks that had been added to the rat mom's job description. Modifications in the connections located in the hippocampus, a brain area involved in learning and memory, seemed to play a role. Compared to virgin rats, lactating rats had more spiny connection points, known as dendritic spines, in the hippocampus. This brain upgrade likely played a significant role in the changing contingencies occurring in the maternal rats. And, not to leave out the dads, when we investigated how paternal experience affected the male brain in a wonderful little paternal rodent known as the California deer mouse (*Peromyscus Californicus*), similar foraging enhancements and hippocampal modifications were also observed.[10] It is interesting that only about 5 percent of all mammals exhibit paternal behavior, but when they do it looks like they are affected in similar ways as the moms. Thus, it appears that nature is an equal opportunity brain game-changer when it comes to making adaptations to care for helpless offspring.

Even when maternal rats are in their twilight years (or twilight months, considering rats' two–three year lifespan), the maternal-induced benefits persist. When maternal rats were placed in a competitive task requiring them to ignore the presence of two additional rats, maternal experience counted—this time in a dosage effect. The females with the experience, or contingency, capital, of raising two litters won most of the competitive Froot Loop matches, with the females having a single experience of being a mom coming in second, and the virgin rats winning virtually none of them.[11]

Turning our attention toward emotional responses, research focusing on emotionally charged areas of the brain, namely the fear-sensitive amygdala, confirmed that maternal experiences dampened the emotional responses of female rats in tasks that didn't involve the welfare of the pups, such as exploratory tasks.[12] Emotional responsiveness in the form of maternal aggression is heightened, however, if an intruder threatens a mother rats' pups. Maternal aggression reaches its height about the end of the first week of lactation, then drops off considerably by the end of the second week, as the pups become more mobile. Yes, this is about the same time that the cocaine starts to look a lot more appealing to these rat moms.

Perhaps a toning down, or mellowing, contingency correction comes on the scene prior to offspring adolescence to preserve the sanity of the maternal brain. Personally, this is about the time my daughters, perhaps seeing that my own mellowing response was not kicking in during their adolescent years, frequently told me to take a chill pill. There seem to be times during our lives that we don't need to accurately calculate all relevant contingency outcomes, and the time associated with parenting adolescents certainly seems to fall in this category. Our brains may not be equipped to handle the stressful reality of realizing just how many ways our increasingly independent offspring can make a decision with devastating consequences. In the infamous words of Colonel Jessep, Jack Nicholson's character in the 1992 movie *A Few Good Men*, parents likely "can't handle the truth!" Yes, during these parental challenging times, when a cocaine chamber isn't an option, maybe we should just take a chill pill and be happy in our partial state of contingency denial.

Although these parental recalculations in rodents are interesting (at least for me), it's time to look a little closer at how these research findings translate to humans. Human moms may not be out catching crickets to provide much-needed sustenance to nurture their brood, but they share many of the same maternal brain circuits with the rodents.

Scanning Parental Recalculations in Human Parents

Just how similar are the human maternal brain circuits to the rodent mom brain circuits I had been investigating? I wanted to see . . . for myself. My colleague, Craig Kinsley, and I packed up our spouses and kids to drive south to the Medical School of South Carolina to visit Jeffrey Lorberbaum, a psychiatrist-researcher who shared our interests in the maternal brain. Jeff had designed several studies in which mothers listened to baby cries, either from their own or from another mother's baby. The design was a simple one and, Jeff told us, was suggested by a brain pioneer whom we both admired, Paul MacLean. Among other accomplishments, MacLean is known for naming the *limbic system*, an area of the brain involved in emotions.[13] MacLean had written extensively about the maternal brain and had communicated with Jeff that it would be fascinating to put moms in a brain scanner and have them listen to babies' cries to see what areas would light up. Jeff's subsequent studies were designed to do just that.

By the time I arrived at Jeff's lab in the beautiful Southern city of Charleston, South Carolina, he had already collected valuable data on this topic.[14] For example, in one study he placed first-time moms who were still breastfeeding in a scanner to obtain functional magnetic resonance images (fMRIs) of their brains when they heard their babies cry, and compared these results to standard control groups with generic background noise or no sound. He found that the usual maternal brain suspects identified in the rodent literature were differentially activated to the baby cry sounds—that is, the hypothalamus and basic brain reward areas were activated. Further, supporting MacLean's earlier ideas that a pathway from a brain area in the center of the brain (the thalamus) to the more recently evolved cortex was involved in maternal behavior, Jeff found that the moms' thalamus and various cortical areas were activated in their brains. In fact, I was so intrigued by MacLean's writings about the maternal brain that I designed an image reflecting the evolution of the maternal brain from reptiles to mammals (Figure 11). Getting back to Jeff's research, considering that cortical areas such as the prefrontal, orbitofrontal, and cingulate areas are involved in multiple cognitive and emotional responses, the baby cries had a strong impact on the maternal brains—as the moms attempted to devise a plan to get to those crying babies as soon as possible!

So, how did my brain respond to the baby cries? Well, since my daughters were already beyond the baby cry stage at that point, I was more interested in experiencing the study from the standpoint of the mothers serving as participants. Indeed, it was intense listening to the shrill cries (of other babies, in this case); however, in full disclosure, I made a serious error before entering the scanner. After drinking my morning coffee, I neglected to visit the restroom before climbing into the scanner. Once tightly secured in the scanner, with absolutely no way to escape until the scanning time was complete—with my two colleagues, Craig and Jeff, watching my brain activation patterns with interest—I was obsessed with the strong desire to break out of the scanner and run to the restroom. Lessons learned for future brain scanning adventures!

James Swain, another psychiatrist-researcher currently at Stony

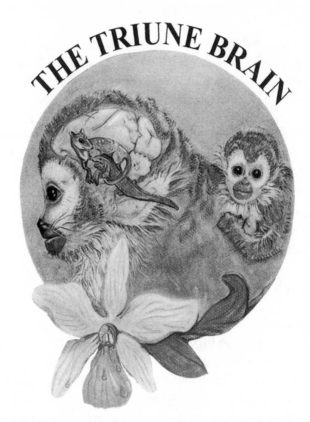

Figure 11. Nurturing the Maternal Brain. *As described by Paul MacLean, the triune brain has components of earlier evolved brains such as reptiles and ancient mammals. Although this synopsis may be overly simplified, it is clear that, while the more recently evolved primate brain shares a brain stem with reptiles, the cortical complexity is unique to mammals. The reptile shown here depicts the brain stem, the small mammal (paleomammalian species) depicts the hippocampus (especially the curved tail) in the rich emotional system named by MacLean, and the squirrel monkey cortex represents advanced responses, including play, language, and nursing, that characterize mammalian maternal behavior and may have influenced the evolution of caring and nurturing. I designed this image when I was a young mother and asked my daughter's talented caregiver, Jacqueline Berry, to bring it to life so that I could present it to Paul MacLean in a special symposium devoted to his research insights about parenting. (Image courtesy of Lambert Neuroscience Laboratory, University of Richmond)*

Brook University, has continued Lorberbaum's work in fascinating ways. Swan and his colleagues have shown that certain brain areas involved in maternal reward and motivation such as the hypothalamus exhibit structural growth when assessed three to four months following delivery.[15] That's right, even though lots of mothers have scoffed at our rat research, singing the praises of more complex maternal brains because they felt anything but "smart" during this time, we now have evidence that this is happening for human moms as well.

In the course of observing such dramatic changes in the mom's brains, Swain also became interested in investigating activity patterns in fathers' brains. Whereas increased activity in a few of the brain areas previously associated with maternal responses such as the hypothalamus and prefrontal cortex were observed between about 3 and 15 weeks following their baby's birth, some puzzling decreases in a few cortical areas such as the orbitofrontal cortex were also recorded. This is indeed a head-scratcher; however, inverse, negative correlations between paternal depression and growth in a few of the brain areas were also observed, indicating that fathers with more brain responsiveness were less likely to suffer depressive symptoms as they became fathers.[16] At this point, it's clear that fathers' brains change with the arrival of offspring, but more research is necessary to determine how brain plasticity is different between mothers and fathers— and if this information may be useful as we consider *best practices* for maintaining healthy parenting strategies.

Although I haven't assessed human parental brains, my colleagues, students, and I have investigated the impact of parenting in two wonderful monogamous species of monkeys, the cotton-top tamarin and the owl monkey. I have been fortunate to conduct noninvasive field research with several primate species in collaboration with the DuMond Conservancy in Miami, Florida. Since these two primate species contribute to the 5 percent of paternal mammalian species, we were anxious to see if both the moms and the dads would be more efficient foragers as we had observed with the rodents. We constructed a foraging tree on which we placed marked rubber change purses containing various amounts of rewards—for example, purses with vertical stripes had two pieces of sweet treats, horizontal stripes indicated one piece, and a pentagram design indicated no rewards. When these purses were hung on ventilated shelving, similar to pieces of fruit hanging from a tree, we simply stood back and recorded the foraging strategies exhibited by the animals. Sure enough, the primates of both species with parental experience went for the high-value purses more often than those who had not been parents.[17] Further, research conducted with Massi Bardi revealed that urine samples from the owl monkeys that were parents had more resilient profiles of stress-related hormones, suggesting that, similar to the rodents, these nocturnal monkeys also experience emotional resilience in the midst of their parenting journey. Thus, parents from across the animal kingdom should be happy to learn that evidence from rats, humans, and monkeys confirms that parenting indeed reprograms contingency calculations, especially contingencies related to searching for food and maintaining efficient emotional responses.

Neuroeconomics of Parenthood during Turbulent Parental Times

Although a tsunami of brain changes occurs to prepare a female for the changing contingencies accompanying motherhood, this elegant transformation can't always withstand physical, emotional, and environmental challenges that some mothers face. I always emphasize to my students that the bulk of our research focuses on animals with all of their needs met—food, water, safety, comfortable temperature, etc. Sure, being in a laboratory cage isn't wonderful, but most of the natural threats faced by rodent moms in nature are removed. When the resources start to become scarce, then the maternal rat needs to take care of the offspring while keeping herself alive as well. If ever there was a case of essential downsizing and redistribution of resources, it's when a mother is trying to save her offspring during challenging circumstances.

If rats are given limited resources in the form of a wire mesh floor and little to no bedding, but still given sufficient food and water, the rat moms' ability to care for offspring is severely compromised.[18] Recently, a group of my students designed a version of this type of maternal resource study. They tried to simulate a low socioeconomic status (SES) environment by exposing animals to their normal cage bedding, just one-half inch instead of one and a half inches, and one strip of paper towel for nest building compared to the standard three strips. The typical one and a half inches of bedding with three strips of paper towels represented what we called the high socioeconomic status condition. In my opinion, the low SES group didn't represent a very impoverished condition compared to the normal resource condition (high SES), but for this student group project it was worth exploring. I was fortunate to be in the lab one morning after a rat in each SES group had delivered its litters the previous evening. The differences in these two animals were evident. The high SES mother had her pups organized into one group positioned in a neatly constructed nest of paper towels. She was positioned over them in the typical arched-back nursing posture, with everything appearing very organized. The mom in the low SES group seemed confused. Small strips of paper towel were strewn across the cage and, even though most of the pups were grouped in a single huddle, one pup was across the cage all alone. The mother didn't seem to notice, or at least wasn't responding to that lone vulnerable pup— hairless newborn pups can't thermoregulate and are dependent on warmth provided by the mom and other sibling pups to survive. It was looking like limited resources had restricted the appropriate maternal contingency calculations. We are currently exploring these maternal SES data further.

Another finding in that initial pilot study was unexpected. For a more thorough understanding of the effects of the poverty-induced maternal care, I asked the students to record pertinent physical measurements of the pups, kind of like a laboratory rat version of the Apgar Scale, to determine the trajectory of their growth patterns. Interestingly, the low SES pups had shorter tails—by about 20 percent. I know, tail length was certainly not a component of our children's Apgar assessment. But isn't this interesting? As we are typically focused on the brain, this effect on the tails was quite surprising. But once we considered that finding, we realized that the tail size may be a bit of a luxury when growth resources are limited. When we checked the past literature on this topic we found that we weren't the only lab that had noticed this effect. In Nepal, anatomy professor Shaligram Dhungel, noted that the removal of the mom from the nest during certain parts of the day resulted in reduced tail length, along with reduced body length and head size. It's not clear what exact function a rat tail serves, but there is speculation that it regulates temperature and facilitates balance.[19] Regardless, when resources are compromised (even bedding resources), the physiological and survival bells and whistles provided by a nice, long tail may be compromised to provide more essential functions.

In humans, limited resources may be even more detrimental to the development of our children. You'll recall from Chapter 5 that parental socioeconomic status and education level had significant compromising effects on the surface area of the child's cortex.[20] An additional study of children in France indicated that, in addition to cortical shrinkage, the hippocampus, involved in learning and memory, was smaller in children from lower SES households. And, focusing on specific cognitive effects, language seems to be the most vulnerable cognitive ability in low SES children.[21] These compromised language abilities reinforced the prior findings of Hallum Hurt, a neonatologist at the Children's Hospital of Philadelphia. She and her team found that the four-year-old children of parents who were able to provide more resources in their homes, such as books, music playing devices, and social nurturing, had stronger language and memory scores, along with a larger hippocampus. The number of words children are exposed to appears to be critical for building their cognitive reserves so that they can engage in effective contingency calculations as they develop. For example, another study found that children of parents with a higher SES profile (e.g., college educated) heard approximately 2,200 words per hour, whereas lower SES children heard only approximately 600 words per hour—a difference of about 30 million words by age four.[22] Rich and engaging conversations, therefore, may be a significant factor in the development of healthy brains, regardless of actual SES status. Language, of course, is a critical component of a child's growing contingency and experiential capital.

One interesting program of research suggests that restricted maternal care changes the offspring's genetic blueprint and output via a natural genetic phenomenon known as epigenetics. Epigenetics is a popular field of study focusing on environmental factors that alter the degree to which genes are turned on and off. Thus, environmental and behavioral conditions can alter the expression of the genetic blueprint that was once thought to be carved in stone. McGill University's Michael Meaney and other researchers such as Columbia University's Frances Champagne have conducted valuable research on this topic. Specifically, pups that receive a lot of parental attention in the form of licking and grooming exhibit more emotional resilience and healthier brains as adults compared with pups receiving little such attention. Thus, the inherited genetic blueprint can be tweaked by relevant factors in a young animal's environment.[23] Although some researchers aren't convinced these changes are totally explained by epigenetic changes, it's an intriguing idea with impressive empirical support.[24] These potential epigenetic changes to the stress response likely result in lifelong changes in contingency calculations for these animals.

Thus, in the context of neuroeconomics, well-placed investments in maternal care result in long-term returns on parental investments in the form of healthy, thriving offspring. As fascinating as the neuroeconomics and decision-making prowess of motherhood are, the paternal investments of male blue-footed booby birds provide perhaps the most dramatic example of neuroeconomics in parenting. Like most birds, the booby birds are biparental, with the dads incubating the eggs, feeding the chicks, and defending them when necessary. In fact, these dads spend about six months with the brood. Researchers observed the parenting investment in young and old blue-footed booby birds on Isla Isabel in Nayarit, Mexico, a volcanic island sometimes referred to as Mexico's Galapagos Island due to its diverse wildlife. In a clever test of long-term contingency calculations in the bird brains of this species, the researchers gave the young and old dads a dose of a bacterium, lipopolysaccharide (LPS), a bacterium that would make them feel weak and sick for a period between a few days and a couple of weeks. Would the paternal responses be similar between the young and old dads?

Compared to healthy controls, the sick young dads were a bit more neglectful of their brood, ending up with 16 percent fewer hatchlings and 59 percent fewer fledglings (that is, birds that could successfully leave the nest—the bird version of leaving for a job or college). Remarkably, the old dads played their reproductive cards a little differently. Compared to healthy controls, they produced 59 percent more hatchlings and "graduated" an astounding 98 percent more fledglings. This observation likely reflected the fact that, for these birds over 10 years of age, this was very likely the last blue-footed booby bird brood (that's quite a tongue twister!). So, all parental resources were invested in this final brood. The younger birds, however, after recovery, could produce many more broods, so attending to their own health likely resulted in the long-term outcome of increased hatchlings and fledglings. The evolutionary biologists refer to this phenomenon as the terminal investment hypothesis. This dramatic change in parenting behavior provides beautiful support for the transformation from *self-attentiveness* to *other-attentiveness*. Although it's more pronounced in mammals, there is certainly strong evidence of these effects across the animal kingdom, especially in the biparental birds.[25]

I'll close this section with another rat example of changing neuroeconomics accompanying parenthood. I often show my students a video of a rat mom who has her nest along the edges of an urban underground sewage system, a nice dry spot close to food-carrying water that is released from the houses and apartments from above. During a flood, however, everything changes and the mother and pups often find themselves in peril. The video I show my students features a rat mom grabbing a pup gently in her mouth and carrying it to safety—navigating the rising water along the way.[26] One might conclude that having one safe pup would suffice for the maternal rat and that, once she and the pup were out of harm's way, she would stay put on dry and higher ground. But she kept returning, each time with the threat probability rising, to retrieve her pups—her genetic investment—so that they would all be in the safe, new area. It's fascinating to ponder the changing neural circuits that contributed to this once self-oriented rat to the current others-oriented maternal rat, a transition that occurs over the short duration of her three-week pregnancy. We see examples of such selflessness in human parents all the time. Nurturing and love directed toward others appear to be grounded in our neural circuits. It should come as no surprise, however, that when nurturing is compromised in a child's life, the neural circuits responsible for healthy brain functions break down on many levels.

When the Childhood Contingency Accounts Are Frozen:
Lessons from the Romanian Orphans

Twentieth-century Romanian dictator Nicolae Ceausescu's plan to "grow" the population of his country ignored important information about families and healthy development of our society's greatest resource—children. Consequently, his plan to enhance the power and greatness of Romania backfired as he planted the seeds for a national brain crisis. According to Ceausescu's uninformed line of thinking, if he coerced women to have more babies, there would be a larger base of citizens, enhancing the strength of Romania. Accordingly, he taxed women for not having more than five children and implemented the "menstrual police" to make sure healthy young women were menstruating and on the path to getting pregnant. Women who had seven or more offspring were awarded the title of "Order of Maternal Glory." Family units gave way to "worker" units, as young adults moved to cities for work, away from their extended families. As families had more children than they could support, a situation exacerbated by Romania's failing economy, they were forced to leave their children in institutions. Although many parents viewed this gut-wrenching decision as temporary, it was rare for the financial conditions to improve enough to bring their children back home.[27]

After Ceausescu's execution in 1989, the world got a glimpse of the conditions of the institutions that served as homes for approximately 170,000 children. It was reported that the caregivers for these children worked in three shifts, and a single caregiver may have had the responsibility of attending to up to 15 children. Basic needs were met—food was provided, along with a crib—but they received little social contact or sensory/motor stimulation. Television crews filmed children as they stared passively at ceilings and walls, the unfortunate residents of what looked very much like a child factory. The images captured the blank stares, repetitive movements, and stunted growth of these unresponsive children, and produced a collective gasp across the world and an intense desire to help.[28]

Neuroscientist Charles Nelson, currently at Harvard University, and his colleagues Nathan Fox and Charles Zeanah set out with an ambitious plan of learning from this horrific situation. They hoped to acquire information that would help the millions of children around the world who continue to live in institutions. The key to their research program, later named the Bucharest Early Intervention Project (BEIP), was a fundamental statistical trick known as randomization of subjects. This basic component of research requires researchers to test the effects of a particular manipulation, such as those of a particular diet, by starting with a group of similar individuals and then randomly assigning each individual to a specific experimental or control group. For the diet example, a group of similarly sized individuals would be randomly assigned to either a diet group or a nondiet group. Ideally, the only difference between the two groups would be the type of diet assigned, which helps to ensure that any differences after the implementation of the manipulation— that is, the particular type of diet—are due to the manipulation and not to existing differences in the study's participants such as different starting body weights or varying metabolic rates, or growing up in a culture that prefers high-fat foods.

Refocusing our attention on the children, past research had already indicated that such impoverished conditions were associated with a plethora of developmental delays. However, in these real-world situations, it was always difficult to tease out the potentially confounding effects of other variables because there was no randomization of participants. For example, prenatal conditions, or the notion that the child may have already possessed characteristics that prompted the parents to abandon them or leave them at institutions, could have been factors in past investigations. With so many children in the Romanian institutions, the plan for the Bucharest project was to establish a foster care system and randomly assign children to the foster care group or to a group that remained in the institution (which they referred to as the "care as usual group"). The ethical dilemmas were intense—these were human children, not laboratory rats. The researchers took great pains to keep the best interests of the children in mind at every step—acquiring consent from their parents, placing siblings in the same home, and enthusiastically supporting the adoption of children in the care as usual group when the opportunity arose.[29]

When Nelson and his colleagues first visited the institutions, they were struck by the silence. Unlike the children in rowdy preschools in the United States, these kids were hauntingly quiet. Nelson reported that this was typically seen in neglected children. Most of us are used to day care centers filled with the sounds of children—laughter, endless chatter, crying. This is because children growing up in responsive environments learn that there are consequences to these various forms of communication. When you cry, someone comes running. However, that wasn't the case with these children. They had learned the absolute saddest of contingencies: "If I cry, no one will care or come to check on me . . . so, why bother?" This is the emotional scar of neglect, and it is invisible—there are no bruises or broken bones clearly indicating that a trip to the emergency room is necessary—just learned contingencies that the children's responses don't lead to desirable outcomes. Consequently, Nelson has suggested that childhood neglect is among the most damaging of the various forms of childhood maltreatment, including physical abuse.

Did the researchers associated with the Bucharest project find that the institutionalized children could be rescued by foster care placement? The multiple years of assessments suggest that foster care helped move the children's growth and intellectual scores closer to the children raised by their parents (the community control group); however, the foster children never quite reached the level of the community group. And, the greatest gains were seen in children adopted by the time they were two years old. Also encouraging were the brain electroencephalogram (EEG) data that the researchers collected by placing something akin to a shower cap on the children, with sensors strategically placed throughout the cap. Institutionalized children's EEG results were characterized by lower output in higher-frequency brain waves (i.e., alpha and beta, typically associated with more arousal) and more output in the lower-frequency brain waves (e.g., theta) typical of lower levels of arousal. Children in foster care who were placed in homes by the time they were two years old, however, had EEG patterns that were indistinguishable from the children raised by their parents when they were tested at eight years of age. Foster care also reduced the brain tissue deficits (identified with magnetic resonance brain imaging) that were observed in institutionalized children. Once these results were made public, Romania began a more formal foster care system. Hopefully, with an estimated 8 million children institutionalized around the world, these findings will continue to shape policies surrounding the care of these kids.[30] In the United States it has been reported that the cortex (the outer layer of the brain) of children who were adopted from institutions overseas and tested as teens was smaller than that of children raised by their biological parents. This deficit was especially apparent in the prefrontal area that is so important for gaining the ability to form new contingencies to solve problems and make smart decisions. Further, the longer the child was institutionalized, the smaller the volume of the hippocampus, another brain area involved in learning and memory.[31]

Nurturing Contingency Capital: The Historic Behaviorist Parenting Debacle and the Informed Views of Maria Montessori and Carol Dweck

In the course of singing the praises of behavioral perspectives throughout this book, I have been cautious about a few select theories espoused by J. B. Watson, a noted pioneer in the establishment of behaviorism within the discipline of psychology. As mentioned in Chapter 2, the insights of the early psychologists with behaviorist perspectives were intriguing, as they captured the value of understanding our responses and movements. There's no doubt that the contributions of the behavioral pioneers—Pavlov, Watson, Skinner, etc.—had a huge impact on the field of psychology and the emerging field of neuroscience. However, Watson's ideas about parenting and nurturing children certainly didn't fall in this category. Although I recently served as chair of a psychology department for 17 years and have always respected the principles of behaviorism, I can't give this famous psychologist a pass in the "understanding parental responses" category.

When Watson was at Johns Hopkins University, he was well known for his infant studies in which he recorded their reflexes and responses to various stimuli. Yes, he would take infants who were only a few days old and force them to hang from a bar to determine how long it took them to drop. In 1920 he told the president of Johns Hopkins, Frank Goodnow, that he wouldn't be satisfied until he had a "laboratory" in which he could raise children from birth to age three.[32] In what would be his last official "scientific" publication, he and his young protégé, Rosalie Rayner, proudly described their work with a nine-month-old infant infamously known as Little Albert. After establishing that the infant had no fear of a white rat, they established a "conditioned fear" by pairing the rat with an extremely loud noise made by hitting a metal pipe with a hammer. After several pairings of these rat stimulus-response contingencies, Little Albert wasn't too happy about seeing that rat. Additionally, his fear generalized to other stimuli in his environment such as white fluffy rabbits. Voila! Watson and Rayner had created a conditioned fear in a helpless toddler.[33]

After rereading Watson and Rayner's famous article describing this case study, I found myself thinking about how substandard this study was on many levels. Using only one subject, and implementing such tactics as "refreshing the reaction" when it appeared that the emotional phobic response was waning, were far from the methodological ideal. Ethical matters aside, an undergraduate student of mine would receive an incomplete at best for such work lacking in appropriate experimental rigor. And I haven't even mentioned the fact that the child was not "unconditioned" so that the conditioned fear would be diminished. For all we know, he may have been impacted by this study for the rest of his life. To make matters worse for the necessary follow-up of this study, Watson had an affair with his student, Rosalie, who was half his age, while they were conducting this experiment. The resulting scandal culminated in Watson's firing, and he never worked in an academic institution again. Young Rosalie, who was not allowed to complete her degree at Johns Hopkins, later married Watson.

In his 1928 book *The Psychological Care of Infant and Child*, Watson advised against the "mawkish and sentimental" behavior of coddling one's child. In stark contrast to what we have learned since from studies of institutionalized children, his book argued that infants should be raised by a series of rotating "parents" and nurses—going so far as to say that traditional family life was detrimental to the development of a child's independence and individuality. And it gets better (well, actually worse) with this admonition: "Never hug and kiss them, never let them sit on your lap. If you must, kiss them once on the forehead when they say good night. Shake hands with them in the morning. Give them a pat on the head if they have made an extraordinary good job of a difficult task. When you are tempted to pet your child remember that mother love is a dangerous instrument. An instrument which may inflict a never-healing wound, a wound which may make infancy unhappy, adolescence a nightmare, an instrument which may wreck your adult son or daughter's vocational future and their chances for marital happiness."[34] In contrast, recall the work of Harry Harlow discussed in Chapter 2 indicating the importance of touch and nurturing, what he referred to as love, in his rhesus monkey subjects.

It's difficult to imagine the suffering that occurred in the children whose parents read this book by the former Johns Hopkins authority. When Watson guaranteed he could raise a child to qualify for any profession—including doctor, artist, or thief—he admitted that he was going beyond his data or, facts, as he called them.[35] By this time he had been ousted from Johns Hopkins and now was applying his behavioristic views at his job in a Manhattan advertising firm. Although out of his familiar academic surroundings, he remained influential; for example he created new trends, such as a coffee break that would increase the consumption of coffee. But, being far enough from the halls of academe that he need not worry about empirically supported theories, he loosened up his scientific rigor as he espoused his ideas about parenting. It was John B. Watson *unplugged* by this point, but that didn't minimize the negative impact on children raised under these faulty parenting principles. The lives of his own two sons with Rosalie, raised under the couple's behaviorism principles, demonstrate the harmful nature of these principles. One son, James Watson (Jimmy), wrote in adulthood that his dad's behaviorism beliefs compromised his ability to respond effectively to human emotions, contributing to his poor self-esteem and other emotional crises, and, likely, to his brother's suicide as well.[36] Watson's granddaughter, actress Mariette Hartley, born to Watson's daughter from his first marriage, freely wrote about the toxicity her grandfather's parenting principles had on her mother and, ultimately, herself.[37]

As I have reviewed Watson's work related to parenting, it has become increasingly apparent that his controversial research and writings mark a tragic misstep in the history of psychology. Interestingly, other early behaviorists didn't fare well in the child-raising category. In the 1940s, for example, Harvard psychologist B. F. Skinner was criticized for his "Skinner Air Crib," which provided a constant temperature for babies, freeing them from the need of heavy clothes and blankets for warmth. In fairness to Skinner, though, there were few negative outcomes associated with this approach; in fact, from the few air cribs that were sold, mostly positive experiences were reported.[38]

In contrast to Watson's distorted view of a child's developing brain, Maria Montessori espoused a different perspective about the most effective enriching and nurturing environments for children. While Watson's influence has waned almost entirely (the lone exception may be the use of the term "time out"), Montessori's child-rearing ideas, which were emerging just a few years prior to Watson's work, are still vigorously discussed in the field of child development and education. Practical evidence of her influence is the continued popularity of the Montessori educational system; more than 5,000 schools in the United States use the Montessori method. These schools include multiage classrooms, specialized self-paced educational materials, self-directed preferences of task selection, and a diminished emphasis on structured tests and grades. With this system, there's no passive contingency building; the cognitive and experiential inventories are self-initiated and maintained in this style of learning.[39]

Born in 1870 in Chiaravalle, Italy, Maria Montessori was the first woman to receive a medical degree in that country, finishing with an emphasis on neuropathology. Her early work with mentally handicapped children reinforced her belief that these children still had needs and desires, and she set out to reach them at their level in order to maximize their educational experience. Whereas others may have directed these developmentally delayed children to institutions so they could focus attention on the development of healthy children, Montessori listened and learned from these children. How could she build their behavioral contingency repertoires? Her observations and research pointed her in the direction of sensory stimulation—especially after seeing the children use their hands and sensory systems to explore their restricted environments. Perhaps their brains needed more of this type of stimulation.[40]

As Montessori set out to develop educational programs for all children (not just delayed children), she balanced her respect for both scientific principles and the well-being of the children. There were most certainly no babies hanging from pipes nor were there loud clanging noises designed to generate phobias in children on Montessori's watch. Instead, she emphasized independent learning and discovery by designing learning activities in which each child guided his or her own experience by working with the various sensory and motor-rich tasks, such as feeling different grains of wood with eyes closed, smelling different floral odors, and stacking blocks in an incremental tower that could balance. My oldest daughter went to a Montessori preschool where I was able to volunteer to help with the children one day every week or so, and I was amazed at how diligently the children *worked* on their tasks—no annoying music in the background, no loud voices, no piles of toys to distract them. The interesting tasks were enough to attract and maintain their attention.

Although Maria Montessori emphasized the importance of the scientific process in evaluation of educational and enriching opportunities for children, she didn't produce much in the form of scientific data to support her theory-driven ideas. Her personal stories and anecdotes were powerful, but data are also required to make final judgements. More recently, however, the Montessori educational program was evaluated formerly through a scientific lens. In a study conducted by psychologists Angeline Lillard and Nicole Ese-Quest of the University of Virginia and the University of Wisconsin, respectively, subjects weren't randomly assigned as they were in the Bucharest Project. However, a large number of parents who wanted their children to attend a Montessori school in Milwaukee, Wisconsin, were targeted so that the children who won a lottery to attend the Montessori school could be compared to children who were not selected and were subsequently placed in mainstream schools. Using the lottery group assured the similarity of the parents, since they all wanted them to attend the Montessori school. At five years of age, the Montessori children were more likely to use higher reasoning levels to persuade another child to share an object. For example, they were more likely to speak of justice and fairness compared with the mainstream-schooled children. At 12 years of age, the Montessori children wrote essays that were scored as being more complex and creative. At five years of age the Montessori children also scored higher on standardized types of tests, but this difference waned at the assessment at 12 years. Finally, the 12-year-olds exhibited more assertive responses and exhibited a greater sense of community than did the mainstream-educated students.[41]

Thus, it appears that Montessori's approach to building the experiential contingencies in children had cognitive and emotional payoffs. Another researcher, Stanford University's Carol Dweck, has emphasized the importance of being mindful of building experiential and cognitive contingency repertoires throughout our lives. She has distinguished between "fixed" mind-sets, in which children felt that their cognitive abilities had little room for change regardless of effort building cognitive capital, and a "growth" mind-set in which children understood that, with hard work, their cognitive abilities could become more efficient and sophisticated. When she taught middle-school children the values of a growth mind-set, their math scores improved more than those of the control group, who learned simply about effective study strategies. Thus, adopting a mind-set enabling us to build our contingency repertoires throughout our lives may be the best source of mental vitamins for maintaining healthy brains.[42] Although some parents may want to control the life contingencies of their children to minimize heartache and distress, the best gift we can give them is the independence to understand that they and only they are the captain of their neural journeys. With the appropriate effort and reflection about the success of that effort, new and improved contingencies are formed throughout our lives—the contingency gift that keeps on giving.

Although the unfortunate Bucharest reports suggest that there are indeed critical windows for certain aspects of nurturing to take place, I recently met a man who suggested that it may never be too late to give the gift of self-contingency building. To learn more about this, however, we have to go to prison.

Parenting Our Prisoners: You Be the Judge

Regardless of their parenting experiences, the contingency calculations of certain individuals lead them to make the wrong choice, a choice with consequences that can be as dire as being sent to prison. In the traditional prison setting, the growth mind-set that Carol Dweck speaks of is severely restricted, as others make most of your decisions each day—when and what to eat, what to wear, where and when to sleep. Regardless of where inmates were in their cognitive contingency development, prisons rarely prepare individuals to make the best decisions to keep them out of prison once they're released. In the United States, recidivism rates are 77 percent within five years of release, meaning that the prison experience isn't changing the contingency calculating abilities and subsequent outcomes for prisoners when they are released.[43] Because past research suggests that one of the worst things you can do to a rat's brain is to raise the animal in an impoverished environment, the notion of rehabilitating prisoners by putting them in the equivalent of an impoverished rat cage appears less than ideal.

When I was researching the plight of prisoners in various programs, I ran across a news video describing a unique drug rehabilitation program for prisoners in Texas, a state known for its no-nonsense, tough-on-crime approach. Thus, Texas is a big state with a big prison population. I was so impressed with the judge directing the program featured in the news story that I contacted him to ask if I could visit his court for a day. He agreed, and I was off to Dallas to meet Judge Robert Francis and his impressive team at his unique Drug Court. Little did I know the impact this man's vision and dedication would have on my own mind-set as a scientist, parent, citizen, and all-around person.[44]

To provide a little history, Texas has been very successful at directing offenders, mostly drug offenders, to prisons but not so successful at rehabilitating them so that they don't return to prison. Judge Francis conveyed that he considered himself just a cog in the prison machinery of Texas, more of a "housing relocation specialist" as he shuffled offenders from one lockup experience to the next. He was even recognizing them as they came through for repeat visits— evidence that something wasn't working.[45] At a time when Judge Francis was seriously contemplating leaving his bench to start his own plant nursery—yes, the simple contingency of nurturing flora and seeing the fruits of his labor in strong, healthy plants—there was some interest in giving offenders with addiction problems an alternative path. Even if one had no compassion for the actual humans in this system (though Judge Francis certainly did), the cost of the ineffective program was substantial. A 2007 budget projection indicated that, on its current trajectory, Texas would require approximately 17,000 additional prison beds in five years—costing upward of $1 billion over those five years.[46]

The obvious failure of the existing prison system prompted the state legislature to earmark $217 million for drug rehabilitation programs that included mental health treatment, job training, and specialty courts. In 2009 Judge Francis received funding from this legislation that enabled him to set up a full-time staff of 20, including drug probation officers and counselors (he currently has 27 people on his staff). The initial results are impressive. Instead of building new prisons for much-needed beds, Texas has closed three prisons, as well as a few juvenile detention centers. Additionally, the state saw a 13 percent drop in the crime rate between 2005 and 2010, along with a 27 percent drop in parole revocations in 2007–2008, and a 30 percent drop in 2008–2009. Regardless of a person's political perspectives about criminals and incarceration, these preliminary results are encouraging.[47]

As I learned during my Texas visit, those in the program don't find it easy. Participants are subject to random drug tests, required to show up at specific times for meetings, and expected to attend counseling and employment sessions and interviews. Failed drug tests or failure to attend or to produce documentation of attendance at required meetings result in three days in jail. The judge tells them that there are two things he doesn't tolerate: running or lying. If a participant messes up and admits it, Judge Francis is more tolerant than if the person tries to lie to him about it. And this supportive judge doesn't hesitate to send participants back to serve their full sentences in prison after they screw up a few times. In a recent interview, Judge Francis described the program as a "job—if you work hard, if you go to work, I will give you a paycheck. I will reduce your community service hours, I will reduce your fines and court costs, I'll help you get off probation early, I'll write a letter to the guy you're having an interview with to help you get a job. But if you come in here and you earn 20 years in prison, I'm going to sign that paycheck, too."[48] It was clear that Judge Francis was emphasizing contingencies in his court—this time giving the participants of the program an opportunity to control their own life contingencies.

As part of my visit, I observed the weekly gathering of all of the participants in the program at that time—about 40 individuals who had committed a felony and had been identified as having a drug problem. Prior to bringing the participants into his small courtroom, Judge Francis's staff allowed me to sit in on their weekly meeting, during which any and all concerns were raised about the program participants—that is, any concerns that may become an obstacle to compliance with the program's expectations and the participant's ultimate graduation. Achievements were also discussed and celebrated. I wondered if the behavior of students in the most elite of private schools is ever discussed with the concern and interest that I observed at that meeting. These former inmates were no longer a number—they had a name, a story, and, best of all, the potential of a future. I felt like I was in the middle of one of the most interesting documentaries I had ever seen.

The most fascinating part of that meeting was the discussion of one participant who had strayed. It was the very person who had won the coveted gold star the week before. Yes, I'm still talking about adults who had recently served time in prison. In the most perfect of stimulus-response contingency-building worlds, these former inmates valued winning a gold star above and beyond money, cigarettes, or other tangible awards. The gold star was valuable because it could be redeemed for two very valuable experiences: pride for being recognized for positive, rather than negative, decisions and actions, as well as the opportunity to share a barbeque lunch with the judge. The infrastructure of contingencies appeared to be changing in the program participants, from tangible real-time rewards to experiences that boosted intangibles such as self-esteem and pride.

As to the previous week's gold star winner, this particular participant confessed that he had not attended his employment session; instead, he had forged the signature of the supervisor. He told his caseworker that, after winning the gold star and seeing how proud the judge was of him, he felt terribly guilty for misleading everyone. Even though his deception would likely go undetected, he nevertheless admitted his misstep fully aware of the consequences. As I watched Judge Francis as he listened to this story, I could tell he was impressed with this participant's sense of accountability. The man would indeed have to suffer the consequences, but he would do so knowing he had eventually made the right decision.

I had to stop and regroup. A former inmate who had bamboo-zled the entire 27-member team, including the judge, had risked all of this glory because he was tormented with a sense of guilt. Some-thing was changing about this participant's values and his desired response outcomes. The contingency rules were being restructured. No longer was it about the immediate outcome; it was now about the circumstances surrounding the outcome or the reward. Trust and honesty among friends was important. Being accountable for one's actions was taking top priority. This had all the makings of a contingency-calculating game changer. Even as an adult, it wasn't too late. My mind raced imagining what areas of the brain were changing . . . which neural networks were responsible for building accountability, pride, and integrity?

Once the staff meeting ended, it was time for court. The partic-ipants slowly filed in and found a seat among the wooden benches as Judge Francis entered, dressed in jeans and a button-down shirt along with his signature boots. No formal black robes, no unintelligible legal speak, no arrogant, condescending attitudes. Even though I was definitely outside of my college classroom comfort zone, it was ob-vious that a lot of learning was taking place under the tutelage of the judge. He called each of the participants by name and, in a genu-inely interested tone, asked how he or she was doing. How did that job interview go? How did that meeting with a troubled family member go? What really happened at that party last weekend? The questions weren't that different from those asked by loving parents checking into their child's life . . . making sure everything was on track. This imagined documentary was getting better and better.

At one point a participant who was new to the program intro-duced himself, and his words reminded me that, regardless of a per-son's past contingencies, everyone searches for hope—even in seem-ingly hopeless situations. He shared that he dropped out of high school in the tenth grade and hit the streets doing all the wrong things. He had been in and out of prison ever since, missing the birth of his two sons. He said that he had never completed *anything* in his life and was hopeful that this program would be the *first thing in his life* that he successfully completed.

What are the consequences of completing the program? A grad-uation ceremony, of course—music, robes, and all the expected pomp and circumstance. Family and friends are invited, and the judge individually acknowledges each graduate as the person steps up to receive his or her certificate and hear his inspirational words. The smiles on their faces reflect the pride they are experiencing.

Wanting to learn more about participants' individual stories, I interviewed a graduate of the program, Laniqua Pittman, during my visit. In 2011 Laniqua was in court facing a theft charge with up to a 25-year sentence. She was offered the option of six months in the Substance Abuse Felony Punishment Program, a program she described as prison with counseling. Following this she entered Judge Francis's program. Until she took that step, she told me, she had no control over her life . . . she had no routine other than just sleeping, eating, and seeking drugs. Her destructive cycle had to change if she were to complete the judge's program successfully. She told me that the program had given her, at the mature age of 35, the life skills to cope with everyday challenges. And then came that word again: she conveyed that she was no longer wallowing in her horrible life situations and that she had developed a sense of *hope.* Two years out of the program she still harbored this hope and had channeled it into the decision to complete her associates degree in chemical dependency counseling. She told me that her days in prison were a thing of the past. "I don't want to wear anybody else's underwear. I don't want to eat commissary food. I don't want someone telling me what I can and cannot do. I don't want to drink this dirty, nasty water that no one else in this city drinks but us. I said I'm done with that life, and I made that decision, and what his [the judge's] staff does is help us with that decision."[49] Her past contingency calculations were now outdated and were being replaced with updated response-outcome probabilities. She was gaining a sense of control over the outcomes of her life.

Laniqua and a few others I interviewed described Judge Francis as paternal and, using a religious analogy, their angel who was sent from God to help them. After court, the judge and two of his staff members took the time to join me for lunch, where we continued conversations about the Drug Court Program. Judge Francis acknowledged that most of the individuals who entered his court didn't have the nurturing parents that he had, or the nurturing that he provided for his children. Maybe it wasn't too late for a little tough love

in the form of parental nurturing. Further, he reminds the participants how rewarding it is to be on the other side of the nurturing
parental fence by being an attentive, loving, and present parent to
their children. Judge Francis pulled out his phone and shared a picture of his precious niece, whom he refers to as "Dumplin'." He
conveyed that he showed the participants this picture and reminded
them what they would be missing if they were using drugs or in
prison. It simply wasn't worth it.[50]

So there you have it. This tough on crime judge opted for genuine concern, vigilant monitoring, well-earned rewards, and, yes, stories of his precious Dumplin' to model the most rewarding aspects
of humanity. I had indeed learned a lot in Judge Francis's court classroom that day. This Texas field trip reminded me that, even though
there are important critical windows for nurturing social interactions, it may never be too late to make incremental or, in the case of
the initial outcomes of Judge Francis's drug court, monumental improvements in more effective contingency calculations.

As described in this chapter, various aspects of parenting alter
the contingency calculations of both those being parented and those
doing the parenting. Regardless of variations in parenting and childhood conditions, some individuals enter this world with a predisposition for altered mental functioning. Psychiatric illnesses such as
schizophrenia, depression, and obsessive-compulsive disorder drastically change the brain's ability to form authentic contingency calculations. The unfortunate footprint that mental illness leaves on
one's ability to make informed decisions about future responses and
their associated outcomes is the subject of the next chapter.

CHAPTER EIGHT

Calculating Effective Strategies
for Treating Mental Illness

W ITH THE UNFORTUNATE ONSET of psychiatric illness, distortions of thoughts and emotions begin to emerge in various forms of reality-distorting brain bubbles. Patients diagnosed with schizophrenia, for example, experience a fabricated reality that expresses itself in the form of hallucinations, especially voices, that are completely realistic to the patient. These hallucinations and accompanying false beliefs, known as delusions, appear to be generated by faulty brain processing. With obsessive-compulsive disorder (OCD), reality is distorted so that minor threats are exaggerated, compromising a person's ability to live a functional life. An unrealistic fear of germs, for example, can lead to hours of compulsive hand washing due to false beliefs (known as obsessions) about the toxicity of germs. In depression, the reality distortion tilts toward the negative accompanied with an aversion toward risk and uncertainty so that the consequent brain bubbles compromise a person's motivation to work toward his or her existing goals.

Schizophrenia, OCD, and depression are just three examples of psychiatric illnesses associated with brain bubbles that distort reality in ways that disrupt a person's thoughts, emotions, and behavior. This compromised ability to calculate real-world contingencies makes it increasingly difficult to get through life's everyday ups and downs. With increased knowledge of the importance of maintaining accurate contingency calculations for optimal responses, the most effective treatment strategies should focus on bursting existing brain bubbles so that the brain can, once again, return to an ability to filter authentic information from both the external and the internal environments. If these individuals could gain or regain the ability to engage in realistic decision-making skills and effective contingency calculations, the more realistic brain filters would go a long way toward mitigating mental illness.

As described in Chapter 1, Nobel Prize–recipient John Nash, the subject of the biopic *A Beautiful Mind*, reported working on his mathematical formulas for years following his schizophrenia diagnosis—rebuilding his cognitive capital in the Mathematics Department at Princeton University.[1] Before his symptoms began compromising his academic productivity, he generated the previously mentioned Nash Equilibrium Theory, a game-type theory that had applications for economics and decision-making—and contingency calculations! Nash preferred his self-prescribed problem-solving treatment strategy to antipsychotic medication and induced comas that his doctors recommended when he was initially diagnosed. His attendance at the Nobel ceremony to accept his award was a testament to the progress he had made in his fight against the disease that threatened the very brain areas that enabled him to make the discoveries that earned him the award in the first place.[2]

Aside from Nash's self-prescribed treatment strategy, an emphasis on rebuilding the contingency-calculating circuits in the fight against mental illness generally hasn't been the go-to approach. In fact, it's a stretch even to use the word "strategy" when describing the introduction of many popular treatments for psychiatric illnesses. Many of these approaches arrived on the scene by accident rather than via strategic, informed hypotheses. The fact that we haven't seen the expected decline in the number of cases of mental illness confirms that little progress is being made on this front. With approximately 11.5 million American adults suffering from debilitating mental illness—affecting their personal happiness as well as their ability to hold down jobs and support themselves—there's no question that progress has been slow. It has been estimated that the mental health costs in the United States, including medical costs, lost wages, and social services to provide necessary support, approach $500 billion each year.³ As I tell my students every semester, these patients deserve better. The rather haphazard past needs to be replaced with more strategic treatment options that will not only relieve symptoms temporarily but place the patients on a long-term path to recovery. Although the origins of mental illness vary from genetic to environmental to everything in between, there is still hope among both researchers and clinicians that individuals diagnosed with various psychiatric illnesses can be restored to a functioning level.

Throughout this chapter, we'll explore past and current therapies for mental illness, considering the role of accurate contingency-calculating functions along the way. First, I will introduce you to an extreme case in which a psychiatrist very meticulously diminished a patient's ability to perform contingency calculations. Without strategic processing, this patient lost the ability to interact effectively with the world around her as she became increasingly dependent on the therapist.

Sheri's Contingency-ectomy

Several years ago I received an email from Sheri J. Storm, a patient of Kenneth Olson, a psychiatrist who, at the time, was practicing in Milwaukee, Wisconsin. I had written about another of Olson's patients, Nadean Cool, in a clinical neuroscience textbook as an example of how damaging a so-called psychiatric treatment could be when it hadn't been sufficiently investigated to determine its effectiveness. I learned about Nadean's case through researching newspaper stories and seeing an episode of *60 Minutes* that covered Olson's treatment for Nadean's symptoms.

I contacted Nadean myself, and during our interview she shared that she had visited Olson to treat anxiety related to a trauma experienced by her daughter. She had no way of knowing the nightmare she was about to experience. She was diagnosed with Multiple Personality Disorder and told she had over two hundred personalities (including the bride of Satan and an animal or two); she was "treated" with hypnosis and a litany of psychoactive drugs, along with excessive hospitalizations that maxed out her insurance—including one stay that included an exorcism, complete with a fire extinguisher on hand in case she self-combusted during the session. The absurdity of this therapeutic strategy eventually became apparent, and Nadean filed a lawsuit; she eventually agreed to settle with Olson for $2.4 million.[4]

Enter Sheri, who was upset that the case was settled after Nadean's lengthy, often humiliating stream of legal depositions following weeks of intrusive questioning by Olson's defense team—but before Olson was subject to the same scrutiny. Most important to Sheri was the fact that the settlement meant that Olson wouldn't be held legally accountable for his actions; she had hoped for a trial and a guilty verdict. Sheri had read an article I had published in the little known *Journal of Undergraduate Neuroscience Education* about a textbook in which I discussed Nadean's case, and she had noticed an error: I had incorrectly stated that Nadean received a court-determined settlement, when of course the settlement occurred outside the court.[5] Sheri was understandably frustrated with my less than accurate legal reporting. I was a little frustrated myself for the reprimand, but I then read on to learn that Sheri had also been one of Olsen's patients. I rewatched the *60 Minutes* segment about Nadean and, sure enough, Sheri was there, interviewed as another patient of Olson's (along with three other of his patients with similar stories). My heart sank—another person affected by this fiction-inspired therapy. I conveyed to Sheri that I was very sorry for what she had been through and asked her to tell me more about her story. I told her that I was a neuroscientist, not a clinician, but I could listen and also share some of the existing knowledge about responding to trauma and its impact on neural functions and mental health.

Sheri agreed, and her story generated a river of emotions. I experienced disgust and anger as I learned more about what she had gone through. I regretted that someone would provide such an ill-supported "therapy" and felt genuine remorse that a field that I was even remotely associated with hadn't definitively denounced such harebrained therapeutic strategies. But I'm getting ahead of myself . . . I'll start from the beginning of Sheri's story . . .

Sheri had been experiencing anxiety and insomnia as she tried to juggle a high-pressure radio sales job and a divorce following 13 years of marriage. She initially spoke to a mental health counselor to help her through her emotional challenges. Although her issues were certainly problematic, her counselor confirmed that Sheri's symptoms were certainly not out of the ordinary for individuals going through similar experiences. Her contingency calculators were still functioning, directing her toward the most appropriate help so that she could reduce her anxiety and move forward with life. Even so, she was advised to see a psychiatrist, who, unlike counselors, could prescribe medication to facilitate a normal sleep pattern. She ended up in the office of Kenneth Olson. From the beginning Sheri was impressed with all of his academic credentials—diplomas from universities and a medical school, an extensive medical library on his shelves—all evidence that she was in the office of a highly trained professional who had a prestigious reputation at the local hospital. She felt certain that he would take care of her. She felt safe.

The sessions became a little confusing when Olson diagnosed her with multiple personality disorder and began "recovered-memory therapy." This treatment consisted of excessive hypnotherapy sessions in conjunction with prescriptions for several psychoactive medications. During hypnotherapy he interrogated her after she was given sodium amytal (a purported truth serum). He recommended that she remain isolated from her family during her therapy, and to facilitate this arrangement she was hospitalized in a mental ward on multiple occasions—all this in response to her original symptoms, which were anxiety and insomnia coinciding with life transitions in the forms of a new job and a pending divorce.

Sheri doubted Olson's accounts of what happened during the hypnotherapy sessions, and so he then began to videotape them. Sheri sent some of those videos to me (after being obtained from her lawyer) so I could view them. They were difficult to watch. Sheri was so drugged that she literally had to be propped up by a nurse as Olson asked her bizarre questions such as clarifying whom he was talking to. Yes, you read that correctly: although Sheri provided no evidence to represent herself as anyone other than herself, Olson would identify an *alter* (an extra personality that inhabits a person) and start to ask questions of the supposed alter. Unless I missed something in one of my psychology or biology courses, I don't understand how another person or personality could inhabit another person. Exactly where in the brain would these mind-mates reside? I realize this sounds more like fiction than a twentieth-century psychiatry case study but it unfortunately happened to Sheri and to many other patients. The following exchange I recorded from one of the videos provides a flavor of these sessions as sodium amytal is administered:[6]

SHERI STORM (SS): How does this [sodium amytal] operate with the brain? I mean, is it like alcohol?

KENNETH OLSON (KO): Yeah, I imagine.

SS: So, does this mean I won't remember this part?

KO: [inaudible]

SS: It's on tape, oh.

KO: I think the first question that Sheri wanted to ask, and probably the most important one, is did it really happen?

SS: [inaudible]

KO: Did it really happen? And I'll encourage you to talk to the camera as if you were talking to Sheri.

SS: Did what really happen?

KO: She wants to know if she was really abused. She's confused and thinks she's making it up . . . Is there anybody who'd like to come forward and answer that question? For Sheri? Hi. Who's here?

SS: I don't know.

KO: *I don't know* is here?

SS: Must be.

Sheri conveyed that Olson told her a five-year-old alter emerged during her first such session (not videotaped) and declared that she had been sexually abused. Sheri countered that she didn't believe that such a thing had occurred, and she told me that he told her repeatedly that our minds are similar to a computer that holds all memories of our lives in pristine and complete form. In view of the initial statements in this chapter, and the theme throughout the book, which reinforces the notion that the brain needs a good dose of REALITY to facilitate effective contingency calculations to reach its top functioning capacity, it becomes difficult to understand the rationale behind this "recovered-memory therapy." Alternatively, bringing real-world experience to the mental treatment table in the forms of cognitive and experiential capital-building activities provides the fuel for the reemergence of these important abilities. I'll let you be the judge whether the administration of "truth serum" and other psychoactive drugs, coupled with hypnotherapy and blatantly leading questions, is an appropriate way to engage relevant contingency calculations that will lead to sustained recovery. Just as you can't rehab a strained muscle with painkillers, sedating the brain and leading it into a fairy tale world isn't the way to activate its functional circuits. A muscle requires actual physical effort to facilitate recovery, and a brain requires the appropriate gathering and processing of information to maintain functioning neural networks and enable it once again to engage in proper decision-making mode.

If contingency calculations are indeed important for mental health, then Sheri's treatment, whereby her psychiatrist created a context in which she didn't even have control over which PERSON was occupying her mental space (for lack of a better term), should have severely compromised her level of functioning. That is exactly what happened. Although she initially fought Olson's diagnosis, his extended "therapy" sessions led her to accept that she would get worse if she didn't continue with the recovered memory therapy. Using the ultimate fear-inducing tactic, Olson told her that her so-called alters would harm her children if she terminated her therapy. Her diminishing world of reality filters clashed with her fabricated therapy-induced brain bubbles one memorable morning when she sat at a McDonald's and opened the *Milwaukee Journal Sentinel* to the headline: "Malpractice Lawsuit: Plaintiff Tells Horror of Memories." In a seemingly unbelievable coincidence, another patient (Nadean) at the local hospital had similar recovered memories of child abuse, over 200 alters, and a diagnosis of multiple personality disorder while in treatment with the same psychiatrist as Sheri's. (Also about this time, the American Psychiatric Association dropped the diagnostic category of multiple personality disorder, and replaced it with the slightly different diagnosis of dissociative identity disorder.)

Emory University clinical psychologist Scott Lilienfeld and I wrote an article about Sheri's case for *Scientific American MIND* titled "Brain Stains."[7] The title refers to the fact that, years after her "therapy" had ended, Sheri's brain had remnants of Olson's psychiatric handiwork as a result of the fears the sessions ignited—including the fear of being abused as a child and the fear of harming her children (which she never did). I invited Sheri and Scott to speak to my students about the importance of evidence-based therapies in the field of mental health, and the class was riveted by Sheri's story while also confused and baffled about how a medical specialist in the United States in the late twentieth century could botch a case so badly.

Slowly Sheri is recovering from her contingency-ectomy. She is gaining experiences through work and relationships, but her progress has been slow. Her brain stains continue and make her hyper-vigilant about the intentions of others in her foggy but slowly clearing reality. If a one-time trusted psychiatrist can turn your world upside down, what might others do to you? This was the strongest contingency her brain learned during her time with Olson's "therapy," as she currently finds it difficult to trust the intentions of others. But life goes on, and she recently sent me a text with a picture of her new therapy: an adorable puppy, Titus (Figure 12). I asked her how puppy therapy compared to the therapies of her past. She replied, *"There's no comparison. Your dog might cause occasional damage to your property—but the joyful endorphins they induce via unconditional love, comic relief and devotion make you forget all about your favorite shredded afghan and initially unblemished carpeting."*[8] What a wonderful response! It was evident that Sheri was gaining control of her experiences, response outcomes, and emotions . . . way to go, Titus!

I wish I could say that recovered memory therapy for multiple personality disorder is a rare, ineffective blip on the radar screen of therapies for mental illnesses, but logic is missing from other past and present therapies as well. Further, an effort to enhance contingency-calculating functioning to protect against emerging brain bubbles is present in only a few therapies. For the most part, rehabilitation of diminished reality processing hasn't been a focus of mental illness therapies.

The Contingency Void in Psychiatric Therapies

I love sharing science and medical stories with my students, because I am always interested in their responses to the sometimes unbelievable stories of mental illness and our feeble attempts through the years to treat it. It's important to tell these stories to the next generation

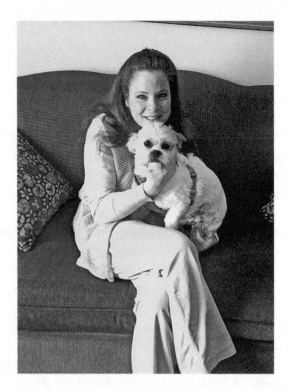

Figure 12. Conditioned Canine Therapy. *After enduring misguided treatment for "multiple personality disorder," including multiple psychoactive drugs and extended hypnotherapy sessions, Sheri reports that the real-world contingencies of caring for her pet dog, Titus, have resulted in more positive outcomes than she experienced with the approaches dispensed by her psychiatrist. (Photo courtesy of Sheri J. Storm)*

of medical doctors, researchers, counselors, teachers, and parents so that the trajectory of these sad stories may one day change, perhaps even ending happily for once. There's no question that, for the millions of individuals suffering from mental illness, finding little to no relief with existing therapies, they deserve better.

One damning characteristic of past mental health therapies is a clear lack of theoretical guidance throughout the process of identifying causes of various psychiatric illnesses. These therapies have ranged from prefrontal lobotomies, in which holes were drilled in skulls so that brain tissue could be damaged or disrupted, to extensive psychoanalysis sessions in which patients learned that their subconscious urges influence their thoughts and emotions. The most popular contemporary treatment is the psychopharmacological approach, in which a particular drug is administered to treat a so-called chemical imbalance.

Indeed, several therapies that exist today are products of serendipity.[9] In the 1930s, for example, the rights for a purple dye synthesized from coal tar were purchased by a drug company after discovering that it had antihistamine properties. Coincidentally, in an early clinical trial of this antihistamine conducted at a French hospital, the population of patients that was used in the study consisted of individuals diagnosed with schizophrenia. The medical staff reported that the schizophrenia symptoms (delusions and hallucinations) were more subdued in the patients receiving the drug, similar to patients who had received a lobotomy. For this reason, the effects of this (and similar) drugs were sometimes referred to as a "chemical lobotomy." This drug was also referred to as a neuroleptic drug (*leptic* is Greek for seizure), as it also produced effects that were similar to therapies that involved inducing seizures (e.g., electroconvulsive shock therapy) to treat the malfunctioning brain. Variations of this drug, now known as chlorpromazine, continue to be used in the twenty-first century—with disappointing success rates and disturbing side effects.[10] The neuroleptics were responsible for the acceptance of the dopamine theory of schizophrenia suggesting that, if a drug that blocks the activity of the neurochemical dopamine reduces the symptoms, then schizophrenia must be caused by having too much circulating dopamine. This work describing the role of dopamine in healthy and unhealthy brain functions won Arvid Carlsson the Nobel Prize for clarifying the neurobiological effects of these drugs. But research today suggests that the role of dopamine in the expression of schizophrenia symptoms is more complex. To use the same logic that was applied in the chlorpromazine case, if homemade chicken soup makes me feel better when I have a cold, is my cold the result of a chicken soup deficit?

In the treatment of depression, a drug used to address tuberculosis symptoms caught the attention of nurses who noted that the mood of patients appeared to be lifted after being given this drug, known as iproniazid. Another drug used in the treatment of depression, imipramine, was initially prescribed as an antihistamine. It turned out that these drugs increased the levels of the monoamine category of neurochemicals in synapses, which are the tiny gaps between neurons. For depression the chemical imbalance was characterized as a deficit since a drug that increased the neurochemical in the synapse was associated with diminished symptoms, spawning the mono-amine theory of depression. A few decades later, the drugs became more specific as they targeted just one neurochemical, serotonin, and were just as effective yet with fewer side effects. One of the early forms of this serotonin-selective receptor inhibitor (SSRI) was the wildly popular drug marketed as Prozac.[11]

Although it appeared that drugs offering perfectly good medical treatment for mental illness were coming on the scene at a time when scarier treatments such as stays in asylums, induced comas, and shock therapies were the most popular options, these drugs fell short of representing true progress when it came to providing long-term relief and recovery from the symptoms. For example, studies tracking the long-term outcomes of patients with schizophrenia who remained on neuroleptics indicated no improvement after 20 years of pharmacological therapy. Interestingly, although it's difficult to control the necessary variables across cultures, long-term outcomes of schizophrenia are better in less-developed countries such as Nigeria, where medications aren't traditionally used for treatment.[12] This *outcomes paradox*, in which the richest, supposedly most-developed countries have worse outcomes with psychiatric illnesses such as schizophrenia compared with less-developed countries, may be due to several factors; for example, high recovery rates in India may be the result of a greater dependence on family and social support for recovery.[13]

My students often are less than impressed with the haphazard process that characterizes our knowledge about effective treatments for psychiatric illness. When they learn that the efficacy/success rates of the drugs they have heard about and trusted all of their lives are actually low, and that the drugs sometimes have an unacceptably high probability of multiple side effects, they are concerned. The truth is that many students are taking some version of these drugs themselves— or drugs related to anxiety, sleep, or learning/attention problems. At a conference in Virginia for college counselors, Ira Birky, director of counseling services at Lehigh University, read a letter he received from a student who shared her story of mental illness. This student needed to take a yearlong hiatus from college and had been feeling guilty about her behaviors leading up to the break: her excessive drinking, minimal scholastic effort, and negative attitude about life. But after speaking with a psychiatrist, she learned that she had a condition that predisposed her to a chemical imbalance, and she was diagnosed with depression. She was relieved that her actions at school had nothing to do with her current mental health challenges. Her psychiatrist told her that she was destined to have a mental breakdown regardless. In addition to the student's sense of relief, her newfound faith in her medical diagnosis brought her prescriptions for four psychotropic medications: the antidepressant Lexipro, sleeping aid Seroquel, mood stabilizer/antiseizure medication Lamictol, and ADHD medication Focalin.[14] It's difficult to comprehend the effects so many drugs must have on an individual's existing neurochemistry and neurophysiology.

Now that we've considered the therapeutic paths that haven't worked so well, let's engage in a thought experiment about the best treatment strategies for mental illnesses such as depression, schizophrenia, and various anxiety disorders. And let's start with an overarching theory emphasized in this book—that we function at optimal levels when our brains gather experiential capital and, in real-time, receive, filter, and process relevant signals from the environment. According to this line of reasoning, these abilities are critical for sharpening our contingency calculations in order to make the best decisions for healthy and desired outcomes. With this theoretical structure in mind, brains diagnosed with a mental illness should stay clear of treatment approaches that generate brain bubbles that will compromise processing of valuable information necessary for making the most informed life decisions. Since there is no unequivocal evidence indicating that chemical imbalances associated with psychiatric illnesses such as depression actually exist, it's a little scary to prescribe drugs or chemicals that may interfere with necessary functioning. As neuroplasticity pioneer Michael Merzenich and his colleagues recently wrote, "The behavioral clinician sees such approaches as necessarily crude . . . treat a patient with a wounded or dysfunctional brain by chemically RE-distorting it? How can that provide correction in the key deficits underlying the disorder, when hundreds of chemical processes have been altered as a consequence of the wounding or the disease?"[15]

As an alternative to chemical therapeutic strategies, Mike Merzenich has extended his neuroplasticity research from rodents and monkeys to humans, with very interesting results. He is co-founder and chief scientific officer of Posit Science, a company that has developed cognitive training software to sharpen sensory, cognitive, and decision-making skills—all designed to enhance and prolong mental health. Based on successful preclinical work with patients diagnosed with schizophrenia, this therapeutic approach is currently undergoing trials by the U.S. Food and Drug Administration to assess its effectiveness and safety.[16] We will have to stay tuned for the final outcomes, but the thought of contingency-building software in the absence of traditional medications and surgeries is very exciting.

Using our working theoretical structure to restore accurate contingency calculations, treatments such as surgeries that disrupt the brain's tissue when no known specific structural abnormality exists, as well as pharmacological approaches that may throw the neurochemicals off-kilter, should be ruled out as the most effective therapeutic approaches. Frontal lobotomies are a thing of the past—thank goodness—replaced with what was viewed as the more sophisticated pharmacological therapy in the 1960s. Unfortunately, despite a nearly twofold increase in the use of antidepressants from around 1995 to around 2005, depression rates continue to rise.[17] It's true that some individuals get better after some time has passed, but those success rates are sometimes as low as 20 to 30 percent, and the placebo effects aren't too far behind with their success rates (more about the fascinating area of placebo effects to come in Chapter 10). Even with the modest success of antidepressant drugs, side effects sometimes create more problems than those caused by the disorder itself, and relapse rates are unacceptably high, even when patients are continuing their medication therapy.[18]

Whereas it is easy to rule out less-than-effective therapies retrospectively, it is difficult to identify therapies with the most potential moving forward. Using the "improved contingency calculations" criterion, however, a few treatment strategies emerge as potential candidates. Such treatment approaches emphasize patients' ability to rehabilitate contingency-building circuits and enhance the experiential and cognitive inventory in order to get their brains closer to a normal functioning status. It's interesting that the most effective psychological treatment, exposure therapy or systematic desensitization therapy, does just that. This therapy consists of building patients' accurate contingency calculations by exposing them repeatedly to a fear-generating stimulus (such as a spider) that in the past stopped them in their tracks. There is ample evidence for the effectiveness of this approach for mental illnesses such as phobias. In one study, approximately 90 percent of patients still benefited from the therapy four long years after this rather short therapy.[19] The contingent response outcomes are simple with this technique, even if a therapy consisting of confronting one's greatest fears isn't always welcomed by the patient. In essence, the patient is learning that there is no negative outcome associated with exposure to the spider (in the case of a spider phobia), so the repeated response-outcome trials eventually leave the patient free of the impending fear. Of course, exposure to other fears such as public speaking, test taking, or heights could also be treated with exposure therapy.

Another form of therapy, cognitive-behavioral therapy (CBT), has been used mostly for depression, although it has been effective for other disorders as well. This therapy is based on the premise that the symptoms of depression are due to faulty cognitions, or thoughts. In other words, this therapy views brain bubbles as different forms of faulty reasoning that interfere with the processing of authentic information. CBT involves therapist-guided interventions that reshape the cognitive framework of the patient so that desired life outcomes can once again be obtained. The focus is more on symptom reduction that leads to remission, regardless of identifying the exact neurobiological causes of the disorder. In CBT, patients have to play an active role in the pursuit of testing the validity of their current thoughts and beliefs in addition to assessing new thoughts about how desired behaviors can be acquired. Although conducting a perfect study with any of these techniques to determine their success rates is next to impossible given the extensive life histories of study participants seeking and receiving treatment, CBT does appear to be more effective than antidepressant therapies based on several outcomes including lower remission rates, less-severe side effects, and lower costs.[20]

Although current behavioral therapies appear innovative and promising, they don't represent the first version of a noninvasive therapy that required active participation of the patient. (Here non-invasive refers to no instruments being introduced inside the body to deliver a therapeutic agent.) In the early nineteenth century the Quaker strategy was to treat the mentally ill with respect, providing an engaging environment with classes and gardens that invited the patients' active participation. Records indicate that the patient recovery rate at the Institute of Pennsylvania Hospital, which was run by Quaker physician Thomas Kirkbride, was 50 percent, rivaling the best of any treatment for mental illness conditions today (except for exposure therapy)—and this was during an era when virtually nothing was known about the brain or the causes of mental illness. Transitioning from the insensitivity of the seventeenth century, when "lunatics" were placed on public display, to the dignified hospitals in the nineteenth century, when patients received humane treatment, represented a dramatic change in the treatment of the mentally ill. The name given in 1813 to the first private hospital maintained by the Philadelphia Quakers is wonderful: the Friends Asylum for the Relief of Persons Deprived of the Use of Their Reason.[21] It is very sad that, in the twenty-first century, with the exception of a few promising approaches on the treatment horizon (discussed below), little to no progress has been made that rivals this early nineteenth-century approach. We must do better.

Thus, our thought experiment suggests that treatments that aren't characterized by the patient's active participation (such as surgeries and drugs) have a lower probability of rehabilitating the brain compared to the more active and participatory treatment strategies. In the next section we'll focus on depression therapy, a research area in my own lab that I have been thinking and writing about for decades. Through the years I have learned that it's important to keep revising our thoughts about this disorder and its treatment as new information is generated. Thus, I continually update my own contingency calculations about the best therapeutic approaches for desired outcomes in depression. As current information is considered, however, a treatment known as behavioral activation therapy checks both the theoretical and the empirical evidence criteria boxes that are so important for identifying effective therapies.

Point in Case: Blue's Clues

Even when my daughters were young I wasn't a huge fan of children's television shows—they seemed so unlike real life, and I found the silliness a bit annoying. However, there was one show, *Blue's Clues*, that seemed interesting even though, at the time, I wasn't extending anything about the show to my professional interest in another version of "blues," that is, depression. My respect for this show has grown considerably over the years, and I would argue that the producers were laying the groundwork for their preschooler audience to develop thought processes that would make them champion contingency calculators in the future. Thus, in retrospect, *Blue's Clues* provides clues about building resilience against the emotional blues.

So, what about the *Blue's Clues* format led to this potential resiliency-building education for the students? The producers studied the children's education research literature and decided to use a format that invited the children's participation as they viewed the show. Wow, this is aligning with our "best practices" for emotional resilience. Thus, this show was more like an entertainment version of cognitive-behavioral therapy—BEFORE an actual need for the therapy. Additionally, the show's innovative strategy of repeating the same episode for five consecutive days was instituted once the producers discovered that their preschooler viewers were asking to see the pilot episode over and over. In each episode a mystery was first presented about a dog named Blue, and then the show's only live character, Steve, guided the process of collecting clues about Blue's mystery. Once all the information was gathered and systematically recorded in a handy dandy notebook, Steve invited the children to help solve the mystery topic for that day. That's right—contingency calculations for preschoolers!

Did the show have a positive impact on its viewers? One study indicated that the repeated presentation of the same episode enhanced viewers' comprehension and problem-solving strategies. Over time *Blue's Clues* viewers also developed enhanced information-gathering skills, allowing them to be more efficient at problem-solving.[22] Even though the research was sponsored by Nickelodeon, the show's cable network, and therefore it may have been a bit self-serving, the results are promising, reinforcing the idea that the brain should be trained to be the most efficient contingency calculator from early childhood.

We don't have a version of *Blue's Clues* for adults, but a therapy program that is an extension of cognitive-behavioral therapy stands out, providing valuable clues about treating depression. Mentioned earlier, behavioral activation therapy (BAT) was formally introduced in 1990 by Neil Jacobson at the University of Washington, and it extends the notion of active participation in the therapy process much more intensely than a television show can accomplish.[23] In essence, he teased this approach out of the more-traditional cognitive behavioral therapy to determine if it would be just as effective as the broader therapy. BAT requires patients to work with their therapist-coaches to identify activation strategies that once again will lead them to positive consequences. In my opinion, and based on research in this area, the positive emotions associated with desired outcomes serve as nature's purest form of antidepressant therapy. In this type of therapy, current patterns leading to avoidance, passivity, and withdrawal that serve only to exacerbate the negative outcomes fueling the symptoms of depression are identified so they can be diminished. Thus, BAT represents a transition from an individual illness model, in which the focus is on some dysfunction within the individual, to what is referred to as a functional model that focuses on how the organism establishes connections between behavior and the environment. This strategy gives patients more control over their response outcomes. There's no denying, however, that it's also important to understand the neurobiological mechanisms related to optimal environmental interactions—which is exactly what we're doing in the lab with our effort-based reward contingency building. What is changing in the brain as an individual gains more control over his or her environment and becomes more equipped to make optimal decisions leading to desired response outcomes? Of course, our patients are rats, not humans, but they engage in complex behaviors, so it's a good place to start our pursuit of strategic therapeutic approaches with translational value in humans.

As previously described, the effort-based (or effort-driven) reward model allows rats to "earn" Froot Loop rewards by learning to dig them up in small mounds of bedding. After training, they exhibit flexible behavior in the form of multiple search strategies when their expected reward is nowhere to be found. The enhanced search strategies and heightened resilience found in the animals receiving this rat version of BAT suggest that, when it comes to experiential capital for the brain, rats aren't very different from humans.

The uncertainty, presented in the form of prediction errors, in our rodent behavioral task when the coveted Froot Loops are removed may be an important key to understanding susceptibility to anxiety and depression. As discussed throughout this book, quite often uncertainty arouses anxiety. When the outcomes to our response choices aren't clear, some of us may delay responding out of fear of making the wrong decision. According to our rodent model, this contingency-calculation anxiety can be reduced by gaining experiential capital, a goal of BAT as well. In fact, one common characteristic of several different psychiatric illnesses is an intolerance of uncertainty.[24] Consequently, life experiences and therapeutic approaches that build a sense of control over uncertainty will be effective approaches. This isn't surprising since it fits within our overarching theoretical approach about the key role of contingency calculations in the maintenance of healthy brains. Accordingly, I was interested to hear from Canadian researcher and author Stephanie Westlund, who has reported preliminary evidence that active, outdoor activities such as gardening and farming are effective in reducing posttraumatic stress disorder (PTSD) symptoms when the traditional therapies aren't sufficiently effective.[25]

What about brain disorders that are more typically categorized as neurological—that is, conditions such as brain tumors or Alzheimer's disease that are accompanied by visible neuroanatomical changes? Does the contingency-building theory apply in those conditions as well? More study needs to be done in this area, but recent research utilizing previously mentioned brain-training exercises suggests that this more virtual form of contingency building sharpens decision-making skills, evidence that contingency calculations are being influenced. For example, a recent study conducted by Jerri Edwards at the University of Southern Florida using a brain-training computer exercise known as Double Decision concluded that the module reduced susceptibility to Alzheimer's disease. The software, which is offered by Posit Science, features two types of vehicles, such as a truck and a car, and participants are challenged to identify the vehicles as their images alternate randomly in the center of the screen. The pace of the "game" gets faster and faster as the vehicles are flashed on the screen ever more quickly, and they also increasingly resemble each other so that they are more difficult to differentiate. And, there's more—at the same time the person ALSO has to determine where in the periphery of the visual field a Route 66 road sign is presented. Add to this a background that becomes more distracting as users try to locate that pesky Route 66 sign and you will begin to understand how much attention this module requires. There are no pills, needles, surgical tools, or electrodes utilized in this type of therapy. The fascinating aspect of the particular study that tracked approximately 2,900 healthy participants ranging from 65 to 94 years of age over a period of 10 years was the minimal amount of participation necessary to achieve protection against the onset of the disease. Completing 10 one-hour sessions over five weeks resulted in a 33 percent decreased risk of contracting Alzheimer's over the subsequent decade, and adding a booster session after the first and fourth years resulted in a 49 percent reduction.[26] These rates are even more impressive considering the low cost and, for good or bad, the lack of necessity for a medical professional to dispense the treatment.

Thus, it is difficult to look back at the history of mental health therapies and declare that significant progress has been made. In retrospect, the early approach utilized by the Quakers appears to be the most promising of all the early therapies, although sophisticated research is required to tease out the most important aspects of this multifaceted approach. What are the exact mechanisms fueling the benefits associated with providing engaging surroundings for the patients? The contingency-training rodent model has identified potential markers of emotional resilience that are associated with more active interactions with the environment and the likely success of behavioral activation therapy. CBT and BAT, along with the promising new brain-training computer interventions, are providing formal laboratory methods to understand more about the link between brain activation in various forms and brains that process information in healthy ways. In a sense we are coming full circle with these approaches that emphasize an active role of patients in their therapeutic journey. Recent findings confirm the importance of patients reaching a place where they are not just devoid of symptoms but also no longer deprived of their *use of reason*—a place where their reality-based contingency circuits are finely tuned for successful contingency-calculating futures.

Merging Magnetic and Contingency-Building Fields

Although progress has been slow in identifying effective treatments for psychiatric illnesses, research has been chugging along at a steady pace—much of it in exciting and innovative areas. Genetic markers are being explored as well as various forms of brain treatments ranging from deep brain stimulation to optogenetics (see Chapter 4). Semester after semester, I make the statement in class that, with all this exciting research, we are past due for some transformative treatments.

In my opinion, outside of the behavioral therapies, one of the most promising brain treatments involves gently perturbing the brain's electrical fields from an external force—a very large and very strong magnet. This therapy, known as repetitive transcranial magnetic stimulation (rTMS), offers benefits with minimal risks—the desired formula in this maze of mental health therapies. rTMS has been shown to be effective in the treatment of depressed patients who fail to respond to pharmacological therapy—patients referred to as treatment- or medication-resistant. Roughly half of these medication-resistant patients respond to rTMS, with about 33 percent experiencing remission.[27] Because the magnet can be used to target various sections of the brain, clinical neuroscientist Jonathan Downar and his colleagues at the University of Toronto are focused on finding the most relevant brain targets for this therapy. Identifying the most-effective brain locations will maximize the effectiveness of the treatment—that is, it will produce the fastest response and remission rates with minimal side effects.

The prefrontal cortex, with its integrated neurocircuitry serving as a nexus for emotional and cognitive functions, has been a target of rTMS. More recently, Downar and his colleagues have focused on the dorsomedial prefrontal cortex as a specific area that is most closely associated with improvement with this technique. Further, when this area is damaged, an 80 percent risk of depression is observed, with less risk observed when the most popular target of rTMS, the dorsolateral prefrontal cortex, is lesioned.[28] Extensive research is being conducted to ensure the safety of this procedure and to high-light the parameters such as duration of stimulation and number of treatments to streamline the costs, side effects, and time associated with this particular treatment. As previously mentioned, thus far this noninvasive therapy is showing promise as an effective therapeutic strategy, especially for treatment-resistant depressed patients. Inter-estingly, the improvements have been associated with improved at-tention and enhanced processing speed. Hmmm . . . that sounds familiar. Perhaps both the brain training and rTMS approaches are stimulating similar brain circuits and influencing similar response outcomes, just in very different ways.[29]

You may be thinking that, according to our criterion for thera-pies including an active role of the patient, a limitation of rTMS is that the patients' role is extremely passive. That's exactly my con-cern. However, if rTMS is tuning up brain areas that facilitate the processing of contingency calculations when the patient leaves the treatment facility and engages in real-world activities, then that's helpful. But what if the more-active cognitive behavioral therapy could be combined in some way with rTMS? Perhaps a more spe-cific fine-tuning of the brain's attention and contingency-calculating circuits could be achieved. This strategy was used on one patient, a 26-year-old married woman who had suffered from depression; her various antidepressant medications were scarcely effective. She was provided with an earpiece so that the therapist could communicate with her about her thoughts and associated responses at appropriate times during her rTMS session. Upon reflection, this patient con-veyed that, compared to receiving rTMS only, this combined thera-peutic approach enabled her to recognize her more toxic, negative thoughts in time to "work" to diminish them.[30] Adjunctive therapies such as this hold much promise. Just as a physician needs to educate patients about lifestyle changes that should accompany prescribed medication for certain medical conditions, real-world interactions are critical for bursting brain bubbles that could lead to debilitating mental illness.

I look forward to seeing the results of additional studies combin-ing various types of noninvasive therapies. Because the brain needs authentic experiences to fine-tune the contingency-calculating brain circuits, an active type of therapy such as CBT or BAT approaches is extremely valuable in achieving mental health. Additional therapies, such as brain training, rTMS, or even self-subscribed active programs involving new hobbies or jobs, can further reinforce the activation of the necessary circuits to pull the patient out of the brain bubble fog to a clearer reality.

Whereas most of the research in this chapter has focused on treating existing illnesses AFTER they emerge, the more important question is whether the likelihood that a mental illness ever becomes a reality can be diminished. Are there preventive strategies that can protect us against the development of mental illness?

Brain Whispering

The traditional way to conduct neuroscience research is to use past research and experiences to generate a hypothesis that points to a particular brain area of interest for a particular research question. Which brain area(s) will enhance responding in animals when an expected reward is not where it should be?. . . produce effective coping in the midst of chronic stress?. . . generate more active and strategic responses during uncertain conditions? Once the literature is consulted and past findings in our own lab are considered, the studies are conducted and the brains are processed to determine the accuracy of the hypothesis. This is the story of my lab year after year, student project after student project—slowly we gather apparent truths that lead to interesting theories, such as our theory about strategic contingency calculations being an important function of the brain. And I am always anxious to see the results of these studies to determine if the hypothesis was supported—it's like a suspense thriller each time. Additionally, for each study I just can't help but revisit the microscope slides that contain a very thin cross section of the brain mounted on microscope slides, and look all over the tissue to see what stands out. Similar to a pathologist conducting an autopsy in search of clues that shed light on an individual's demise, I can't wait to examine all the nooks and crannies of the brain to detect any cells or neurochemicals that may have played key roles for building resilience in the rodents' brains. My students and I call this *brain whispering*, and it has put us on interesting paths of discovery as we design the next interesting study.

In a recent series of studies related to identifying neurobiological markers of resilience that may protect against the emergence of depression symptoms in rats, my whispering habit has identified two brain areas that seem to be speaking out—the lateral habenula and the insula (Figure 13). Their interesting activation patterns during an emotional threat has forced me to learn more about how these brain areas may be involved in emotional resilience and building authentic contingency calculations to avoid unnecessary brain bubbles. It turns out those rat brains were onto something very interesting— our research is now featuring these brain areas more prominently in our investigations. And, it turns out that these areas are already targets of clinical research and may be important keys to developing new therapeutic strategies to fight the unacceptably high rates of mental illness. I'm not suggesting they are independently contributing to contingency-confused brains diagnosed with various mental illnesses; rather, they are critical components among targeted neural networks necessary for mental health.

Let's start with the lateral habenula. Once my attention was directed to this area, we incorporated it into our emotional regulation studies, and it appears that the most vulnerable animals have revved-up activity there. To provide a little brain background, the lateral habenula is a small structure that mediates responses to stress, anxiety, sleep, reward, and pain. It also has connections to areas that influence the neurochemical circuits that utilize the monoamine neurotransmitters that have been implicated in emotions and depression (i.e., serotonin, noradrenaline, and dopamine). Although we most often consider more activity to be good, in this case hyperactivity of the lateral habenula has been associated with depressed symptoms in both animal models and humans. When this area is damaged in animal models, an antidepressant effect is observed; that is, the animal is less likely to be stopped in its tracks.[31] Further research suggests that the lateral habenula is keyed into potential aversive outcomes to behavior, so it could bias contingency calculations to direct an individual to avoid uncertain circumstances to diminish the likelihood of experiencing unwanted outcomes.[32] We've found that more of the brain-derived neurotrophic factor (BDNF) is in the lateral habenula of animals that receive no contingency training, that is, the contingency-challenged group. In other labs, increased activity of this brain area

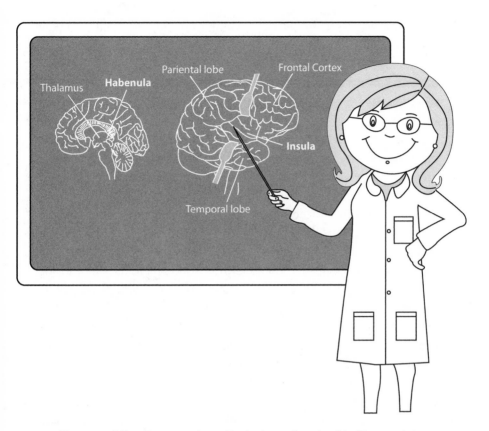

Figure 13. New Lessons about Brain Areas Involved in Depression.
*Ongoing research in my laboratory and beyond suggests that, in addition to
other brain areas involved with emotional processing, the habenula (involved
in suppressing movement in fearful conditions) and insula (involved in integrated
feelings throughout the body) may play critical roles in the emergence of mental
illnesses such as depression. (Image by Bill Nelson)*

has been associated with helplessness—behavior that is viewed as
"giving up" and just accepting the circumstances as if nothing the
animal can do will change the circumstances. Thus, the lateral habenula appears to play a role in assessing threatening situations and
determining that the best response is no response.[33]

Indeed, at times no response is best—an animal may be better
off being very still in a nest than being active and running around
drawing attention to itself, especially in the presence of a predator.

However, there are limits to how long an animal should hunker down and wait out the emotional storm. While an animal is in the stress-induced quiescent state, other animals are getting mates as well as food and other resources. Thus, if hyperactivity of the lateral habenula has been associated with learned helplessness and depression symptoms, this area should be targeted for various types of brain therapies such as deep brain stimulation, an invasive technique that requires the implantation of electrodes into the brain area of interest. There's likely to be noninvasive ways to inhibit exaggerated lateral habenula brain activity as well.[34]

What about the other brain area my whispering pointed out in our studies—the insula? Neuroanatomist Bud Craig, who conducts research at the Barrow Neurological Institute in Phoenix, has uncovered the most information about this brain area. His explorations led him to associate this area with a sensitivity he has labeled *interoception*, a type of processing of relevant information related to the body. Just as thermoreception refers to monitoring body temperature, and proprioception to monitoring limb position and movement, interoception monitors sensations originating in the body's interior. When someone asks you the generic question "How do you feel?," it's likely that the insula is involved in your subsequent interoception to provide a response. The insula also has ties to neuroeconomics, or strategic decision-making linked to survival and success, as this brain area monitors the body's expenditures associated with various potential responses. According to Craig, research focused on this brain area indicates that the brain uses interoception to represent the energy-related costs and benefits for various responses. Thus, the process of interoception generates our feelings or emotions that guide us to the most efficient responses. Similar to a monetary system, aversive emotions and feelings (sadness, fear) represent a disproportionately high energy cost (or physiological price tag) that prompts us to avoid the situation, whereas positive emotions (joy, happiness) lead us to make the responses that will likely produce the desired benefits. This action-specific valuation, as Craig refers to it, is critical in helping us make decisions and engage in responses that don't outstretch our safety zone of energy expenditure.[35] Beyond this neuroscience technical language, Craig suggests that the insula helps us decide if certain actions are worth carrying out . . . if the outcome will be worth the physical and emotional effort. That sounds like contingency calculating to me!

Research suggests that the insula is important for neural processing related to the emotional response known as disgust, which typically forces a person to avoid whatever is triggering the response, as it will likely be too costly or dangerous. Depressed patients display impaired recognition of faces exhibiting the disgust responses and, accordingly, less gray matter in the insula. This suggests that their insula may not be sensitive enough to guide responses toward the most adaptive decisions, compromising contingency calculations.[36] On the other hand, in our rodent models, when rats profiled as flexible coping rats are presented with a prediction error—that is, an expected reward isn't there—these animals with higher emotional regulation, and exhibiting strategic information-gathering tactics to fix the problem, have less neural activity in this brain area. It appears that these flexible coping rats aren't as affected by uncertainty as are the animals with other coping strategies.[37]

The insula is being seriously considered as a target for depression therapies. In one fascinating study, patients with differential response rates to medical treatments and cognitive behavioral therapy for depression received a brain scan to regulate glucose metabolism (this test is known as a positron emission tomography, or PET, scan). Interesting differences in the insula were observed. Patients who had a low metabolism response in this area responded more positively to cognitive behavioral therapy, whereas patients who exhibited a hyperactive metabolic response responded more positively to antidepressant medication. These results suggest that too much self-awareness of internal functions is calmed by the medication, whereas cognitive behavioral therapy seemed to be providing a needed kick start to the insula in the low metabolic group.[38] In another study that utilized a different brain scan, fMRI in this case, participants were shown a threatening picture that stimulated activity in the insula, then, based on their training, they were able to appropriately upregulate the insula's activation to process the threat and appraise the response.[39] Thus, this brain area can be influenced through basic learning/behavioral interventions.

As you may have concluded, the likelihood of finding a single magic bullet brain area that is involved in the onset of psychiatric illnesses such as depression is not likely to happen. However, the lateral habenula and insula represent two additional zones to add to our arsenal of critical brain areas—in addition to the executive functioning prefrontal cortex, brain structures sensitive to neuroplasticity such as the hippocampus, and other emotional areas such as the amygdala, which is involved in fear. All of these brain areas are likely integral components of relevant neurocircuitry, fueled and modified by neurochemicals, that allows us to make the most informed decisions day after day.

Based on several different research approaches, there is ample evidence suggesting that treatment strategies geared toward fine-tuning the brain's ability to take in relevant information, process it, and respond in an effective manner represent an encouraging development in mental illness therapies. The days of trying to replace nonexistent chemical deficits or disrupt neurocircuitry that doesn't clearly show damage are becoming a thing of the past. Even so, it's interesting how slow the psychiatric industry is to embrace nontraditional medical approaches such as behavioral activation therapy and brain/cognitive training. As Mike Merzenich has suggested, it's because these are *disruptive therapies* in the sense that they conflict with the current mind-set of the industry—take a pill, attend a counseling session, prepare for surgery. There's no denying that lots of money can be made from these more traditional medicinal approaches, and money is important in dictating the approaches that will receive the most attention. However, it's time for the mental health industry to recalculate the response outcomes associated with these traditional therapeutic approaches so we can provide the most effective therapies to get individuals with debilitating psychiatric diagnoses back in the contingency-calculation game—back to the point where they have the cognitive and the emotional capital to trust their decisions and, consequently, once again be satisfied with their interactions with the world around them.

Contingency Paths to Preventive Mental Health Prophylactics

When it comes to mental health, effective treatment strategies haven't come along as quickly as they have for other medical conditions. Why is this? According to Tom Insel (introduced in Chapter 1), who recently served as the director of the National Institute of Mental Health, the focus of mental health has been on the treatment of symptoms. This doesn't sound like a bad strategy except that the time point is pretty late in the process of neurobiological decline if the behavior has already been modified sufficiently to generate the unwanted symptoms. Just think how far behind we would be with the treatment of cardiovascular disease if we had to wait until a person had a heart attack before treatment was considered. In the area of cardiovascular medicine, as is the case for many medical conditions, emphasis has been placed on risk factors such as high blood pressure, irregular heartbeat, or high cholesterol levels so that the risk factors can be addressed BEFORE heart attack occurs.[40] Thus, more emphasis needs to be placed on prevention of mental illness by identifying biomarkers and addressing them before a full-blown psychiatric illness emerges.

Given what we know about malfunctioning brains needing to use real-time responding to recalibrate network structures tipping toward a diagnostic category, why is it taking so long to translate these findings into real therapies that reduce suffering in humans? Merzenich states that these new approaches represent an example of disruptive technology in which the new medicine may be delivered in nontraditional ways, via computers or apps on "smart" devices, rather than by medications or surgeries. New therapeutic strategies such as behavioral activation therapy don't necessarily require someone with a medical degree to dispense the "treatment," which is another aspect of these new approaches that society has been slow to embrace. It's interesting that even Insel, who was recently the top authority of mental illness in the United States, and perhaps in the world, joined the Google unit known as Alphabet Life Sciences upon his resignation from NIMH. He was frustrated with the slow pace of effective treatments for mental illness. In a recent interview he commented, *"Biological science hasn't had that many successes against depression or schizophrenia, despite the NIMH's $1.5 billion a year in grants and research spending. Psychiatric drugs haven't improved much in recent decades, and searches for the genetic causes of common forms of mental illness haven't yielded clear answers either. . . . In the future, when we think of the private sector and health research, we may be thinking of Apple and IBM more than Lilly and Pfizer."*[41]

Of course, as we learn more about risk factors and biomarkers, tracking of mental health can be done in a way similar to that of other illnesses such as diabetes and cardiovascular disease. Additionally, as more people understand the plasticity of our neural networks and how they can be recalibrated for more optimal functioning without the use of invasive techniques, our lifestyles should be adapted to avoid increasing mental illness susceptibility. I believe that we all can agree that, when it comes to psychiatric illness, it isn't likely that a magic bullet in the form of a pill is in our immediate future. Neurological illnesses, such as Parkinson's disease and multiple sclerosis, that are associated with documented neurochemical and neuroanatomical abnormalities are more responsive to traditional medical therapies, but even so, experiential therapies can be important supplements to the existing medicinal approaches.

Although mental illness affects many of us, fortunately more of us are mentally healthy than mentally ill. The topic of the next chapter pivots to a topic that affects a majority of us—work! We'll consider how we can put our emerging understanding of the brain's contingency-calculating functions to work for us to contribute to more meaningful and productive careers.

CHAPTER NINE

Getting Down to Business

Putting the Contingency Calculators
to Work

I F A REALISTIC VIEW is critical for our brains to manage our interactions with the surrounding world, is the same true for an
individual working in various types of business organizations?
Can the emergence of reality-distorting brain bubbles compromise the performance of employees, managers, and corporate
leaders?

The world of work is more in the wheelhouse of my husband,
Gary, who is an industrial/organizational psychologist. He has tried
to educate me about the value of assessing an applicant's appropriateness for a job by administering a battery of tests such as the famous Myers-Briggs personality test. As part of my "education," he
has recruited me to take these tests throughout the years as he prepared to use them as tools on various assignments. I always groan
when I'm forced to select which of the response options best describes
me . . . because no option seems to accurately capture my thoughts.
"Don't overthink it, Kelly," my husband has told me on multiple
occasions. I think *overthinking* is the most characteristic descriptor
of my so-called personality—making me the anticandidate for these
assessments.

My true interest extends beyond my personal personality profile (or lack thereof) to the bigger question of the importance of realistic feedback among all the players in particular business ecosystems. Consistent with my past research journeys, I would be more comfortable investigating this topic in the controlled environment of the laboratory. However, I can't hire little rat employees and managers and study their neurobiological responses to yearly evaluations or critical management crises in the nice controlled environment of the laboratory. Or can I? To a very limited degree, I have attempted a study of workplace training when I trained rats to "work" for Froot Loops and, as described previously, found that the work had neurobiological benefits. Thus, this attempt at rat career training suggests that work contributes to a sense of self-efficacy, or self-agency. Although I find our rat career data interesting, I'm not sure this is a story for the *Harvard Business Review* . . . yet!

To understand the importance of avoiding brain bubbles in the business world, I was forced to extend my laboratory observations to the human research world, as well as to relevant case studies and survey research, for a more complete picture of the role of authentic information to promote success in the business world.

Driven to Success: The Case of Overnite Transportation Founder Harwood Cochrane

In the early 1930s, when young Harwood Cochrane was delivering milk from his horse-drawn wagon to the Richmond Commonwealth Club, a nineteenth-century private gentleman's club, he could not have imagined that he would one day enter that same establishment from the main entrance and enjoy the company of wealthy peers whose affluence paled in comparison with his eventual self-made fortune. No, that wasn't a strong possibility for someone who was expelled from high school for punching the principal. His first real-world work experience was equally unimpressive; he was fired after brief employment as a mechanic—apparently turning a repaired vehicle back over to the owner without asking for payment was frowned upon by the management.[1]

Eventually, Harwood landed his job delivering milk (and ice blocks). As an unauthorized perk, he could slug down some of that cold milk when he didn't have enough money for lunch, telling his boss a bottle had broken along the way. A job with a built-in meal plan . . . this was the beginning of Harwood's business journey.[2]

While on his dairy route, Harwood saw the value of transporting goods in a timely manner and decided to supplement his dairy job with the delivery of other items. He and his brother saved their money and purchased a few trucks. His goal was to deliver goods faster than the freight giant of that time, the mighty railroad. Despite horrible roads, a lack of mechanics, and no truck stops along the way, a truck was still more flexible than a train when time was of the essence. Harwood was onto something—fast deliveries could lead to more frequent paydays. In the early days he hauled household goods and fertilizer, and he even took local Richmonders on hayrides.[3]

A few years later, Harwood branched out and started hauling sugar and writing tablets (paper, not computer) up and down the East Coast. During these early days, truckers were very much the cowboys of the roads, and it was an uncomfortable life; they never knew where they could sleep or get a meal, and the challenging road conditions meant they could count on breakdowns. Harwood and the other drivers would carry tools so they themselves could repair whatever broke down: tires, axles, batteries—the list went on and on. This profession certainly required an extensive stash of truck repair experiential capital. One route, from Roanoke to Bristol, Virginia, required drivers to drive through a riverbed. These adventurous early deliveries were plagued with ongoing challenges, failures, and frustrations. However, Harwood kept his eye on the goal of overcoming these challenges so he could get the goods to the customer. It was clear from the beginning that Harwood was an outcomes kind of guy.[4]

Harwood's experiences led him to start his company, Overnite Transportation, in 1935. Apparently, a company called *Overnight* Transportation had already been established, so a quick modification of the spelling was needed. In contrast to the topic of emotional depression that was the focus of the previous chapter, the Great Economic Depression was a challenge for Harwood. This was certainly not an ideal time to start a new business. Even so, it didn't seem to faze Harwood; it was merely one bump on one road among many bumps on many roads that he would have to overcome.[5]

As his business grew, Harwood had to take on many new responsibilities—hiring employees and keeping them happy, and staying abreast of, and even anticipating, new legislation related to the fast-growing trucking industry. These were all challenging bumps along the way and, even though he lacked a prestigious college degree, or even a high school diploma, his experiential capital, which he had acquired by understanding the trucking company from inside out through driving trucks and working on loading docks, helped Harwood form realistic contingencies to keep the business growing. Perhaps the most persistent road bump was Harwood's commitment to avoiding unionization. He felt that being unionized would decrease his flexibility, which would decrease his business edge. One of his prized possessions was a check from Jimmy Hoffa after Overnite successfully sued Hoffa's Teamsters Union for harassment.[6]

As Overnite grew, Harwood managed to stay grounded, strategically trying to save money any way he could. For example, even after achieving success later in his career, once when a particular route was in question, he jumped in the cab of a truck with an Overnite executive to investigate the route by simply driving it. When they were required to stop for the night at a modest Holiday Inn, Harwood and his executive shared a room. Following this entrepreneur's logic, if you could sit in a five-foot-long cab all day together, you could sleep in the same room. This is just one example of the frugality that characterized Harwood's management of his company. His business frugality added to the value of the company and, in his opinion, a return on his investment extended to his "family" of workers. By avoiding unionization, Harwood paid less than standard salaries. He justified this by stating that the resulting flexibility kept the business viable. The Overnite community seemed to find unity in being the only trucking company of its size that wasn't unionized. He found other ways to keep his employees happy, such as extending an invitation to them and their spouses to visit him in his office for career milestones, and allowing them to purchase stock. Consequently, he was described as humanizing his company.[7]

Just how successful was Harwood's trucking company? In the 1980s Union Pacific saw value in adding a trucking company, especially a company that had exploited the need for carrying less than a truckload (viewed as increasing speed and flexibility of delivery schedules). Although resistant, Harwood agreed to sell his business for

$1.2 billion to Union Pacific, which later sold it to United Parcel Freight, now known as UPS Freight—not bad from the humble beginnings of a horse and wagon.[8]

I am fortunate to live in the beautiful Virginia countryside in the western part of Hanover County, in a little place known as Rockville. I know Harwood's story because he built his prized manor home in this area in the 1950s and, even though he was frugal when it came to his business, his philanthropy was extravagant. Thanks to his generosity, Rockville has a beautiful library, community center, and several other contributions from the Cochrane family—as do several institutions throughout the Richmond area, including the Virginia Museum of Fine Arts, the recipient of his largest philanthropic gifts.

Based on the neurobiological information presented thus far in this book, you're probably seeing some behind-the-scenes contingency-calculating strategies that bolstered Harwood's success. He built experiential and cognitive capital by working all aspects of his business and never losing touch with the day-to-day challenges. This experiential capital enabled him to make informed contingency calculations about choosing where to build new terminals and where to buy property along the emerging interstates, and about developing the best strategies for managing his employees. His persistent resilience in the face of constant threats and challenges presented by the Teamsters enabled him to remain vigilant concerning the changing details of his business. And although he became very wealthy, he remained grounded, keeping a firm grasp of the reality experienced by his employees. As described earlier, privilege and celebrity typically present significant challenges in maintaining this sense of reality and avoiding the emergence of distorted realities. To some extent, a wealthy person's reality will be different, but Harwood and his wife, Louise, made an effort to keep it real. He told his biographer, "One fine day we realized we can afford anything anyone could desire. Then we had to look at ourselves in a strong light and realize it is important to . . . keep our feet on the ground, remember from whence we came. We don't ever forget . . . we don't regret the fact we had nothing."[9]

Thus, I didn't have to look far beyond the green rolling hills extending from my country home in Rockville to find an example of how healthy contingency calculations can potentially lead to a successful business. And, as we'll see later in the chapter, the factors that led to Harwood's business success likely led to his excellent health and feeling of well-being. As I was writing this chapter, Harwood passed away at the age of 103, seven months after the love of his life, Louise, died just a month before her hundredth birthday. From my research it seemed these two had quite a good time throughout their lives—raising their three children, sharing their wealth with the community, and hosting friends and family for memorable parties at their estate. Their 81-year marriage is literally one for the record books; according to Wikipedia, they're likely in the running for the 25-longest marriages in the United States. All this in little Rockville, Virginia!

Gallup-ing through Business Success

One of the largest studies of effective management was conducted by the well-known Gallup Organization and described by Marcus Buckingham and Curt Coffman in the popular book *First, Break All the Rules*. This analysis consisted of responses from 80,000 managers at various levels, and in organizations of varied sizes. The top characteristics of the strongest organizations determined by various objective outcomes rather than mere opinion reflected a work environment that enabled employees to hone their skills and work performance—a positive effect for both the managers and the employees. What exactly are these top characteristics? As you'll see in the following list, they foster the likelihood of optimal performance by building the employee's work-related experiential capital to generate the most informed responses, based on accurate contingency-calculations.

1. Do I know what is expected of me at work?
2. Do I have the equipment and material I need to do my work right?
3. At work, do I have the opportunity to do what I do best every day?
4. In the last seven days, have I received recognition or praise for good work?
5. Does my supervisor or someone at work seem to care about me as a person?
6. Is there someone at work who cares about my development?[10]

"Wait a minute," you may be thinking. "What about having the most competitive pay scale? Benefits? Training program to develop similar skill and talent in all employees?" Those were indeed the old industry standards for successful organizations. These new standards were hitting some of the environmental/behavioral points introduced in Chapter 2 and would have likely made the pioneer behaviorists applaud with delight. Environmental resources, clear expectations about optimal performance, real-time feedback about performance, and personalized development fall in the behavioral realm of contingency building in the workplace.

Another accepted rule that the survey proved to be false related to hiring what business leaders have often referred to as "talent" for a job. I cringed when I read this because I have had an aversion to this word ever since I wasn't allowed to join the gifted and talented program at my middle school in Pell City, Alabama, because I was perceived to study too much (at least, that was the feedback I received). This perception seemed to suggest that my academic abilities weren't natural . . . that I needed to actually work to appear intelligent. Although it was true that my grades indeed benefited from studying, it was never clear to me how that was a bad thing. Regardless, the situation stripped any notion that I had an ounce of academic talent. Of course, such a message forces a child to doubt her ability—as certainly happened in my case. Since those middle school days, I haven't embraced any form of academic or cognitive labels, focusing more on the task at hand and the path to master it successfully. Even after I was ultimately allowed in that gifted program following a couple of additional assessments, I have never been a fan of exposing our children to loose academic categorizations and labels.

It was refreshing, however, to read the definition of "talent" used in this extensive analysis of managers. This version of the word wasn't presented as an ability that emerged with no training or practice but was instead "a recurring pattern of thought, feeling, or behavior that can be productively applied."[11] Thus, a propensity for characteristics such as achievement, stamina, competence, discipline, or creativity represents the types of talent the Gallup researchers emphasized. These talents represent broader interests since it's believed that the more mundane skills and knowledge relevant for a particular job can be taught fairly easily. On the other hand, a strong sense of self-discipline or stamina is harder to teach. Consequently, if creativity is important for a particular job, it is advisable to interview candidates for this characteristic and to refrain from thinking you can teach these core personal characteristics.

According to the Gallup survey results, another rule to break is the notion that managers need to focus on treating everyone the same, and training everyone to act the same way. It's okay to realize that different individuals have different strengths and act accordingly. And, finally, the immediate social environment outweighs long-term benefits of working for a particular company. A strong future consisting of stock options and opportunities for advancement are trumped by a feeling of comradery, acceptance, and nurturing. Having no long-term benefits outweighs going to work day after day and dreading seeing your coworkers.

Our case study, Harwood Cochrane, had the foresight to break many of those rules by not fixating on offering the highest salaries. He was, however, interested in the well-being of his employees and referred to his organization as the Overnite family. He made a point of taking the time to get to know his employees, as well as their spouses. The measures of success in his business were clear—the successful delivery of a truck's contents at a predicted time and cost. When asked about the success of the company, Cochrane pulled out data sheets—emphasizing the hard reality in spreadsheets rather than vague generalizations and opinions. There was little mystery surrounding his criteria for success or his company's achievement of success.

Thus, the Gallup Organization's large-scale research project has revealed interesting insights about the core characteristics of successful manager-employee relationships. Considering that the book written about this survey was a best seller, this news should be familiar to the current population of managers. As complicated as it is for the brain to manage most of the processes in a single individual, managers and corporate leaders have to manage several, often hundreds, of different individuals—all contributing to the viability of the company. Regardless of whether organisms or organizations are being maintained, success is often related to the generation of contingency calculations.

Once the contingency capital has been obtained, what happens when the individual who has accumulated all this valuable experience tries to pass this knowledge down to a second generation to run the family business? Success in these situations is definitely not a given.

Passing Contingency Capital to the Next Generation

Theoretically, if gaining experience over a lifetime contributes to one's success in business, then passing all of that information on to the second and third generations should result in even more success. Right? Many of the business powerhouses are indeed family-controlled businesses—Walmart, Hyundai, Samsung, and Ford, just to name a few.[12] Sometimes, however, a few bugs get into the family business system.

For the most part, bugs have been good to the Rollins family of Atlanta, Georgia. When Wayne Rollins learned that Otto Orkin was interested in selling his pest control business in the mid 1960s, Rollins saw a lot of potential in the established, money-making company. The notion was that women hated roaches and would pay each month to keep them away. The purchase of Orkin, which at the time had annual sales of $40 million, was a financial stretch for Rollins and required him to enlist the financial assistance of an investor. In 2014, annual revenue was about $680 million—a nice, steady increase. Wayne's sons, Gary and Randall, had worked with their father and were appointed as the next leaders of the company. Wayne was content that he had left the company in good hands when he died at age 91.

It turned out that Wayne Rollins had made a few mistakes that would threaten both his family and the business. In an apparent attempt to rule the family from the grave, he established guidelines for dispersing the family funds, an empire currently worth $8 billion. The grandchildren had to provide evidence they were doing "meaningful" work in order to get annual payoffs. This practice was taken a step further after the Rollins patriarch died. The second-generation Rollins businessmen stepped up personal accountability by declaring that private investigators would provide reports about their lives, complete with random drug tests, to determine if each grandchild was worthy of his or her annual payments from the family business. This was too much for one set of siblings, including Glen Rollins, who was serving as CEO of the Rollins Corporation. He and his siblings sued their father and uncle, prompting Gary's termination from the extermination company. After that, a huge family mess ensued.[13]

It probably comes as no surprise that a controlling hand from the grave—as well as from living relatives—compromises the ability of subsequent generations to thrive as managers of a family business. Even though one could imagine that, in the best circumstances, an individual may have an early start gaining experiential capital for a certain family business, the reality is that approximately 70 percent of family businesses don't make it to the second generation. A mere 10 percent survive as third-generation family-owned businesses, and only about 3 percent make it to the fourth generation. One contributing factor to the failure of family-owned companies is the lengthy tenure of the first family CEO—about a quarter of a century, compared with six years for non-family CEOs. The extended leadership may result in a lack of flexibility to change in accordance with fast-paced changes in technology and business models.[14]

Extended leadership also deprives the next-generation leaders of essential knowledge that the founding family member gained through on-the-job experience and real-time responses to business failures. Further, if the second generation feels confident that joining the family business is always an option, this choice becomes more of a fallback plan, and proper training isn't a priority. Entering the business without proper training and experience, of course, threatens the viability of the business. Recognizing these concerns, some families are emphasizing that a job with the family is not an entitlement, and if a family member is considering this option he or she needs to earn a university degree appropriate for the job, gain adequate experience in a relevant work environment outside of the family business, and, when job openings come up within the family business, they must compete with qualified candidates.[15]

Of course, even if a family figures out how to pass the family business to the next generation successfully, it's almost impossible for the business to grow fast enough to accommodate a growing family. If the founding family has three children who marry and eventually have their own children, the family could easily grow from 2 to 25 or more people in three generations. It would be difficult to provide jobs for all these family members![16]

Family businesses that have survived, however, have played a critical role in the global economy. In the United States alone, family-controlled businesses employ 60 percent of the workers. Often family members continue to own a significant portion of the company's equity, as is the case for about 40 percent of the top 250 firms in France and Germany.[17]

Thus, with family-owned businesses, it is possible that subsequent generations may be in a better position than others to take advantage of gaining more experiential capital in that specific business area. However, this process is often disrupted by privilege, entitlement, and limited opportunities associated with the ruling generation. This makes it difficult to jump into the business and learn the contingency calculations firsthand by experiencing both failures and successes. When this happens, the second and third generations are stifled by compromised contingency-building opportunities, a disadvantage that likely leads to the emergence of reality-distorting brain bubbles related to one's resilience and management abilities. The value of experiencing failures in the process of building expertise in a career is eloquently captured by Thomas Edison, who, when reflecting on his many failures when trying to create the lightbulb, noted, "I have not failed 10,000 times—I've successfully found 10,000 ways that will not work."[18] Another innovative and successful company, Google X, rewards teams who identify failure in a proposal before an exorbitant amount of money is devoted to it—quite a different culture from most businesses that reward success only.[19] No doubt that Edison and Google X prioritized the role of embracing failure in building experiential capital, a process necessary to fine-tune the prized contingency calculators along the eventual path to success. With multiple-generation family businesses, it is difficult for subsequent generations to have an opportunity to benefit from highly valued failure.

Building Business-Minded Brains

If running mazes is considered a business model for laboratory mice, one aspect of the work environment that poses a considerable threat to optimal performance is stress. As part of a standard laboratory work environment, for example, mice in a study conducted by Ohio

State University neuroscientist Jonathan Godbout learned that, when running the maze, there were strategically placed mouse hole exits in case a crisis ever occurred in the maze. The mice easily learned this maze contingency and ran for the nearest exit hole at the first sign of a looming threat. However, when these standard run-of-the-mill mice were psychologically stressed by the presence of larger, bullying mice for several weeks, they lost their ability to think on their four feet/paws and scrambled around the maze, forgetting about their exit strategy training.[20] Apparently, stress formed a bit of a brain bubble—clouding the brain's access to all the valuable contingency calculations of the past. This is no surprise to most neuroscientists, as stress greatly compromises the executive-thinking prefrontal cortex as well as the hippocampus (involved in spatial memories), even restructuring essential connections among the vast network of neurons.[21]

Although it's not clear if Godbout's mouse employees could be categorized as managers or nonmanagers, human investigations of decision-making have provided interesting evidence that, if indeed the mice were managers, they may have fared better in the face of those big mouse bullies. When given familiar types of decision-making tasks in which the human participants were forced to select specific word choices, managers exhibited activation in the subcortical brain area known as the caudate nucleus. You may recall from Chapter 3 that this brain area is involved in habit learning and, in the case of managers, may suggest more secure foundational hardwiring of certain responses. It is likely that these fundamental and familiar responses would be less vulnerable to stress—enabling humans and mice alike to find the proper escape routes in a crisis situation.[22]

Making decisions in times of emotional crises has been referred to as making "hot" decisions in the human version of employees in the workplace. It's fairly easy to make the right decisions when everything is calm in the absence of emotional involvement, a task referred to by Barbara Sahakian at the University of Cambridge as "cold" decision-making. But what about hot decision-making when a good bit of risk is involved, making the situation very emotional? Sahakian and her colleagues explored these emotionally laden decisions in intelligence and aged-matched business employees in an attempt to get at this question. The subjects varied in their business experience, with half categorized as entrepreneurial and the other half identified as having no entrepreneurial experience. An example of a cold decision could be making decisions related to the design of a new branch for the company with plenty of time and resources to move forward with the plan, whereas a hot decision could be related to making the decision to terminate a multi-billion-dollar business venture requiring cutting the company's losses and moving on at precisely the right time to avoid the financial demise of the company.

What did Sahakian find? Both the entrepreneurs and the non-entrepreneur managers scored similarly on the cold decision task. In the hot decision task, the differences between these two groups were unmistakable. The managers were more conservative in their decisions whereas the entrepreneurs exhibited more risk-taking, a finding that was pretty surprising for a group of 51-year-olds who traditionally become more risk averse as they age. Of course, the point of the game isn't always to be risk takers in the face of adversity but to make the best decisions in the face of adversity. In today's business climate, possessing a brain that can regulate itself in the midst of hot decisions, regardless of the risk involved, is of critical importance. Perhaps it's most accurate to describe the most successful entrepreneurs as calculated risk takers who incorporate the appropriate contingency calculations into every decision.[23]

When the brains of entrepreneurs and managers are explored in fMRI scanners, different brain operating systems begin to emerge. In one study, the participants were confronted with two types of innovative tasks—exploitation tasks that required the participant to search for novel ways to optimize performance of existing work practices, and explorative tasks that required the participant to dissociate him- or herself from the current state of affairs to consider alternative options to achieve existing goals. In both types of tasks, the entrepreneurs and managers had to exhibit flexibility in their thinking as they were asked to step outside of their work environment comfort zones. Interestingly, when the managers performed these innovative tasks, especially the explorative task, they primarily used the left hemisphere area of their problem-solving prefrontal cortex. You'll recall that this hemisphere is known as the logical, rational decision-making hemisphere. Entrepreneurs also exhibited increased activation of the right portion of the left hemisphere's prefrontal cortex, as well as enhanced activation in the right hemisphere of the prefrontal cortex, a prefrontal area more closely associated with creativity and high-level executive functions. Thus, in this study the entrepreneurs incorporated both logic and innovation in their decision-making abilities—an ability that may make a difference between creating and running a business, and managing an existing business.[24]

Dopamine is a neurochemical that may be relevant in the work-related arena. This neurotransmitter has already been discussed previously in several contexts in this book—with its putative involvement in attention, detection of reward saliency, and even psychiatric symptoms pertaining to schizophrenia. In general, dopamine systems invigorate responses to enable an individual to tolerate challenges, including failure, to achieve goals in the most adaptive ways. When goals are actually pretty far in our future, dopamine softens the psychological distance, helping us to perceive that the goal is indeed within our reach.[25] Extending from its more classic and outdated role of being essential for experiencing reward, dopamine has been upgraded to playing a role in *wanting*, rather than *liking*, a reward.[26] It's not absolutely clear in this case if dopamine is creating or diminishing brain bubbles; regardless, it keeps us working toward our goals.

Rodent studies suggest that a depletion in dopamine around the brain's reward area shifts the rats' motivation to work for a more desirable treat. With lower dopaminergic activity, they exert less effort to obtain the more mediocre rodent chow as opposed to working harder for a yummy sweet treat.[27] In a recent study, Stan Floresco and his colleagues at the University of British Columbia found that increased phasic responses of dopamine in the ventral tegmental area of the brain prompted the animals to opt for a high-risk choice in a response task that pitted uncertain desired rewards against the sure thing—that is, definite payoffs that are low-reward versus a more uncertain higher desired reward.[28] The higher tolerance for risk associated with entrepreneurs suggests that dopamine may indeed have a seat at the executive table of potential brain factors related to successful business ventures.

The Evolution of Work

As interesting as it is to differentiate managers, nonmanagers, and entrepreneurs, a more basic question about the human brain is whether it is hard-wired to work. Further, in comparison with other species, are humans more likely to work? If work is important for various species, are there any repercussions for taking extended hiatuses from work?

As anyone who follows animal behavior knows, work isn't unique to humans. Beavers spend an inordinate amount of time serving as ecological engineers as they build effective dams to create the ponds that are necessary for their well-being. In one case, an injured beaver that had been caged during rehabilitation and therefore far removed from its dam-building environment reportedly tried to claw its way out of the cage each time it heard running water from a flushing toilet.[29] Raccoons appear to be predisposed to working in water.[30] They often forage for food by running their forepaws along the bottom of a stream or other accessible water source. When raccoons are caged and simply given food, they resort to dumping their food in the water bowl as if they are trying to recapture the act of working for their food. As described in Chapter 2 in the discussion of instinctual drift, the predisposition to search for food in water, and to associate water with food, leads them back to water when they are merely given food without having to work for it.[31] In my opinion, the award for most impressive work—with a flare for design—goes to the male bowerbird, which spends countless hours building not only a functional nest, but a complex and innovative nest complete with themed decorations such as blue flowers and shells to make it more visible to the female bowerbirds. Even after the construction process, the male bowerbird's work isn't done as he is required to dance for his ladies in order to attract their attention.[32]

What about us? Isn't it considered the ultimate dream to never have to work a day in our lives? According to the U.S. Bureau of Labor Statistics, individuals work outside of their homes approximately eight hours each day. Additionally, work in the home can take up to two hours. Thus, in general, work constitutes a large part of our waking hours. Is this hardwired or just the necessary effort to get by?

If my work with the trust fund rats holds any truth for humans, a buffer against the toxicity of stress may be lost if the opportunity to manipulate the environment to gain resources (i.e., work) is lost. This rodent research suggests that working with the environment to produce desired outcomes is actually good for healthy neural processing, perhaps creating a sense of self-agency, or self-control, in a chaotic world with few guarantees that the necessary resources for sustained living will be realized.

An article in the *Atlantic* entitled "A World Without Work," concludes that the possibility of humans creating a world that no longer requires us to work is very real. In the past, when the workforce was revolutionized, for example, from agricultural to the industrial age, the number of jobs didn't change, just the nature of the work. However, with the technological revolution that we're currently experiencing, humans are successfully putting themselves out of work. Thanks to our past successful contingency calculations, we now have checkout screens instead of checkout clerks in the grocery stores, flying drones instead of pilots surveying target land areas, driverless cars that are less likely than humans to cause accidents, and little robots scurrying around warehouses packing boxes more efficiently than humans awkwardly climbing up ladders in search of boxes with specific product numbers. Wow . . . we may have just successfully ended work as we know it.

If work is indeed "overrated," then its slow deletion from our lives should be a welcome change. After all, a 2014 Gallup survey indicated that up to 70 percent of Americans feel less than engaged at work. If this is the case, it may indeed be time to move on and perhaps use our time more efficiently . . . raising our children, caring for the ill, learning new hobbies, protecting our planet. Current research, however, suggests that individuals without jobs typically don't find themselves engaging in these worthy endeavors; instead, they spend their days watching TV and sleeping.[33]

As I mentioned earlier in this chapter, there aren't controlled laboratory studies that suggest how dramatic changes in the nature of our work may affect our brain and well-being. However, in my opinion, when the convergence of various human and animal studies is considered, it gives us reason to pause . . . and rethink the ultimate contingencies of deleting work from our daily lives. The multiple layers of reinforcement in the forms of achievement, meaningful engagement, skill and knowledge mastery, and social cooperation create a powerful motivational force for keeping humans in the workforce. We're not programmed to respond specifically to running water or colorful shells, but our complex and flexible brain appears to be tuned into the process of manipulating the environment in optimal ways to provide resources necessary for survival. I have argued that, when this environmental interaction is compromised, our brain may also become compromised, resulting in conditions such as depression or anxiety, as mastery over the world around us appears to be slipping from our grasp.[34]

According to political philosopher and motorcycle mechanic Matt Crawford, losing a grasp of the world around us—in the form of changing work conditions that no longer require work involving our hands—may have dire consequences. Matt has written about his own aspirational journey to obtain an advanced degree and become a knowledge worker. After earning his PhD in political philosophy, he landed a job in scientific writing and, eventually, at a think tank in Washington, D.C. Attending the best universities and obtaining a white-collar job represents the typical American dream, but this career path wasn't reinforcing for Matt. Ironically, in comparison with his previous jobs, he felt that his cognitive engagement was stifled in his new knowledge-worker job, as he reported losing the satisfying feeling of meaningful work and problem-solving. So, he opened a motorcycle shop in Richmond, Virginia, and, as he described in his book *Shop Class as Soul Craft*, he found that working with his own hands and seeing positive, tangible outcomes as customers proudly drove their well-running motorcycles out of his shop seemed to provide the necessary neurochemicals to fuel his own neural motivational engines.[35] Matt's story is interesting in light of the fact that U.S. manufacturing jobs have fallen by 5 million (30 percent) since 2000.[36]

Thus, as the nature of the behavioral and cognitive aspects of work changes in the twenty-first century and beyond, we need to be aware of the impact this has on our capacity to maintain physiological and mental health (Figure 14). Matt's story suggests that brains need to interact with the surrounding world in some meaningful capacity to maintain their mental and physical well-being. Thus, ironically, brains need to engage in work to keep working! Even so, there are likely large individual differences in the types of work that keep our brains chugging along.

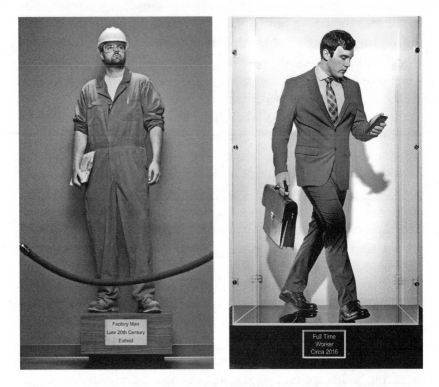

Figure 14. The Evolving Door of the Workplace. *As humans have become increasingly efficient with contingency calculations, we have generated technology that no longer requires the traditional effort of human workers. Consequently, the need for factory workers has greatly diminished (left), and the evolving nature of the office is changing the typical idea of an office worker (right). (Photos courtesy of Adam Levey)*

I-Spy: Reverse-Engineering the Brain Bubble

As a parent, I have spent considerable time thinking about the perfect career or lifestyle for my children, which include a daughter who is currently in college and a daughter who recently graduated from college and has entered the workforce. What are the careers that are rewarding, challenging, and engaging . . . all the things you wish for your children's future? The go-to prestigious careers such as doctor or lawyer are typically high on the list for most parents. Or, those who read the frequent internet articles about college majors associated with the highest earnings know that anything with the word *engineer* is a good option. Further, I have often thought about the best contingency-calculating career training that would give me confidence that my daughters were ready for life's challenges so that I would know that they could always take care of themselves—even when I'm no longer around.

For years, I have been drawn to the one profession that seems to yield the strongest and most self-sufficient individuals. Espionage! Being able to read a situation and anticipate an outcome before anyone else, being physically strong and agile, and developing a sharp, flexible mind would certainly ensure that my girls could handle anything life threw at them. Of course, there are the issues of danger and social isolation associated with this line of work. If those downsides could be deleted from the picture, a spy would certainly be high on my list of optimal careers for my kids.

Since those drawbacks kept me from ever suggesting spying as a serious career option for my daughters, my continued enamor with the virtues of spy training is more of a thought experiment. As I have increasingly considered the danger of reality-distorting brain bubbles, however, and the importance of realistic contingency building, it has become increasingly obvious why I find an espionage career so appealing. As effectively depicted in the undercover spy training film created in the 1940s by the U.S. Office of Strategic Services, a successfully trained spy requires superhuman contingency building, with absolutely no room for error, and no room for emerging brain bubbles.[37]

This classic film describes two spies in training. As the assignments are given, the contrasting approaches become evident. Spy A is confident and impulsive, perhaps not too different from the cinematic version of the ideal spy, James Bond. Unlike in the movies, however, Spy A's confidence compromised his abilities as a successful secret agent. For example, his overconfidence kept him from completing the necessary background research for his assignment. He thought he could handle any situation as an undercover agent, unaware that there was no way he could succeed without appropriate contingency building for his "test" assignment. Working on a fishing boat during his assignment, Spy A needed to know the exact knots tied in that particular culture as well as the emotional demeanor of the typical fishermen—pessimistic and close to hopelessness in this case—in order to convince the locals he was one of them. Spy A's lack of training prior to his assignment eventually led to him blowing his cover and compromising both his life and the mission.

Spy B, on the other hand, had sufficient confidence that, with appropriate research and training, he would be able to infiltrate his targets successfully and be perceived as one of the group. Actively participating in his coaching process, he learned about the importance of wearing clothes with local manufacturing tags only, the appropriate haircut, expected hand gestures for the target culture, and a smoothly practiced life story explaining why he had suddenly appeared in the target area. His situation also required him to learn mechanic skills to acquire a local job to enhance his cover. Thus, a career as a spy requires the trainee to relearn everything—how you talk, gesture, think, feel—for each new assignment. A contingency makeover is required for each new assignment. That requires a superflexible brain! Further, lifelong memories are reshuffled so they are temporarily replaced with fabricated childhood, family, and life experiences. Even habits such as humming a song have to be rewired—humming a song from the spy's native culture would be a clue that he or she is indeed an imposter. Spy B's vigilance through training, as well as his well-placed self-confidence, kept his brain in high alert throughout his successful assignment.

A key element of success in this spy training film was the trainee's ability to consider all possible contingencies in order to avoid an undesirable, possibly deadly, outcome. This career certainly requires the trainees to be on their contingency toes—with no room to let down their guard during an assignment. Forget to remove a pocketed ticket stub to a concert in the trainee's homeland? Busted! Fail to develop a story for that scar on your hand that is in alignment with your assignment? Leave a residue of a hair product that isn't available in the assigned culture? Show ignorance of the meaning of a common slang term in that culture? Busted, busted, busted! Imagining contingency calculations that could potentially come into play on a future assignment is necessary on-the-job training for spies. As these potential contingencies are deconstructed and rebuilt to align with the new assignment, the survival contingencies of the trainee become considerably higher.

Even though, in the end, I didn't push spy careers for my daughters, I remain convinced that a highly functioning spy may indeed possess the most impressive contingency calculating abilities on the planet. In retrospect, a few summer spy camps for my daughters may have been a good idea! In reality, although most employees don't have to worry about blowing their covers if they miss a key contingency calculation, if each employee, manager, and executive becomes more mindful of contingency forecasts for his or her respective business and career endeavors, success would likely be more prevalent in subsequent business outcomes.

Regardless of our chosen careers, it appears that various modes of work, and the accompanying contingency requirements, provide an important fuel for neural engines. As the nature of careers changes in the coming years, it will be interesting to determine the effects on our collective mental health. In the next chapter, accurate and authentic contingency calculations that have been emphasized throughout the book thus far will be relaxed just a bit. The effects of lowering the accurate contingency-calculating expectations on occasion may stretch the brain's potential beyond our imagination!

CHAPTER TEN

Stretching the
Contingency Limits
New and Imagined Realities

AFTER ALL OF MY lamenting about the necessity for real-world contingency building to establish the experiential capital needed to get through life, in all honesty there seems to be some value for the occasional use of nontraditional, even less authentic, contingency calculations. Contingencies that aren't well-grounded in experience or contingencies that push the limits of reality as we know it are sometimes just what we need to get us through the challenges of life. Well-intentioned brain bubbles introduced strategically throughout our lives can produce very different outcomes from the reality distorting bubbles we have discussed thus far. The imaginary friends that accompanied so many of us in childhood may have facilitated the real world of social interactions; out-of-this-world creative ideas lead to realistic adventures to out-of-this-world destinations such as the moon; and that kiss a mother gives her child who just skinned her knee while learning to ride a tricycle somehow reduces the pain in the absence of any real medicine. Such minor obstructions of reality that produce positive life experiences are far from the more prevalent and persistent distortions of reality produced by circumstances such as addiction, psychosis, or extreme privilege—these all lead to distorting brain bubbles and dysfunction.

How do these imaginary and naïve contingencies keep us from creating distorted brain bubbles that will interfere with our future contingency forecasts? In this chapter, we'll discuss responses that have their roots in some version of an imagined or unknown world but grow into realities that facilitate healthy outcomes, perhaps even protection against looming emotional crashes. Placebos, play, and curiosity all involve a good dose of imagined and creative contingencies, a form of medicinal brain bubbles, as they often contribute to real-world outcomes that are critical for our well-being. First, however, we'll return to behavioral conditioning 101, this time with a strange new player.

Neural-Immune Contingencies: Looking beyond the Textbooks

Twenty years ago my mother started complaining of annoying symptoms—fevers during the day, night sweats that kept her up all night, and chronic fatigue. At first glance, considering that she was about 50 years old, her doctors assumed it was related to menopause. Hormone replacement therapy and other attempted remedies failed to provide any relief for her symptoms. The chronic fever suggested her body was fighting something bigger than menopause. Eventually, she was diagnosed with non-Hodgkin's lymphoma. Although we were all devastated by the seriousness of this diagnosis, we were confident she could beat the disease with effective and strategic treatment. Following her diagnosis, I coped the way I cope with most challenges in unknown territories: by consulting the scientific literature. What were the established treatments? Recovery and cure rates? Experimental treatments? Was there hope anywhere in this massive tangle of studies and statistics? At that time (the mid-1990s), neither the statistics nor the nature of the treatments were encouraging. My brother, a young medical doctor at the time, hit his medical books and network of medical colleagues as I perused the scientific abstracts—an effective treatment had to be out there for our mother.

The treatment course we selected was, in many ways, worse than the disease itself. My mother elected to have what is known as an autologous stem cell transplant, a treatment that required the harvesting of stem cells from her bone marrow so that they could be safely frozen while she received intensive chemotherapy. Essentially, the doctors wanted to kill the tumor cells with toxic drugs without wiping out her immune system, always a delicate dance during the administration of chemotherapy drugs. Once the treatment was complete, the stem cells would return from their hiatus. They were thawed and infused back into her blood, hopefully to take up residence and start producing the much-needed immune cells to keep her body healthy, with or without unwanted tumors.

It was torture watching my mother suffer through this treatment. I'm certain that the side effects are managed more effectively now, but at the time it seemed so barbaric that a treatment for a disease could be so destructive to other parts of her body. Even so, the benefits (that is, the hope of remission) seemed to outweigh the costs. She experienced constant nausea, fatigue, blisters in her mouth, hair loss, mental confusion, fear, and anxiety. All of this was part of the process that we thought would lead to her recovery; consequently, my mother endured the roller coaster of symptoms with a glimmer of hope carrying her through the uncertainty of what was to come. As I sat by her bed, I felt so helpless. Of course, she had my love and attention during that time, but what else could be done to return her life to some form of normalcy?

Many of her immediate symptoms were related to her compromised immune system—soon to be a new, childlike immune system that required time and experience to function normally again. How could we get her immune system back to a fighting level as quickly as possible? During this vulnerable time, my mother's visitors were careful to "suit up" with sterile masks, booties, and scrubs for each visit. If a germ was transported on a shoe or a hand, regardless of the tumor the unwelcome pathogens could be deadly during this time of immunosuppression. Additionally, she also needed an effective immune system to assist in the battle against her tumors if the chemotherapy failed to eradicate them. For so many reasons, she needed those immune cells.

At that time I had been reading about a new, emerging field known as psychoneuroimmunology. Robert Ader, an experimental psychologist at the University of Rochester, had stumbled upon a fascinating finding related to immune contingencies in the 1970s. Working with a colleague, Nicholas Cohen, who was an immunologist, Ader had conducted a pretty straightforward immune study with rats. They were administered an immunosuppressant drug that would ultimately compromise the immune system and make them sick. The substance was mixed with their drinking water and, to make the water more appealing, they added a little sugar. Even with rats, sugar helps the medicine go down. The protocol was followed, the rats were observed, and the data were recorded. The study should have ended there, but the exciting part was yet to come.

When Ader and Cohen subsequently gave the rats the sweetened water with *no* immunosuppressant drug in it, something crazy happened. The rats got sick and, if the water was given to them long enough, they died. But, wait a minute! The rats weren't consuming the immunosuppressant drug at this point, just the sugar water. How could the sugar water have transformed into a poisonous elixir for these rats? If you recall your quick journey through the history of behaviorism in Chapter 2, you have probably already figured this out ... and Pavlov would be proud of you. The only explanation that Ader, a psychologist who had training in behavioral conditioning, could offer was that the sugar water became associated with the sickness symptoms produced by the immunosuppressant drug, just as the caretaker's footsteps had become associated with the delivery of food in Pavlov's salivating dogs. Consequently, similar to the way the footsteps later generated the production of saliva in the absence of actual food in the dogs, the sweet water generated the immunosuppressant response in the absence of the actual drug.

The explanation for the rats' sickness was a bit more complicated than the dogs' situation, however. The sound of the caretaker's footsteps and the sight and taste of the food were sensory signals that entered the brain where they could be easily paired to produce the efficient conditioned response preparing the dog for the predicted presence of the food. The sweet taste of the water coursed its way through the taste receptors and associated nerves to the brain ... but how was that connected to an immune effect? At the time of this surprising finding, Ader and Cohen observed there was no formal evidence that the nervous system had any contact with the immune system. Medical students took their neural systems course and their immune system course with no mention that they influenced one another. According to Ader and Cohen's data, however, they did influence one another.[1] How? Where? Under what circumstances? We're not talking about mere distorted brain bubbles here, we're talking about contingency calculations that shouldn't exist between two systems that shouldn't be able to communicate. It was like scratching your arm to start your car.

The mysteries surrounding these data presented challenges when Ader and Cohen tried to present their intriguing findings to the medical community. It seemed more like magic than science to the clinicians and researchers who had always viewed the systems as separate. Consequently, it looked like this new discovery would simply be swept under the scientific rug. Ader and Cohen persisted, however, and formally called for the creation of a new discipline that investigated communication between the nervous and the immune system. Additional research by David Felten, also at the University of Rochester at the time, provided a mechanism for this fascinating finding. There were nerve fibers extending to various immune organs such as the spleen, lymph nodes, and bone marrow. Later it was confirmed that the neurochemicals that directed activity in the brain were also calling the shots out there in the immune organs of the body. The boundaries between brain and body got a little fuzzier when Felten made those initial observations.[2]

Gradually, the idea of psychoneuroimmunology became accepted by clinicians and scientists. In contrast to the idea of using conditioning to suppress the immune system, the more relevant question in my mind was how this information could be used to ramp up the immune system to fight diseases, such as the disease my mother was battling. Could these new findings lead to immuno*enhancement* as opposed to immuno*suppression*?

I mentioned my interest in immunoconditioning to my mother's oncologist and couldn't believe that I was at one of the few institutions in the world exploring that very question. The team treating her at the University of Alabama at Birmingham (UAB) had previously found that pairing the unique odor of camphor with a drug that enhanced white blood cell production increased the number of days a mouse could survive with an implanted tumor . . . longer than the survival rate with just the drug. In the strange world of conditioned immune contingencies, camphor and its psychological associations had a medicinal value. When the camphor was presented without the drug, it enhanced the immune response so that the mouse experienced immunological boosts when the drug was administered as well as when the camphor was administered—increasing the impact of the drug alone. Low cost, no side effects . . . it seemed that this team was onto something. As it turned out, Russian researchers had investigated this question following Pavlov's Nobel Prize–winning research with his dogs at the turn of the twentieth century. If Pavlov's research suggested that the nervous system could extend its learning and conditioning abilities to the digestive system, why not the immune system? The early Russian research led to fascinating results supporting the neuro-immune connections; however, these exciting findings failed to have an impact in the scientific community.[3]

What exactly did the Russian scientists do? In the 1920s, Sergey Metalnikov set out to determine if it was possible to boost the immune system, Pavlov-style. In a program of research with guinea pigs, he warmed their skin prior to giving them an injection of a small dose of bacteria that activated the immune system to defend it against the pathogen intruders. Then he cleverly gave the preconditioned guinea pigs, as well as condition-naïve guinea pigs, a lethal dose of bacteria, *Vibrio cholera*, while he warmed their skin. The condition-naïve animals died within 8 hours, whereas the preconditioned animals made it to 36 hours, with a few of them recovering completely. In this case, heat had actually saved their lives.[4]

I had heard enough. Where did I sign my mother up for this immune boosting therapy? No human trials were in existence at the time. But who needed a sanctioned human trial since there didn't appear to be any risks with this line of research? She was continuing with her more traditional therapeutic approach, so no compromises were being made on her medicinal front. I learned that my mother had been prescribed daily injections of a drug known as filgrastim (Neupogen in this case), which is given to chemotherapy patients with a compromised immune system in order to activate the production of white blood cells—immunological soldiers in the war against impending infections. The injections were painful and expensive and limited to one each day. Could I extend the effects of this drug by borrowing some insight from the Russian scientists working with guinea pigs decades earlier? Or, closer to home, from the oncology researchers working with the mice in the same building at UAB? I briefly mentioned a hypothetical scenario to her doctor and proceeded to run to the drugstore to purchase some lemon drops. All I needed was a noticeable sensory experience, so taste would do the trick (at least that was my thought). I checked that my mother didn't regularly consume lemon drops to ensure that the experience would be unique and somewhat novel, and easily paired with the immune modification that would be occurring concurrently.

The next day, about a minute prior to her filgrastim injection, I gave my mother a lemon drop. As she was experiencing that bitter taste, her immune cells were being activated with the drug. The next day she repeated the lemon drop–filgrastrim combination. Then, beginning on about the third day, she continued to suck on a lemon drop during her morning filgrastim injection, but also sucked on a lemon drop each afternoon. I was hoping to double the impact of the filgrastim injection with one actual dose and one imagined dose. Of course, this is a case study, but her doctors enthusiastically reported an upward blip in her daily white blood cell count once we started the lemon drop conditioning. I'm not sure if my mother thought I was crazy or a genius, but we both found a spark of hope with this lemon drop endeavor . . . a positive experience in the midst of fear and uncertainty.

Even though her white blood cell count was encouraging and kept her healthy during the treatment—the white blood cells weren't enough for the tumors. A few months later, after my mother incurred the torment of the stem cell transplant, the tumors became more robust than the defenses of her immune system. Late one August evening in 1996, after I had just arrived from Virginia to visit, I rode with her in an ambulance back to the same hospital where she had received her stem cell transplant. She was able to hang on until I arrived, something I will forever be grateful for. After a valiant fight, her immune system was worn down. As I described in my previous book, *Lifting Depression*, the loss of my mother that night rocked my world, instantly recalculating almost every life contingency I had known to that point.[5]

Although it got off to an encouraging start, my personal psycho-neuroimmunology experiment ultimately had a sad ending. However, the scientist in me knew that the communication between the nervous and the immune system opened the door to exciting medical advances. Still, 20 years later the progress has been slow, as this approach still feels too far out of mainstream medicine to be embraced while more traditional therapies have been enthusiastically accepted by the medical community. It's safe to say that the lemon drop therapy has not been adopted in mainstream oncology. This situation isn't unlike the challenges described with behavioral approaches to treating psychiatric illness. We're so much more comfortable with a pill or an injection. The *take a pill—feel better* contingencies are more easily accepted by our neural networks than the *engage in a behavior—feel better* contingencies. We need to work on this contingency distortion in medicine.

When German researcher Manfred Schedlowski began his conditioned immune research in the mid-1990s, he was told that approach was more like art than science. His work has an interesting twist of maximizing the immunosuppressant properties of the drug cyclophosphamide. In some patients the immune system becomes overactive and suppression alleviates symptoms. Patients suffering from extreme allergies or arthritis, for example, have overactive immune systems. Additionally, transplant patients need to take immunosuppressant drugs to minimize the probability of rejecting the transplanted tissue. Following pairing the drug with sweet water, similar to Ader and Cohen's research, Schedlowski implanted a second heart into rats' abdomens and simply gave them doses of sweet water with no immunosuppressant drug. Animals with prior conditioning experience with the drug survived three days longer than the control group, which had received the drug with no sweet water pairing prior to the transplant. When a low dose of the drug was added to the daily sweet water administration, the survival time extended to about a month, with 20 percent surviving the entire experimental period.[6] This approach suggests that immunoconditioning may be used as an adjunctive type of therapy with traditional immune drugs.

As intriguing as conditioned immune responses are, another twist on health-related contingencies is observed in the placebo response.

In comparison to conditioned immune responses, the contingency boundaries get even fuzzier with placebos since improvement is observed in the absence of a drug ever being administered.

The Peril and Promise of Placebos: The Expected Contingency Rx

Whereas conditioned responses use *past* experiences to predict future outcomes, placebos, in the purest sense of the term, rely on *expected* outcomes that may never have been experienced. Technically translated as "to please," placebos challenge the notion of building contingency capital in real time to discern future outcomes. In this case, imagined contingencies become the star players in the response-outcome formula. Although some researchers consider immunoconditioning observed in animals and humans to be a form of a placebo, in my opinion a true placebo response is uniquely human, requiring an awareness of expectations and hope linked to a particular perceived medicinal approach.

In the classic sense, a placebo effect is when a patient is given a sugar pill or some inert substance and told that it is an active drug— or in controlled studies, that it is "possibly" an active drug. Being told by a doctor or another trusted individual that the treatment will improve one's health generates hope and expectations of recovery in the patient. As described below, with or without a drug on board, that expectancy is not lost on the brain.

The term *placebo* was formally introduced to the medical literature in the mid- to late eighteenth century as an act of desperation more than anything else. When a child keeps asking the same question a parent may get so frustrated that he or she will say anything to get the child to be quiet. (I hope other parents have done this.) Well, when patients kept complaining of symptoms for which the doctors had no known medicinal treatment, they fibbed a bit just to get the patients out of their hair. What could be the harm in giving patients a supposed inert substance and telling them that it should relieve their symptoms? Often, the patients were fully satisfied with the seemingly fake treatment. In 1807 President Thomas Jefferson wrote, "One of the most successful physicians I have ever known, has assured me, that he used more bread pills, drops of colored water, powders of hickory ashes, than of all other medicines put together. It was certainly a pious fraud."[7]

The question that fascinates researchers and clinicians today is the degree to which this treatment is a fraud or the real deal. Anecdotes of placebos providing specific healing properties to sick individuals are impressive. Consider "Mr. Wright." He was in the final stages of cancer, with orange-size tumors located in lymph nodes throughout his body. None of the existing treatments had successfully attacked the cancer. In a 1957 report of Mr. Wright's case it was reported that he found out about a new anticancer drug called Krebiozen and became convinced it would cure him. Although he was bedridden when he was given his first injection of the drug, in just three days he was motoring around his room, cracking jokes with his nurses. His test results indicated that the tumors had shrunk by half, news that led to his release from the hospital. When Mr. Wright later read in a newspaper that Krebiozen wasn't living up to its expectations as an anticancer drug and expressed his concern to his doctors, they responded by lying to him and telling him they had received a new and improved version of the drug. In reality they gave him an injection that didn't include any of the drug. Improvement once again continued, and he remained healthy for two months, at which time he read a report that the drug was worthless. He died a few days later.[8]

Of course, it's difficult to know exactly what was going on with Mr. Wright and if the tumors would have returned even if he had never learned that the drug was ineffective. However, in the absence of any effective treatments for certain diseases, the hope associated with these placebo stories is certainly intriguing. After it had become clear that the stem cell transplant hadn't eradicated my mother's cancer, I often thought about an elaborate scheme in which her doctors and I told her that an amazing new drug had been introduced for non-Hodgkin's lymphoma. Would it save her? Give her more time? Was this the last chance to boost her immune system in a more powerful way than the lemon drop immunoconditioning? I'll never know because I couldn't bring myself to lie to my beloved mother. To this day, I question my decision.

The mechanisms of the placebo are not clearly understood, but the connections between the nervous and the immune system that support immunoconditioning are key players with the placebo as well. Further, when placebos are used for neural diseases and psychiatric illnesses, their effectiveness may be more pervasive since the brain is key for recovery. Fascinating revelations about the potent reach of placebos are found in patients with Parkinson's disease. In this neuromuscular condition, cells in an area of the brain known as the substantia nigra start to die, accompanied by a decrease in the neurotransmitter dopamine they produce. Symptoms include muscle rigidity and tremors and an inability to initiate movement. Drugs that replace the diminished dopamine relieve the symptoms, but the window of treatment is often limited as the cells producing this essential neurochemical continue to diminish.

In the 1980s various young adults in California injected some "designer" heroin that been mixed in such a way that it destroyed cells in the substantia nigra in a similar fashion as observed in Parkinson's disease. The effects were faster than those observed in Parkinson's, however, and several of the individuals who were unfortunate enough to use this toxic drug found themselves immediately frozen, completely unable to move or talk. Neurologist Bill Langston served as both their doctor and a medical investigator as he searched for an explanation for the transformation of these active young adults into human statues. He soon traced their stories to the toxic heroin. A few of the patients were considered for a novel therapeutic approach investigated by Swedish neuroscientist Anders Bjorkland involving transplanting fetal substantia nigra neurons into adult brains. This treatment had been conducted on rodents with encouraging results, but it was a stretch to apply the surgery to humans. One of the oldest victims, George Carillo, received the surgery when he was 52 (10 years after consuming the drug) and experienced impressive improvements, so much so that the surgery was conducted in a few of the other patients.[9] It seemed that the fetal transplant cell surgery was the much-anticipated cure for Parkinson's disease. But then there was the placebo effect.

Ongoing ethical concerns over the use of fetal tissue in cell transplants have limited this treatment strategy in the United States. Interestingly, these apprehensions have spurred the discovery of alternative types of cells. For example, Titan Pharmaceuticals introduced an experimental therapy known as Spheramine, which bypassed the need for fetal cells. Specifically, this treatment involves implanting human retina cells that produce a chemical precursor for the missing neurotransmitter dopamine.

Peggy Willocks was just 44 years old when she was diagnosed with Parkinson's disease, and it progressed quickly, forcing her to retire four years later. The promise of this new therapy was very appealing to Peggy, and in 2000 she was the second patient to receive the treatment. The effects were slow but impressive. After about six months she started to feel some improvement, with a drastic improvement in her balance emerging after about nine months. At one year after receiving the treatment, she experienced a 48 percent improvement in motor ability, a result that persisted at her four-year follow up! This treatment seemed to be effective, offering hope to patients.

As part of the experimental study involving both the fetal and the retinal cell treatment, a sham surgery group was included. This important experimental group controls for expectations about the treatment effects by including randomly assigned patients, who receive all of the procedural steps, including anesthesia, holes bored into the skull, etc. An inert substance, however, is administered instead of the cells. It was almost inconceivable that this sham surgery could improve the symptoms of a neurological disease and the accompanying diminishing brain tissue. There were no cells being infused into the substantia nigra . . . no apparent way to enhance dopamine production to treat the movement disorder. However, the trials for the promising new Spheramine treatment were halted in 2008 when the sham surgery group responded in a similar fashion as the true surgery group.[10] Could the expectations that the drug could work (remember, patients did not know if they were receiving the real treatment, so everybody could have hope that they were on the receiving side of the cells) stimulate the dopaminergic system and literally generate more cells?

Similar placebo effects have been described with patients taking antidepressant drugs. Because one of depression's signature symptoms is diminished hope, expectation may also alter neurochemistry to combat the specific symptoms of depression. In fact, the brilliant work of Irving Kirsch (now at Harvard Medical School and Beth Israel Deaconess Medical School) suggests that improvement is observed with *any* drug given to depressed patients—sugar pill, anti-depressant, thyroid medication, you name it.[11] An interesting point made by Kirsch is the necessity for active placebos in pharmaceutical trials. Although patients are thought to be "blind" to the type of drug they are given (drug vs. placebo), they are tuned in to any side effects that an actual drug may have on their bodies. Such an effect, even if it isn't related to the depression symptoms, confirms that they are actually taking a drug—which heightens expectations for improvement. An active placebo doesn't contain the targeted chemical in the drug but does produce generic side effects. Similar to Parkinson's disease, if any of these treatments, drug or placebo, increase hope and expectations—those emotions can affect neurochemistry in ways that can diminish the symptoms of depression. Considering the discussion of cognitive and behavioral therapies for depression in Chapter 8, placebos should also be considered a nonpharmacological treatment for depression.

With these observations, scientists and clinicians are scratching their heads as they contemplate the requirements for adequate placebo controls and, in the case of sham surgeries to investigate placebo effects, whether it is even ethical to submit patients to such invasive techniques.[12] Those questions certainly won't be answered here, but I hope that I have made the case that imagined contingencies can influence actual brain responses and have a meaningful impact on our well-being. It appears that the medical profession would be well served by a strong dose of an understanding of contingency calculations, real and imagined, that affect health outcomes.

Playful Contingencies

Turning to a lighter topic, children invoke imagined contingencies in their wonderful bouts of play. Sure, they are building reality-based contingency capital as they determine how hard a person can push someone before they cry, or identify the highest tree limb from which they can jump to the ground without breaking an arm. This rough-and-tumble play can be considered contingency building on steroids—at a critical brain development window, certainly wonderful fodder for developing brains. In addition to this playful reality, children also utilize imagination in their play as they imagine they are a superhero or that their new puppy is a winning racehorse. As it turns out, both reality- and imagination-based play components contribute to the experiential and cognitive contingency inventory of our growing children.

Interestingly, reality-based rough-and-tumble play isn't unique to humans. As I described in *The Lab Rat Chronicles*, rat play is my favorite among the fascinating rodent behaviors. When my students house young rats individually but then give them "play dates" by placing two rats in a cage for a designated time, the rats immediately run to one another—chasing, wrestling, pulling each other's tails—as if they are making up for lost playtime (Figure 15).[13] It's a true delight to watch. Images of two young human children always come to mind—chasing each other and wrestling, pulling shirttails instead of actual tails.

If play is my favorite rat behavior, then one of my favorite rat researchers has to be Jaak Panksepp, perhaps the world's foremost researcher on the value of play in mammals who sadly passed away during the editing of this book. In the controlled laboratory environment, Panksepp and his colleagues generated data indicating that play is critical for brain development. He also suggested that, as play has been systematically removed from our children's lives (especially during school hours), their ability to mature and focus attention on meaningful variables is compromised. It's interesting to consider if this effect is manifested in the condition referred to as attention deficit hyperactivity disorder (ADHD).[14] Considering that ADHD rates have increased a whopping 43 percent since 2003, this disorder deserves a close scrutiny of all potential contributing variables.[15] Regardless of the cause, contingency calculations are likely compromised in children as they find it difficult to focus on the most meaningful stimulus-response associations and predicted outcomes. Even Plato recognized the benefits of unstructured, free play in *The Republic*, writing, "Our children from their earliest years must take part in all the more lawful forms of play, for if they are not surrounded by such an atmosphere they can never grow up to be well conducted and virtuous citizens."[16]

Play, whether it is physical or imaginative, is characterized by less of an emphasis on realistic outcomes than is seen in other behaviors such as foraging for food, seeking social contact, or building

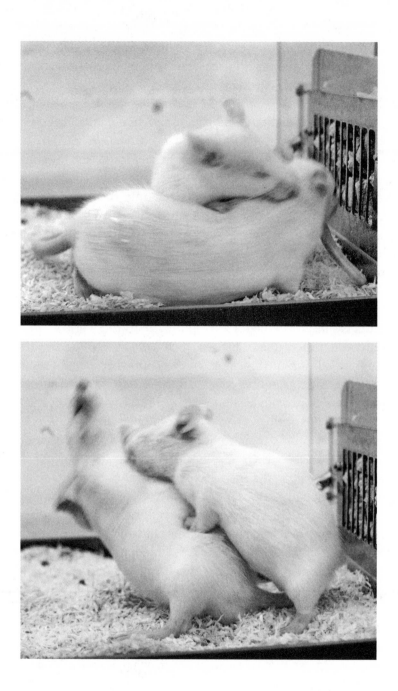

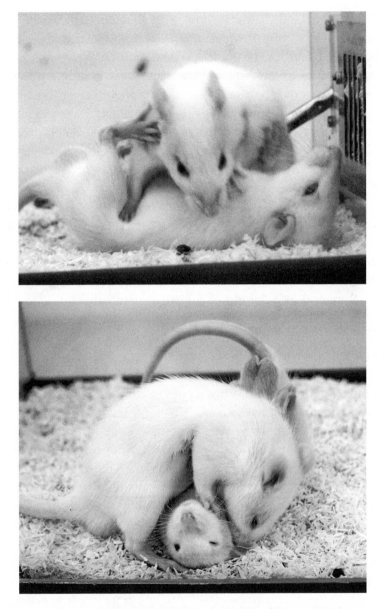

Figure 15. Play-Induced Experiential Capital. *Play behavior looks similar in many different mammalian species, suggesting that it serves an important role in sculpting adaptive neural networks. As these images from the social neuroscience laboratory of Alexa Veenema at Michigan Statue University suggest, play behavior is complex in rodents and serves as a valuable model for investigating play in humans. (Photos by Alexa H. Veenema)*

a shelter. That's the aspect about play that puzzles evolutionary biologists. What purpose does it serve? Energy is expended, risk is encountered, but for what end? We know what the response is— running, jumping, hiding, pushing—but what exactly is the outcome? It's not precisely clear what the actual outcome is other than the gathering of life experiences that may facilitate well-being in the future. I like to think about play as a more open-ended contingency-building strategy, perhaps even a contingency training boot camp for the brain. Children repeat seemingly silly and worthless behaviors that have no immediate tangible outcome just as teens and adults repeat sit-ups for no immediate tangible result. Although we become aware of many benefits accompanying exercises such as sit-ups as we mature, an outsider observing our species would certainly be perplexed about why humans spend so much time expending energy in large buildings called gyms. Regardless, play could be considered the mammalian brain's form of contingency calisthenics.

Beyond the lack of perceivable tangible outcomes associated with play, more immediate outcomes in the brain likely accompany this complex behavior. Although there are no standout specific neural effects that have been observed in playful animals, research has introduced a few themes. When a protein known as fos, which marks active brain areas, is tracked, rats that have recently played exhibit increased neural activity across many areas of the cortex and subcortical area, including the area that processes the neurochemical involved with movement, anticipation, and goals—dopamine. Additionally, play appears to activate the brain's growth factors such as brain derived growth factor (BDNF). BDNF enhances neuroplasticity, which is so important for a developing brain. Thus, the play-induced brain effects appear to be as ubiquitous as play itself. Nonetheless, because animals compensate for lost playtime following social deprivation, it appears that play is a serious ingredient for the development of healthy brains.[17] Further, because an inverse relationship exists between stress and play, with lower levels of stress associated with increased rates of play, a little play may be just what the doctor ordered for adults as well in order to dilute the toxicity of chronic stress that often accompanies the real world of grown-ups.[18]

Although play has been observed in reptiles and birds to some degree, it is much more robust in mammals. Dogs, cats, elephants, and otters all exhibit beautiful bouts of play.[19] Because the mammalian brain is the most complex brain in nature, play may serve an important role in priming all of its complex circuits for more flexible learning and spontaneous responses that are necessary for survival in addition to the more traditional learned associations, habits, and reflexes. Neuroscientists at the University of Lethbridge, including Sergio Pellis, Vivien Pellis, Heather Bell, and Bryan Kolb, have found that play restructures the shape of neurons in the contingency-calculating prefrontal cortex, and even serves as a primer for subsequent neuroplasticity later in a rat's life.[20] Thus, the physical twists and turns that characterize rough-and-tumble play may prepare animals for the unexpected twists and turns that will inevitably present themselves later in life.[21] You'll recall from Chapter 7 that Paul MacLean, a pioneering U.S. neuroscientist, wrote in his book *The Triune Brain* that three behaviors separated mammals from other animals—nursing, maternal-offspring communications, and . . . play.[22]

While the behavioral response-outcome contingencies are a little fuzzy when considering play, all of the traditional elements of behavioral and cognitive associations are thrown out the door when it comes to creativity. Both the process and the outcome are unique and novel. Although classic behaviorists are perplexed by creative endeavors, there's no denying that we spend considerable time cultivating curiosity in our culture.

Curiosity-Driven Creative Contingencies

In one sense, exploration in animals could be considered a form of a curiosity-driven response. What is behind this rock? What is this fruit that fell from the tree? Why is this animal hopping along this path—and where does the path go? Although risky and energy-expensive, exploration of new environments leads to new information and richer experiential capital for calculating future response contingencies. Recall that the two mice that were exploratory in the *Who Moved My Cheese?* parable survived the dreaded moving of the cheese. Although it's difficult to define creativity objectively, it seems to involve the transition of brains from considering "What is?" as associated with curiosity . . . to "What if?"

Creativity is generally characterized as a novel response that produces an idea or product that is perceived to have some value. A creative product could have utilitarian value (an innovative gadget to help the elderly open a pickle jar) or artistic value (a beautiful painting using a novel brush technique). Although no behavior exists in an experiential vacuum, creative responses appear to be a little footloose and fancy-free in the previous experience department. Certainly, past interactions contribute to creative solutions, but the linear trajectory of acquiring the appropriate experiences to generate accurate contingencies outlined by Pavlov, Skinner, and Watson is less clear when it comes to creative endeavors.

When I go to my rodent laboratory, I can certainly investigate exploration, determining when rats are asking "What is?" questions as they venture into new territories or investigate new objects. But I have yet to enter the lab in the morning to find blocks stacked up to create a novel escape route or a gnawed toy used as a tool to knock the rodent chow down from their cage tops. And I have yet to tap my own creativity reserves to successfully design a rodent assessment of creativity. There's no convincing evidence that these laboratory rats ever enter the "What if" phase that we so often associate with creativity. That may be because the most creative endeavors require the generation of an idea that the animal or person has to retain . . . somewhere in their neural networks . . . in order to execute the creative response. I have written extensively about how clever rats are, but I simply don't know if they can hold an idea in their rodent brains or minds.

Over a century ago, Walter Hunter conducted research that informed our ideas about animals having ideas. Hunter's mentor was Harvey Carr, the scientist who took over the animal laboratory at the University of Chicago following J. B. Watson's departure to Johns Hopkins (and we know how that worked out). For Hunter's comparative intelligence study, he focused on rats, raccoons, dogs, and children. After the subjects viewed a three-panel apparatus with three light bulbs, their task was to notice the single light bulb that was illuminated so that, after a specific delay, they could approach that same light bulb and receive a yummy treat. Whereas the rat could retain the information for only a one-second delay, the raccoons could successfully solve the task after 25 seconds. The raccoon performance paled in comparison, however, to the dogs and children, who could easily handle a five-minute delay. It's important to note that subsequent research with more training and sophisticated tasks, such as the delayed-matching-to-sample task, suggests that rats can indeed hold information in their memory, also known as working memory, for much longer than one second, and this ability is likely facilitated by the now familiar medial prefrontal cortex.[23] Being a student of behavior, however, Hunter noticed something else about these animals in this early comparative study. During the delay phase, the dogs and rats stayed oriented toward the direction of the previously lit bulb, so all they had to do was walk toward it when the delay was terminated. The raccoons and children, however, walked around doing other things and, when the time came, easily approached the target stimulus they were supposed to remember. Did the raccoons and children keep an image of the task in their neural networks while they proceeded to do other things? Could this image of the task be considered an idea?[24] Further, when a raccoon approaches your bird feeder, which has been strategically hung from a tree out of the supposed reach of any animal, does the raccoon form an idea that allows it to implement a plan and easily access the birdseed? Perhaps the raccoons can harbor ideas about gaining access to the feeder that escaped the humans, who were trying diligently to keep them out of the bird feeder in the first place.

It turned out that the raccoons' potential to form and maintain ideas may be the reason they were kicked out of the running for the model laboratory animal early in the twentieth century. Herbert Davis wrote that his raccoons "broke out" of the lab one day. He found them in the ventilation system of the lab, apparently headed toward their escape. Maybe the raccoons went to the spy camp mentioned in the previous chapter that I wish I had sent my own kids to! It turned out that it was just too difficult to keep these animals in the lab, perhaps due to their curiosity and creative ideas. When it was later declared that there were great individual differences in the learning ability of raccoons, making it difficult to achieve statistical significance in the experimental investigations, the raccoons were officially kicked out the laboratory door. Robert Yerkes, a well-known comparative psychologist, introduced the next poster mammal for laboratory investigations—the mouse. Mice were small, tame, continuously active, and easy to care for, very different from the raccoons and, in many ways, very different from the humans they were designed to model.[25] Today, it is estimated that both mice and rats are used in approximately 85 percent of all biomedical research.[26]

In addition to the raccoons, glimpses of curiosity and creativity have been observed in other animals, even invertebrates. Octopi have been observed transforming coconut shells into shelters, even developing a fancy walk known as stilt walking to carry their new homes to the final destination.[27] Bowerbirds create elaborate novel nests to attract females, as mentioned in the previous chapter.[28] However, no other species has used its creativity to change the landscape of its habitat to the extent observed in humans. Beavers probably come the closest to achieving this designation, but, even to our detriment, humans are the clear winners. In this case, the "What is?" has definitely been transformed to the "What if?" in the human brain.

One creative endeavor that has been investigated by neuroscientists is an extreme creative behavior known as freestyle rapping. In this hip-hop style of music, the artist improvises rhythmic lyrics to a guiding instrumental beat. That's right, generating novel lyrics that rhyme at the same time—with no prior practice. In my mind, this just doesn't seem possible. Which neural area or network enables a person to generate such a freewheeling response? In one study, the rappers were placed in an fMRI scanner while either freestyle rapping or simply reciting lyrics. It turns out that, in order for the brain to improvise, it has to tone down the activity of the executive function cortical area known as the dorsolateral prefrontal cortex so that another brain area, the medial prefrontal cortex, involved in motivation and incentives, can take command. Turning off an important gatekeeping part of the brain is okay for freestyle rapping, but this may not be advisable for important life decisions such as deciding the best career option or life partner.[29]

An additional way to deconstruct the brain's fully operational status to enhance creativity is to loosen up the neural attentional circuits with a distracting activity prior to generating the idea. This distraction was the emphasis of one study investigating creativity by having one group consciously think about an idea while distracting another group from thinking about an idea, prior to asking the participants of both groups to generate ideas. Although the two groups had no problem generating ideas, participants who engaged in conscious thought about the upcoming idea-generating session were less satisfied with the quality of their creative ideas than the distracted group.[30] Thus, just thinking about ideas starts the brain's filters buzzing in ways that will likely nix the subsequent ideas that don't appear especially relevant—no room for such rational filtering and contingency calculating in the world of creative ideas.

The neurochemistry of creativity is also being explored. Researchers at Tel Aviv University performed a study to assess creativity in people in their early 60s, and a portion of the participants were taking a drug that enhanced dopamine used to treat Parkinson's disease. The results were fascinating. Those taking the drug, even with their neurological diagnosis, demonstrated more creative activity than did the brain-healthy participants.[31] The extra dopamine may enhance motivation and drive, as well as impulsivity, an effective cocktail for creativity. This neurochemical cocktail works within limitations. People with schizophrenia, associated with heightened dopaminergic activity, are haunted with creative thoughts that transform into hallucinations and delusions. Further, recreational drugs that enhance dopaminergic circuits (e.g., amphetamines, cocaine) have been known to produce impulse control challenges and distorted realities. This gets us into the problematic brain bubble territory, suggesting that there is a fine line between the healthy integration of contingency-relaxed thought adventures leading to creative experiences, and full-blown psychosis.

Thus, humans seem to be primed for curiosity and creativity more so than any other creature on the planet. This behavioral and cognitive flexibility has enabled us to leave our comfort zones and explore new territories and make them our own. It has also provided a way to jump-start the areas of the brain involved with motivation and drive, leading to the achievement of goals. Then there's poetry, sculpture, and music. Our brains have been more reluctant to reveal the specific purpose of these endeavors. Although the exact nature of these creative contingencies remains a mystery, there's no denying the reality that they make our life journeys more enjoyable. Maybe the advice of my husband, Gary, about the personality assessment tests described in the previous chapter are appropriate here as well in my feeble attempt to analyze creativity . . . *Kelly, don't over-think it.*

The topics discussed in this chapter—neuroimmune conditioning, placebos, play, and creativity—all push the limits of contingency building in different ways. Stepping outside of our contingency comfort zones results in intriguing and fascinating responses that have enhanced the quality of our lives in many ways. Everything in moderation, however. The healthiest brains need a balance of the more grounded contingencies and occasional relaxed creative contingency detours. In the Epilogue, we'll review the importance of keeping our lifestyles within the proper contingency-building zones to protect us from losing touch with the all too important real-time authentic interactions with our physical and social worlds. If we generate too many shortcuts, we will short-circuit our contingency-calculation efficiency. If these shortcuts are taken to an extreme, we lose touch with the world around us, and, eventually, our lifeline to this world— our brains—becomes compromised.

Redefining Prosperity

From Strategic Champagne Bubbles to Accurately Perceived Life Affordances

I BEGAN THIS BOOK with a discussion of real estate bubbles. Allowed to grow, these bubbles can lead to economic crashes, as we saw most recently in 2008. The 2008 real estate market crash resulted from the fact that the authentic value of homes was distorted, an *irrational exuberance* of the market, as Alan Greenspan has described. As we approach the end of this book, I want to leave you with a more balanced perception of well-placed strategic brain bubbles in the midst of our authentic life views. As described in the previous chapter, conservatively placed brain bubbles in the form of play, hope, and creative ideas add a wonderful texture to the brain's contingency-calculating neural fabric, but are there additional lessons to be learned about bubbles occupying our neural territory?

After borrowing from the real estate literature to make a case against life-distorting brain bubbles, I turn now to the world of champagne bubbles. An innovative physicist and oceanographer, Helen Czerski, may be the world's most informed expert on the physics of bubbles. At University College London she has revealed the delicate relationship between well-placed champagne bubbles and the perceived value of a particular champagne glass. Czerski points out that bubbles don't automatically emerge when champagne is poured into a glass. As the gases are released, a slightly rough surface in the glass triggers the development of bubbles. Ideally, the bubbles will begin their journey from a tiny surface area at the bottom of the glass and stream to the top of the glass in a beautiful, orderly fashion, bursting into celebrated aromas and fizzy popping sounds for your guests.[1] However, if champagne flutes have scattered imperfections such as accumulated specks of dust or nicks in the glass, the bubbles will keep forming, spewing toward the top of the glass and creating a distraction. The continual blast of bubble streams distorts the anticipated beauty of the modest bubbles within the beautifully crafted champagne flutes. Although he was referring to wine, even the Hawaiian singer (and perhaps life philosopher) Don Ho knew the value of well-placed bubbles, as the lyrics of his 1960s hit song suggest. *Tiny bubbles . . . in the wine . . . makes me happy . . . makes me fine.* Thank goodness he qualified the appropriate size of the bubbles leading to emotional well-being.

Although we typically use champagne to toast celebrated life events—weddings, career achievements, the passing of one year and entry into another—it appears that champagne also offers lessons about the placement of bubbles in healthy mental lives. Strategically placed bubbles produced at an appropriate rate enhance the experience of those champagne toasts, but the experience is compromised if distortions in the glass produce too many bubbles in all the wrong places—at least for champagne aficionados. Thus, even with champagne, healthy environments in the form of champagne glasses are critical for maximizing the emotional experience of making those noteworthy toasts recognizing significant life achievements. Similarly, authentic interactions with our environment maximize our emotional experiences—at least for the *life* aficionados among us. A stream of emotional highs or lows coming from the wrong places, such as addiction, poverty, or celebrity, compromises the brain's ability to keep on track with reality and generate authentic contingency calculations for future responses—hopefully leading to celebratory events.

Although there is supporting evidence that our neural circuits can tolerate, in moderation, scaled-down brain bubbles, the most critical criterion for mental health and success is the maintenance of a direct line to the environment that produces accurate perceptions of our surroundings. This practice builds our experiential capital so that accurate contingency calculations can be generated to facilitate informed decision-making. As emphasized throughout this book, when the value of life experiences becomes distorted in the form of disruptive brain bubbles, it becomes difficult to respond in the most adaptive ways. Just as our immune systems need T cells and B cells to defend our bodies against the invasion of pathogens, our brains need authentic experiences to defend our neural networks against the invasion of factors that compromise emotionally rewarding experiences and lead to psychiatric illness. As described in previous chapters, impoverished conditions, stress, and privilege are just a few of these potential experiences known to invade our brains and threaten our mental health.

Extending the enlightening work of the early behaviorists, experimental psychologist James Gibson introduced the term *affordances*, admitting that he just simply made the word up. We all know the word *afford* and think about it often as we contemplate such things as whether we can pay for that new car that has caught our eye. But what did Gibson mean by affordances? He defined the term as the potential for specific actions provided by certain aspects of the environment. A handle on a teapot offers the affordance of picking the teapot up and pouring hot water in a mug; a smile on a colleague's face offers the affordance of a friendship; and the open space in a backyard offers the affordance of a garden and all of its delicious bounty in the form of fresh vegetables.[2]

Gibson also suggested that, throughout our lives, we gain insights about the *invariants* in the world around us. Invariants are the variables that remain somewhat stable and predictable against a background of changes and unpredictable outcomes. For many, cherished relationships, hobbies, meaningful careers, and spiritual beliefs represent the invariants throughout life that, at their best, keep us grounded as opposed to distorting reality. By providing safe harbors, these invariants also have the potential to reduce stress and anxiety as we face life's inevitable challenges. Of course, nothing is absolutely constant in life, and, at some point an invariant in our life will shift to variant status. Losing a loved one, a friendship, or a job will put the brain's contingency calculators in a tailspin requiring a substantial recalibration that is not unlike the recalculations of the betting odds on tote boards at horse races—in the span of a moment, all the payoffs have changed.[3]

Whereas our savings account balances determine what we can afford to purchase from a financial perspective, our experiential investments and accumulated cognitive and social capital determine our perceived affordances throughout life. Accurate contingency calculations keep us on track to maximize affordances, ensuring that we avoid the toxic, life-distorting brain bubbles described throughout this book, and enabling us to take advantage of new opportunities that emerge on life's horizon. Ironically, these very contingency calculators are successfully creating a world that, for those of us living in technologically advanced societies, is characterized by diminished interactions with the environment. We easily press buttons to obtain food, clothes . . . just about anything our hearts desire. More recently, we have relinquished even the minimal effort involved in button pushing to Amazon's intelligent personal assistant, Alexa, for such tasks as ordering takeout or finding the nearest place to get the car washed. As we work less and less to obtain valuable resources we may experience a *contingency conundrum*, in which the brain eventually loses its capacity to generate the most adaptive response options for our emotional well-being. Although introducing shortcuts to desirable resources sounds appealing on many levels, such a world compromises the neural networks that are so critical in guiding our behavior toward the most satisfying responses. Thus, our brain's interpretation of prosperity may be at odds with the contemporary worldview that has emerged in our technologically advanced society. In this Western view of prosperity, limited experiential capital increases susceptibility to emotional crashes.

James Gibson's wife, Eleanor, also an experimental psychologist, wrote in her biography that "every day brings new affordances. Perceiving them makes all the difference, especially when there is more than one that can be acted upon, so choices must be made."[4] As we now know, contingency capital reserves must be stockpiled throughout our lives to enable us to make the most informed choices with the highest emotional payoffs. Without this experiential capital, life's affordances will be overlooked and misinterpreted.

Although it would have been nice to have unlocked the mysteries of the brain and mind when the human genome was sequenced, we shouldn't be surprised that our life outcomes are determined by much more than those sequences of nucleotide bases. Genetic sequences are certainly vital to the brain's operations; however, behavioral and environmental variables are also critical in the determination of responses and outcomes that contribute to one's life experiences. If we remember from Chapter 3 that the most highly functioning brains are more like a soufflé than a casserole, we'll continue to respect not only what we put in our brains in the form of life experiences, but how that key information is administered and monitored throughout the various stages of our lives.

Although there was some truth to behaviorism pioneer B. F. Skinner's comment that "human behavior is perhaps the most difficult subject to which the methods of science have ever been applied," subsequent research in various disciplines such as neuroscience, experimental psychology, and evolutionary biology confirms that the mysteries of the human brain and behavioral output are beginning to reveal themselves.[5] Being astute students of this science will provide more information about how our brains continue to pump out healthy contingency calculations when we're faced with multiple options. In the end, healthy, authentic contingency calculations ensure that we're perceiving, and benefiting from, life's affordances, maximizing emotional payoffs and minimizing emotional crashes.

Notes

Introduction

1. R. Dale, *The First Crash: Lessons from the South Sea Bubble* (Princeton, NJ: Princeton University Press, 2004).
2. M. Udland, "On this day in 1996, Alan Greenspan made his famous speech about 'Irrational Exuberance,'" *Business Insider*, December 5, 2014, http://www.businessinsider.com/alan-greenspan-irrational-exuberance-2014-12.
3. Meredith Gillies, "Stars who save: what we can learn from these modest celebrities," Huffington Post, https://www.huffingtonpost.ca/2012/07/23/celebs-who-save_n_1690249.html, July 23, 2012; "Oprah talks to Michelle Obama," *O! The Oprah Magazine*, http://www.oprah.com/omagazine/michelle-obamas-oprah-interview-o-magazine-cover-with-obama/all, April 2009.
4. *Rolling Stone India*, "Triumph & tragedy: the life of Michael Jackson," August 25, 2009, http://rollingstoneindia.com/triumph-tragedy-the-life-of-michael-jackson/, accessed March 6, 2016.
5. N. Metha, "Mind-body dualism: a critique from a health perspective," *Mens Sana Monographs* 9 (2011): 202–209.
6. L. Mudrik and U. Maoz, "Me and my brain: exposing neuroscience's closet dualism," *Journal of Cognitive Neuroscience* 27 (2014): 211–221.

Chapter One. The Brain's Contingency Calculator

1. *Online English Oxford Living Dictionary*, s.v. "contingency (*n*)," https://en.oxforddictionaries.com/definition/contingency, accessed September 27, 2017.
2. J. Sangalang, "Viera teen lands deal on "Shark Tank,"" *Florida Today*, February 19, 2016.
3. The White House Office of the Press Secretary, "June 2000 White House

Event—National Human Genome Research Institute (NHGRI)," June 26, 2000, https://www.genome.gov/10001356.

4. Hippocrates, *On the Sacred Disease,* in *Great Books of the Western World,* vol. 10: *Hippocrates and Galen* (Chicago: Benton, 1952), 69.

5. D. Ribatti, "William Harvey and the discovery of the circulation of the blood," *Journal of Angiogenesis Research* (2009), available at https:doi.org/10.1186/2040-2384-1-3.

6. S. M. Schneider and E. K. Morris, "A history of the term radical behaviorism: from Watson to Skinner," *Behavior Analyst* 10 (1987): 27–39; A. C. Catania, "B.F. Skinner, organism," *American Psychologist* 47 (1992): 1521–1530.

7. T. Insel, "Toward a New Understanding of Mental Illness," filmed January 2013 at TEDxCaltech, https://www.ted.com/talks/thomas_insel_toward_a_new_understanding_of_mental_illness?language=en; T. R. Insel and E. M. Scolnick, "Cure therapeutics and strategic prevention: raising the bar for mental health research," *Molecular Psychiatry* 11 (2006): 11–17.

8. World Health Organization, "Depression," http://www.who.int/mediacentre/factsheets/fs369/en/, accessed October 2015.

9. M. J. Hawrylycz et al., "An anatomically comprehensive atlas of the adult human brain transcriptome," *Nature* 489 (2012), https:doi.org/10.1038/nature11405; M. E. Raichle and D. A. Gusnard, "Appraising the brain's energy budget," *Proceedings of the National Academy of Sciences* 99 (2002): 10237–10239.

10. K. G. Lambert, "Rising rates of depression in today's society: consideration for the roles of effort-based rewards and enhanced resilience in day to day functioning," *Neuroscience and Biobehavioral Reviews* 30 (2006): 497–510; K. G. Lambert et al., "Contingency-based emotional resilience: effort-based reward training and flexible coping lead to adaptive responses to uncertainty in male rats," *Frontiers in Behavioral Neuroscience* (2014): https:doi.org/10.3389/fnbeh.2014.00124.

11. J. E. Lunshof et al., "Personal genomes in progress: from the human genome project to the personal genome project," *Dialogues in Clinical Neuroscience* 12 (2010): 47–60.

12. D. S. Reisman, H. McLean, J. Keller, K. A. Danks, and A. J. Bastian, "Repeated split-belt treadmill training improves poststroke step length asymmetry," *Neurorehabilitation and Neural Repair* 27 (2013): 460–468; Amy Bastian, personal communication via email, December 8, 2014; Amy Bastian, "Learning and Relearning Movement," (Society for Neuroscience Meeting, November 18, 2014).

13. S. Nasar, *A Beautiful Mind* (New York: Simon and Schuster, 1998).

14. K. Sterelny, *The Evolved Apprentice: How Evolution Made Humans Unique* (Boston, MA: MIT Press, 2012).

15. M. Koerth-Baker, "Boredom gets interesting," *Nature* 529 (2016): 146–148.

Chapter Two. The Brain's Output

1. P. Glimcher, *Decisions, Uncertainty and the Brain* (Cambridge, MA: MIT Press, 2004).

2. I. P. Pavlov, "The reply of a physiologist to psychologists," *Psychological Review* 39 (1932): 91–127.

3. W. James, *Principles of Psychology* (New York: Henry Holt and Company, 1890).

4. D. Hothersall, *History of Psychology* (3rd ed.) (New York: McGraw-Hill, 1995).

5. J. B. Watson, "Psychology as the behaviorist views it," *Psychological Review* (reprinted 1994):101, 248–277.

6. R. J. Herrnstein, "On the law of effect," *Journal of the Experimental Analysis of Behavior* 13 (1970): 243–266.

7. S. M. Schneider and E. K. Morris, "A history of the term Radical Behaviorism: from Watson to Skinner," *Behavior Analyst* 10 (1987): 27–39.

8. W. Timberlake, "Is the operant contingency enough for a science of purposive behavior?," *Behavior and Philosophy* 32 (2003): 197–229.

9. B. F. Skinner, "How to teach animals," *Scientific American* 185 (1951): 26–29; B. F. Skinner, "A case history in scientific method," *American Psychologist* 11 (1955): 221–233.

10. F. A. Beach, *Karl Spencer Lashley* (Washington, DC: National Academy of Sciences, 1961).

11. J. Garcia, D. J. Kimeldorf, and R. A. Koelling, "Conditioned aversion to saccharin resulting from exposure to gamma radiation," *Science* 122 (1955): 157–158.

12. K. Breland and B. Breland, "The misbehavior of organisms," *American Psychologist* 16 (1961): 681–684.

13. D. Hothersall, *History of Psychology* (3rd ed.) (New York: McGraw-Hill, 1995).

14. I. P. Pavlov, "Conditioned reflexes: An investigation of the physiological activity of the cerebral cortex," *Annals of Neuroscience* 17 (1927, republished 2010): https:doi.org/10.5214/ans.0972-7531.1017309.

15. F. C. P. Van der Horst and R. van der Veer, "Loneliness in infancy: Harry Harlow, John Bowlby and issues of separation," *Integrative Psychological and Behavior Science* 42 (2008): 325–335.

16. W. M. Baum, *Understanding Behaviorism: Behavior, Culture and Evolution* (Malden, MA: Blackwell Publications, 2005).

17. D. Kahneman, *Thinking, Fast and Slow* (New York: Farrar, Straus, and Giroux, 2011).

18. S. Finger, *Minds Behind the Brain* (New York: Oxford University Press, 2000).

19. Glimcher, *Decisions, Uncertainty and the Brain*.

20. Ibid.

21. S. M. McClure, J. Li, D. Tomlin, et al., "Neural correlates of behavioral preference for culturally familiar drinks," *Neuron* 44 (2004): 379–387.

22. A. M. Graybiel and K. S. Smith, "Good habits, bad habits," *Scientific American* 310 (2014): 38–43.

23. L. D. Loukopoulos and R. K. Dismukes, *The Multitasking Myth* (New York: Ashgate Publishing, 2009).

24. J. Saarikko, "Foraging behaviour of shrews," *Annales Zoologici Fennici* 26 (1989): 411–423.

25. C. J. Barnard and C. A. J. Brown, "Risk-sensitive foraging in common shrews," *Behavioral Ecology & Sociobiology* 16 (1985): 161–164.

26. Pavlov, "Conditioned reflexes," 291.

27. A. Troisi, "Displacement activities as a behavioral measure of stress in nonhuman primates and human subjected," *Stress* 5 (2002): 47–54.

28. Baum, *Understanding Behaviorism*.

Chapter Three. The Human Brain

1. R. T. Knight and H. J. Heinze, "The human brain: the final journey," *Frontiers in Neuroscience* 2 (2008): 1:15–16, https:doi.org/10.3389/neuro 01.020.2008.

2. P. Mazzarello, *Golgi: A Biography of the Founder of Modern Neuroscience* (New York: Oxford University Press, 2010).

3. J. B. Tuke, *The Insanity of Over-Exertion of the Brain* (Edinburgh: Oliver and Boyd, 1894).

4. S. Finger, *Minds Behind the Brain: A History of the Pioneers and Their Discoveries* (New York: Oxford University Press, 2000).

5. A. L. Alexander, J. E. Lee, M. Lazar, and A. S. Field, "Diffusion tensor imaging of the brain," *Neurotherapeutics* 4 (2007): 316–329; C. Zimmer, "Secrets of the Brain," *National Geographic* (February 2014): 28–57.

6. Zimmer, "Secrets of the Brain," 28–57.

7. B. Burrell, *Postcards from the Brain Museum* (New York: Broadway Books, 2004).

8. Finger, *Minds Behind the Brain*; M. Piccolino, "Luigi Galvani and animal electricity: two centuries after the foundation of electrophysiology," *Trends in Neuroscience* 20 (1997): 443–447.

9. Finger, *Minds Behind the Brain*.

10. M. Shelley, *Frankenstein* (London: Henry Colburn and Richard Bentley, 1831), 57.

11. E. S. Valenstein, *The War of the Soups and the Sparks* (New York: Columbia University Press, 2005).

12. M. C. Fishman, "Sir Henry Hallett Dale and the acetylcholine story," *Yale Journal of Biology and Medicine* 45 (1972): 104–118.

13. E. M. Tansey, "Henry Dale and the discovery of acetylcholine," *C.R. Biologies* 329 (2006): 419–425.

14. S. Ochs, *A History of Nerve Functions: From Animal Spirits to Molecular Mechanisms* (New York: Cambridge University Press, 2004).

15. E. Gould and C. G. Gross, "Neurogenesis in adult mammals: some progress and problems," *Journal of Neuroscience* 22 (2002): 619–623.

16. S. Sorrells et al., "Human hippocampal neurogenesis drops sharply in children to undetectable levels in adults," *Nature* (2018): doi: 10.1038/nature25975.

17. G. Kempermann, H. G. Kuhn, and F. H. Gage, "More hippocampal neurons in adult mice living in an enriched environment," *Nature* 386 (1997): 493–495.

18. G. Kempermann, "New neurons for 'survival of the fittest,'" *Nature Reviews Neuroscience* 13 (2012): 727–736.

19. Kempermann, "New neurons for 'survival of the fittest,'" 729.

20. C. C. Sherwood, A. L. Bauernfeind, S. Bianchi, M. A. Raghanti, and P. R. Hof, "Human brain evolution writ large and small," *Progress in Brain Research* 195 (2012): 237–254.

21. S. Herculano-Houzel, "The remarkable, yet not extraordinary, human brain as a scaled-up primate brain and its associated cost," *Proceedings of the National Academy of Sciences* 109 (2012): 10661–10668.

22. O. Cairo, "External measures of cognition," *Frontiers in Human Neuroscience* 5 (2011): https:doi.org/10.3389/fnhum.2011.00108.

23. B. Anderson and T. Harvey, "Alterations in cortical thickness and neural density in the frontal cortex of Albert Einstein," *Neuroscience Letters* 210 (1996): 161–164.

24. R. O. Deaner, K. Isler, J. Burkart, and C. Schaik, "Overall brain size, and not encephalization quotient, best predicts cognitive ability across nonhuman primates," *Brain, Behavior and Evolution* 70 (2007): 115–124.

25. C. C. Hilgetag and H. Barbas, "Are there ten times more glia than neurons in the brain?," *Brain Structure and Function* 213 (2009): 365–366.

26. S. Herculano-Houzel, "The human brain in numbers: a linearly scaled-up primate brain," *Frontiers in Human Neuroscience* (2009): https:doi.org/10.3389/neuro.09.031.2009.

27. S. Herculano-Houzel, "Brains matter, bodies maybe not: the case for examining neuron numbers irrespective of body size," *Annals of the New York Academy of Sciences* 1225 (2009): 191–199.

28. R. Wrangham, *Catching Fire: How Cooking Made Us Human* (New York: Basic Books, 2009).

29. D. Jardin-Messedu, K. Lambert, et al., "Dogs have the most neurons, though not the largest brain: trade-off between body mass and number of neurons in the cerebral cortex of large carnivoran species," *Frontiers in Neuroanatomy* (December 12, 2017), http://doi.org/10.3389/fnana.2017.00118.

30. Herculano-Houzel, "The human brain in numbers."

31. Herculano-Houzel, "Brains matter, bodies maybe not," 191–199.

32. P. F. M. Ribeiro, L. Ventura-Antunes, M. Gabi, et al., "The human cerebral cortex is neither one nor many: Neuronal distribution reveals two quantitatively different zones in the gray matter, three in the white matter, and explains local variations in cortical folding," *Frontiers in Neuroanatomy* (2013): https:doi.org/10.3389/fnane.2013.0028.

33. A. L. Bauernfeind, A. A. de Sousa, T. Avasthi, et al., "A volumetric comparison of the insular cortex and its subregions in primates," *Journal of Human Evolution* 64 (2013): 263–279.

34. M. Pietrasanta, L. Restani, and M. Caleo, "The corpus callosum and the visual cortex: plasticity is a game for two," *Neural Plasticity* (2012): https:doi.org/10.1155/2012/838672.

35. J. Hanggi, L. Fovenyi, F. Liem, M. Meyer, and L. Jancke, "The hypothesis of neuronal interconnectivity as a function of brain size—a general organization principle of the human connectome," *Frontiers in Human Neuroscience* (2014): https:doi.org/10.3389/fnhum.2014.00915.

36. B. K. Branstetter, J. J. Finnergan, E. A. Fletcher, B. C. Weisman, and S. H. Ridgway, "Dolphins can maintain vigilant behavior through echolocation for 15 days without interruption or cognitive impairment," *PLoS ONE* (2012): https:doi.org/10.1371/journal.pone.004748.

37. L. Shlain, *Leonardo's Brain* (Guilford, Connecticut: Lyon's Press, 2014).

38. J. M. Allman, N. A. Tetreault, A. Y. Hakeem, et al., "The von Economo neurons in fronto-insular and anterior cingulate cortex," *Annals of the New York Academy of Sciences* 1225 (2011): 59–71.

39. M. Santos, N. Uppal, C. Butti, et al., "Von Economo neurons in autism: a stereologic study of the frontoinsular cortex in children," *Brain Research* 1380 (2011): 206–217; C. Butti, M. Santos, N. Uppal, and P.R. Hof, "Von Economo neurons: clinical and evolutionary perspectives," *Cortex* 49 (2013): 312–326.

40. G. Roth and U. Dicke, "Evolution of the brain and intelligence," *Trends in Cognitive Science* 9 (2005): 250–257.

Chapter Four. Building the Brain's Contingency Circuit

1. S. Johnson, *Who Moved My Cheese?* (New York: Putman, 1998).

2. P. W. Glimcher, "Decisions, decisions, decisions: choosing a biological theory of choice," *Neuron* 36 (2002): 323–332; I. Levy, S. C. Lazzaro, R. B. Rutledge, and P. W. Glimcher, "Choice from non-choice: predicting consumer preferences from blood oxygenation level-dependent signals obtained during passive viewing," *Journal of Neuroscience* 31 (2011): 118–125.

3. P. W. Glimcher, *Decisions, Uncertainty, and the Brain* (Cambridge, MA: MIT Press, 2004).

4. A. G. Sanfey, G. Loewenstein, S. M. McClure, and J. D. Cohen, "Neuroeconomics: cross-currents in research on decision-making," *TRENDS in*

Cognitive Sciences 10 (2006): 108–116; P. W. Glimcher, M. C. Dorris, and H. M. Bayer, "Physiological utility theory and the neuroeconomics of choice," *Games and Economic Behavior* 52 (2005): 213–256.

5. Levy, Lazzaro, Rutledge, and Glimcher, "Choice from non-choice," 118–125.

6. L. A. Gutnik, A. F. Hakimzada, N. A. Yoskowitz, and V. L. Patel, "The role of emotion in decision-making: a cognitive neuroeconomic approach towards understanding sexual risk behavior," *Journal of Biomedical Informatics* 39 (2006): 720–736.

7. M. A. Hege, H. Preissl, and T. S. Krunoslav, "Magnetoencephalographic signatures of right prefrontal cortex involvement in response inhibition," *Human Brain Mapping* 35 (2014): 5236–5248; H. Kadota, H. Sekiguchi, S. Takeuchi, M. Miyazaki, Y. Kohno, and Y. Nakajima, "The role of the dorsolateral prefrontal cortex in the inhibition of stereotyped responses," *Experimental Brain Research* 203 (2010): 595–600.

8. A. Tversky and D. Kahneman, "Judgment under uncertainty: heuristics and biases," *Science* 185 (1974): 1124–1131.

9. R. H. Thayer, *Misbehaving* (New York: W.W. Norton and Company, Inc., 2015).

10. P. W. Glimcher, M. C. Dorris, and H. M. Bayer, "Physiological utility theory and the neuroeconomics of choice," *Games and Economic Behavior* 52 (2005): 213–256.

11. D. Hothersall, *History of Psychology* (Boston: McGraw Hill, 1995).

12. D. Engber, "The end of the maze," *Slate*, 2011, http://www.slate.com/articles/health_and_science/the_mouse_trap/2011/11/rat_mazes_and_mouse_mazes_a_history_.html.

13. I. Lee, M. R. Hunsaker, and R. P. Kesner, "The role of hippocampal subregions in detecting spatial novelty," *Behavioral Neuroscience* 119 (2005): 145–153.

14. K. G. Lambert, "Rising rates of depression in today's society: consideration for the roles of effort-based rewards and enhanced resilience in day to day functioning," *Neuroscience and Biobehavioral Reviews* 30 (2006): 497–510.

15. K. G. Lambert, M. M. Hyer, A. Rzucidlo, T. Bergeron, T. Landis, and B. Bardi, "Contingency-based emotional resilience: effort-based reward training and flexible coping lead to adaptive responses to uncertainty in male rats," *Frontiers in Behavioral Neuroscience* (2014). https:doi.org/10.3389/fnbeh.2014.00124.

16. K. Sterelny, *The Evolved Apprentice: How Evolution Made Humans Unique* (Cambridge, MA: MIT Press), 2012.

17. M. Rivalan, E. Coutureau, A. Fitoussi, and F. Dellu-Hagedorn, "Inter-individual decision-making differences in the effects of cingulate, orbitofrontal, and prelimbic cortex lesions in a rat gambling task," *Frontiers in Behavioral Neuroscience* 5 (2011): https:doi.org/10.3389/fnbeh.2011.00022;

M. Rivalan, V. Valton, P. Series, A. R. Marchand, and F. Dellu-Hagedorn, "Elucidating poor decision-making in a rat gambling task," *PLoS ONE* 8 (2013): e82052.

18. O. H. Turnbull, C. H. Bowman, S. Shanker, and J. L. Davies, "Emotion-based learning: insights from the Iowa gambling task," *Frontiers in Psychology* (2014): https:doi.org/10.3389/fpsyg.2014.00162.

19. C. R. Riener, J. K. Stefanucci, D. R. Proffitt, and G. Clore, "An effect of mood on the perception of geographical slant," *Cognitive Emotion* 25 (2011): 174–182.

20. K. Lambert, *The Lab Rat Chronicles: A Neuroscientist Reveals Life Lessons from the Planet's Most Successful Mammals* (New York: Perigee, 2011).

21. Rivalan, Coutureau, Fitoussi, and Dellu-Hagedorn, "Inter-individual decision-making differences in the effects of cingulate, orbitofrontal, and prelimbic cortex lesions in a rat gambling task."

22. G. Schoenbaum, M. R. Roesch, T. A. Stalnaker, and Y. K. Takahashi, "A new perspective on the role of the orbitofrontal cortex in adaptive behaviour," *Nature Reviews Neuroscience* 10 (2009): 885–892.

23. D. Tischer and O. D. Weiner, "Illuminating cell signaling with optogenetic tools," *Nature Reviews Molecular Cell Biology* 15 (2014): 551–558; K. Deisseroth, "Optogenetics: controlling the brain with light," *Scientific American* (2010): http://www.scientific American.com/article/optogenetics -controlling.

24. A. Adamantidis, M. C. Carter, and L. de Lecea, "Optogenetic deconstruction of sleep-wake circuitry in the brain," *Frontiers in Molecular Neuroscience* 20 (2010): https://doi.org/10.3389/neuro.02.031.2009.

25. G. D. Stuber, D. R. Sparta, A. M. Stamatakis, W. van Leeuwen, J. E. Harjoprajitno, S. Cho, K. M. Tye, K. A. Kempadoo, F. Zhang, K. Deisseroth, and A. Bonci, "Amygdala to nucleus accumbens excitatory transmission facilitates reward seeking," *Nature* 475 (2011): 377–380; J. H. Jennings, D. R. Sparta, A. M. Stamatakis, R. L. Ung, K. E. Pleil, T. L. Kash, and G. D. Stuber, "Distinct extended amygdala circuits for divergent motivational states," *Nature* 496 (2013): 224–228.

26. S. G. Hofmann, A. Asnaani, I. J. J. Vonk, A. T. Sawyer, and M. A. Fang, "The efficacy of cognitive behavioral therapy: a review of meta-analyses," *Cognitive Therapy Research* 36 (2012): 427–440.

27. P. Baker, "Rewinding history, Bush museum lets you decide," *New York Times,* http://www.nytimes.com/2013/04/21/us/politics/hitting-rewind -bush-museum-says-you-decide.html?_r=0, accessed March 16, 2016.

Chapter Five. When Life Distorts the Contingency Filters

1. K. Lambert, "Santa on the brain," *New York Times,* December 12, 2013, http://www.nytimes.com/2013/12/22/opinion/sunday/santa-on-the-brain .html.

2. "Triumph & tragedy: The life of Michael Jackson," *Rolling Stone India*, August 25, 2009, http://rollingstoneindia.com/triumph-tragedy-the-life -of-michael-jackson/, accessed March 6, 2016.

3. "The drugs found in Michael Jackson's body after he died," *BBC Newsbeat*, November 8, 2011, http://www.bbc.co.uk/newsbeat/article/15634083 /the-drugs-found-in-michael-jacksons-body-after-he-died.

4. K. G. Noble, S. M. Houston, N. H. Brito, et al., "Family income, parental education and brain structure in children and adolescents," *Nature Neuroscience* 18 (2015): 773–778.

5. H. G. Schnack, N. E. van Haren, R. M. Brouwer, et al., "Changes in thickness and surface area of the human cortex and their relationship with intelligence," *Cerebral Cortex* 25 (2015): 1608–1617.

6. Noble, Houston, Brito, et al., "Family income, parental education and brain structure in children and adolescents," 773–778.

7. N. L. Hair, J. L. Hanson, B. L. Wolfe, and S. D. Pollack, "Association of child poverty, brain development, and academic achievement," *JAMA Pediatrics* 169 (2015): 822–829.

8. Noble, Houston, Brito, et al., "Family income, parental education and brain structure in children and adolescents," 773–778.

9. M. A. Fox, B. A. Connolly, and T. D. Snyder, "Youth indicators 2005: trends in the well-being of American youth," Washington, DC: U.S. Department of Education, National Center for Education Statistics (2005), Table 21, http://nces.ed.gov/pubs2005/2005050.pdf, accessed Jan. 4, 2016.

10. K. Oldfield, "Humble and hopeful: welcoming first-generation poor and working-class students to college," *About Campus* 11 (2007): 2–12.

11. J. H. O'Neill, *The Golden Ghetto: The Psychology of Affluence* (Milwaukee, WI: The Affluenza Project, 1997).

12. R. S. Rosenberg, "There's no defense for affluenza," *Slate* (2013), http:// www.slate.com/articles/health_and_science/medical_examiner/2013/12 /ethan_couch_affluenza_defense_critique_of_the_psychology_of_no_con sequences.html.

13. B. S. Frey, "Giving and receiving awards," *Perspectives on Psychological Science* 1 (2006): 377–388.

14. "The Nobel Prize Amounts," The Nobel Foundation, accessed March 3, 2018, http://www.nobelprize.org/nobel_prizes/about/amounts/.

15. G. J. Borjas and K. B. Doran, "Prizes and productivity: how winning the Fields medal affects scientific output," *Journal of Human Resources* 50 (2013): 728–758.

16. H. F. Chan, L. Gleeson, and B. Torgler, "Awards before and after the Nobel prize: a Matthew effect and/or a ticket to one's own funeral?," *Research Evaluation* (2014): 1–11, https:doi.org/10.1093/reseval/rvu011.

17. D. Kapogiannis, A. K. Barbey, M. Su, G. Zamboni, F. Krueger, and J. Grafman, "Cognitive and neural foundations of religious belief," *Pro-*

ceedings of the National Academy of Sciences 106 (2009): 4876–4881; D. Kapogiannis, G. Deshpande, F. Krueger, M. P. Thornburg, and J. H. Grafman, "Brain networks shaping religious belief," *Brain Connectivity* 4 (2014): 70–79.

18. S. Harris, J. T. Kaplan, A. Curiel, S. Y. Bookheimer, M. Iacoboni, and M. S. Cohen, "The neural correlates of religious and nonreligious belief," *PLoS ONE* 4 (2009): https:doi.org/10.1371/journal.pone.0007272.t001.

19. L. R. Caporael, "Ergotism: The Satan loosed in Salem?," *Science* 192 (1976): 21–26.

20. John Hale, *A modest enquiry into the nature of witchcraft, and how persons guilty of that crime may be convicted: and the means used for their discovery discussed, both negatively and affirmatively, according to Scripture and experience* (Ann Arbor, MI: Text Creation Partnership, 2008–2009), http://name .umdl.umich.edu/N00872.0001.001.

21. R. C. O'Connor and M. K. Nock, "The psychology of suicidal behavior," *Lancet* 1 (2014): 73–88; S. Dracheva, N. Patel, D. A. Woo, S. M. Marcus, L. J. Siever, and V. Haroutunian, "Increased serotonin 2C receptor mRNA editing: a possible risk factor for suicide," *Molecular Psychiatry* 13 (2008): 1001–1010.

22. J. M. Bertolote and A. Fleischmann, "Suicide and psychiatric diagnosis: a worldwide perspective," *World Psychiatry* 1 (2002): 181–185.

23. "Mortality among teenagers aged 12–19 years: United States, 1999–2006," National Center for Health and Human Services (NCHS), NCHS Data Brief, no. 37, May 2010, http://chronicle.com/article/After -6-Suicides-U-of/228095/; J. C. Turner and A. Keller, "American Public Health Association (APHA), leading causes of mortality among American college students at 4-year institutions," Paper 241696, 2011: https:// apha.confex.com/apha/139am/webpogram/Paper241696.html.

24. M. K. Nock, M. B. Stein, S. G. Heeringa, et al., "Prevalence and correlates of suicidal behavior among new soldiers in the US army: results from the army study to assess risk and research in service members (army STARRs)," *JAMA Psychiatry* 71 (2014): 514–522.

25. R. Jacobsen, "Robin Williams: depression alone rarely causes suicide," *Scientific American* (2014): http://www.scientificamerican.com/article /robin-williams-depression-alone-rarely-causes-suicide/; D. Itzkoff and B. Carey, "Robin Williams's widow points to dementia as a suicide cause," *New York Times*, November 3, 2015, http://www.nytimes.com/2015/11/04 /health/robin-williams-lewy-body-dementia.html, accessed January 11, 2016.

26. N. W. Egan, "Perfect student, shocking suicide," *People* (February 2, 2015): 74–78.

27. C. Fabris, "After six suicides, University of Pennsylvania takes a tough look at its campus culture," *Chronicle of Higher Education* (March 3, 2015): http://chronicle.com/article/After-6-Suicides-U-of/228095/.

28. V. Aragno, M. D. Underwood, M. Boldrini, et al., "Serotonin1A receptors, serotonin transporter binding and serotonin transporter mRNA expression in the brainstem of depressed suicide victims," *Neuropsychopharmacology* 25 (2001): 892–903.

29. C. Van Heeringen and A. Marusic, "Understanding the suicidal brain," *British Journal of Psychiatry* 183 (2003): 282–284; C. Van Heeringen, K. Van Laere, et al., "Prefrontal 5-HT2a receptor binding potential, hopelessness and personality characteristics in attempted suicide patients," *Journal of Affective Disorders* 74 (2003): 149–158.

30. M. O. Poulter, L. Du, V. Zhurov, M. Paldovits, G. Faludi, Z. Merali, and H. Anisman, "Altered organization of GABA$_A$ receptor mRNA expression in the depressed suicide brain," *Frontiers in Molecular Neuroscience* (2010): https:doi.org/10.3389/neuro.02.003.2010.

31. S. Erhardt, C. K. Lim, K. R. Linderholm, et al., "Connecting inflammation with glutamate agonism in suicidality," *Neuropsychopharmacology* 38 (2013): 743–752; C. Bay-Richter, K. R. Linderholm, C. K. Lim, et al., "A role for inflammatory metabolites as modulators of the glutamate N-methyl-D-asparate receptor in depression and suicidality," *Brain, Behavior and Immunity* 43 (2015): 110–117.

32. M. Nock, J. M. Park, C. T. Finn, T. L. Deliberto, H. J. Pour, and M. R. Bangji, "Measuring the suicidal mind and implicit cognition predicts suicidal behavior," *Psychological Science* 21 (2010): 511–517.

33. O'Connor and Nock, "The psychology of suicidal behavior," 73–88.

34. L. B. Alloy, L. Y. Abramson, W. G. Whitehouse, M. E. Hogan, N. A. Tashman, D. L. Steinberg, D. T. Rose, and P. Donovan, "Depressogenic cognitive styles: predictive validity information processing and personality characteristics, and developmental origins," *Behaviour Research and Therapy* 37 (1999): 503–531.

35. Egan, "Perfect student, shocking suicide," 74–78.

36. R. Rygula, J. Golebiowska, J. Kregiel, J. Kubik, and P. Popik, "Effects of optimism on motivation in rats," *Frontiers in Behavioral Neuroscience* 9 (2015): https:doi.org/10.3389/fnbeh.2015.00032.

37. H. Shefrin, "How psychological pitfalls generated the global financial crisis," in *Voices of Wisdom: Understanding the Global Financial Crisis*, ed. L. B. Siegel, SCU Leavey School of Business Research Paper, No. 10-04, 2010: http://www.istfin.eco.usi.ch/h_oid_Shefrin09.pdf.

38. M. Lewis, *The Big Short: Inside the Doomsday Machine* (New York: W.W. Norton and Company, 2010).

39. T. Sharot, C. W. Korn, and R. Dolan, "How unrealistic optimism is maintained in the face of reality," *Nature Neuroscience* 14 (2011): 1475; K. Izuma and R. Adolphs, "The brain's rose-colored glasses," *Nature Neuroscience* 14 (2011): 1355–1356.

40. Sharot, Korn, and Dolan, "How unrealistic optimism is maintained in the face of reality," 1475.

41. R. Rygula, H. Pluta, and P. Popik, "Laughing rats are optimistic," *PLoS ONE* 7 (2012): https:doi.org/10.1371/journal.pone.0051959.

Chapter Six. Fine-Tuning the Contingency Calculators

1. J. S. Beer and B. L. Hughes, "Neural systems of social comparison and the "above-average" effect," *Neuroimage* 267 (2010): 2671–2679; J. Beer, "Exaggerated positivity in self-evaluation: a social neuroscience approach to reconciling the role of self-esteem protection and cognitive bias," *Social and Personality Psychology Compass* 8 (2014): 583–594.

2. Beer and Hughes, "Neural systems of social comparison and the "above-average" effect," 2671–2679.

3. Mike Lacey, personal communication, January 2016.

4. J. Leno, *Leading with My Chin* (New York: Harper Collins, 1996).

5. J. Aleccia, "Surgery error leads doc to public mea culpa," NBCNEWS.com, 2010, http://www.nbcnews.com/id/40096673/ns/health-health_care/t/surgery-error-leads-doc-public-mea-culpa/#.VtxFhooUWUk.

6. D. C. Ring, J. H. Herndon, and G. S. Meyer, "Case 34-2010: a 65-year-old woman with an incorrect operation on the left hand," *New England Journal of Medicine* 363 (2010): 1950–1955.

7. J. Downar, M. Bhatt, and P. R. Montague, "Neural correlates of effective learning in experienced medical decision-makers," *PLoS ONE* 6 (2011): 222768.

8. B. Chappell, "Groundhog Day: Punxsutawney Phil did not see his shadow," National Public Radio, February 2, 2016, http://www.npr.org/sections/thetwo-way/2016/02/02/465253970/groundhog-day-punxsutawney-phil-did-not-see-his-shadow; D. Yoder, *Groundhog Day* (Mechanicsburg, PA: Stackpole Books, 2003).

9. J. D. Salamone and M. Correa, "The mysterious motivational functions of mesolimbic dopamine," *Neuron* 76 (2012): 470–485.

10. J. D. Watson and F. H. C. Crick, "A structure for deoxyribose nucleic acid," *Nature* 171 (1953): 737–738.

11. C. B. Merrill, L. N. Friend, S. T. Newton, Z. H. Hopkins, and J. G. Edwards, "Ventral tegmental area dopamine and GABA neurons: physiological properties and expression of mRNA for endocannabinoid biosynthetic elements," *Scientific Reports* 5 (2015): 16176, https:doi.org/10.1038/srep16176.

12. T. E. Robinson and K. C. Berridge, "Beyond Wise et al.—Neuroleptic-induced 'anhedonia' in rats: pimozide blocks reward quality of food," in *Brain and Behaviour: Revisiting the Classic Studies*, ed. B. Kolb and I. Whishaw (Washington, DC: Sage, 2017).

13. Salamone and Correa, "The mysterious motivational functions of mesolimbic dopamine," 470–485.

14. C. De Young, "The neuromodulator of exploration: a unifying theory of

dopamine inpPersonality," *Frontiers in Human Neuroscience* (2013): https: doi.org/10.3389/fnhum.2013.00762.peters.

15.   E. Peters, "Baby steps: helping babies with neuromuscular disorders crawl and explore the world," *VCU News* (2015): https://news.vcu.edu /article/Baby_steps_Helping_babies_with_neuromuscular_disorders _crawl.

16.   K. Russel, "Helping hand: robots, video games, and a radical new approach to treating stroke patients," *New York Times,* November 23, 2015.

17.   K. C. Tweedy and L. Ladin, *Secretariat's Meadow* (Manakin-Sabot, VA: Dementi Milestone Publishing, Inc., 2010).

18.   Penny Chenery, personal communication, February 6, 2016; Tweedy and Ladin, *Secretariat's Meadow.*

19.   M. vos Savant, "Ask Marilyn," *Parade Magazine,* September 9, 1990, 16.

20.   G. Klein, *Streetlights and Shadows* (Cambridge, MA: MIT Press, 2009).

21.   A. Sternbergh, "The spreadsheet psychic," *New York Magazine,* 2008: http://nymag.com/news/features/51170/.

22.   M. Lewis, *Moneyball: The Art of Winning an Unfair Game* (New York: W.W. Norton and Co., 2004).

23.   R. L. Gibb, C. L. R. Gonzalez, and B. Kolb, "Prenatal enrichment and recovery from perinatal cortical damage: effects of maternal complex housing," *Frontiers in Behavioral Neuroscience* (2014): https:doi.org/10 .3389/fnbeh.2014.00223.

24.   M. H. Rosenzweig, E. I. Bennett, and M. C. Diamond, "Brain changes in response to experience," *Scientific American* 226 (1972): 22–29.

25.   K. Lambert, R. J. Nelson, T. Jovanovic, and M. Cerda, "Brains in the city: neurobiological effects of urbanization," *Neuroscience and Biobehavioral Reviews* 58 (2015): 107–122; K. Lambert, M. Hyer, M. Bardi, A. Rzucidlo, S. Scott, B. Terhune-Cotter, A. Hazelgrove, I. Silva, and C. Kinsley, "Natural-enriched environments lead to enhanced environmental engagement and altered neurobiological resilience," *Neuroscience* 330 (2016): 386–394.

26.   M. Bardi, C. Kaufman, C. Franssen, M. M. Hyer, A. Rzucidlo, M. Brown, M. Tschirhart, and K. G. Lambert, "Paper or plastic? exploring the effects of natural enrichment on behavioral and neuroendocrine responses in Long-Evans rats," *Journal of Neuroendocrinology* (2016): https:doi.org /10.1111/jne.12383.

27.   R. A. Atchley, D. L. Strayer, and P. Atchley, "Creativity in the wild: improving creative reasoning through immersion in natural settings," *PLoS ONE* 7 (2012): e51474.

28.   N. A. Geverink, M. J. W. Heetkamp, W. G. P. Schouten, V. W. Wiegant, and J. W. Schrams, "Backtest type and housing condition of pigs influence energy metabolism," *Journal of Animal Science* 82 (2004): 1227–1233.

29.   K. G. Lambert, M. M. Hyer, A. Rzucidlo, T. Bergeron, T. Landis, and B. Bardi, "Contingency-based emotional resilience: effort-based reward

training and flexible coping lead to adaptive responses to uncertainty in male rats," *Frontiers in Behavioral Neuroscience* (2014): https:doi.org/10 .3389/fnbeh.2014.00124.

Chapter Seven. Parenting

1. Q. J. Meng, Y. G. Ji, D. Zhang, D. Liu, D. M. Grossnickley, and Z. X. Lou, "An aroboreal docodont from the Jurassic and mammaliaform ecological diversification," *Science* 347 (2015): 764; Z. X. Luo, Q. J. Meng, Q. Ji, D. Liu, Y. G. Zhang, and A. I. Neander, "Evolutionary development in basal mammaliaforms as revealed by a docodontan," *Science* 347 (2015): 760.

2. M. Numan, "Medial preoptic area and maternal behavior in the female rat," *Journal of Comparative and Physiological Psychology* 87 (1974): 746–759.

3. M. Numan and T. R. Insel, *The Neurobiology of Parental Behavior* (New York: Springer, 2003).

4. C. F. Ferris, P. Kulkarni, J. M. Sullivan, J. A. Harder, T. L. Messenger, and M. Febo, "Pup suckling is more rewarding than cocaine: evidence from functional magnetic resonance imaging and three-dimensional computational analysis," *Journal of Neuroscience* 25 (2005): 149–156.

5. C. H. Kinsley, L. Madonia, G. Gifford, K. Tureski, G. Griffin, C. Lowry, J. Williams, J. Collins, H. McLearie, and K. G. Lambert, "Motherhood improves learning and memory," *Nature* 402 (1999): 137–138.

6. C. H. Kinsley, J. C. Blair, N. E. Karp, et al., "The mother as hunter: significant reduction in foraging costs through enhancements of predation in maternal rats," *Hormones and Behavior* 66 (2014): 649–654.

7. Kinsley, Blair, Karp, et al., "The mother as hunter," 649–654.

8. K. Lambert, *The Lab Rat Chronicles* (New York: Perigee, 2011).

9. K. M. Seip, M. Pereira, M. P. Wansaw, J. I. Reiss, E. I. Dziopa, and J. I. Morrell, "Incentive salience of cocaine across the postpartum period of the female rat," *Psychopharmacology* 199 (2008): 119–130.

10. C. L. Franssen, M. Bardi, E. A. Shea, J. E. Hampton, R. A. Franssen, C. H. Kinsley, and K. G. Lambert, "Fatherhood alters behavioural and neural responsiveness in a spatial task," *Journal of Neuroendocrinology* 23 (2011): 1177–1187.

11. G. Love, N. Torrey, I. McNamara, M. Morgan, M. Banks, N. W. Hester, E. R. Glasper, A. C. DeVries, and K. G. Lambert, "Maternal experience produces long-lasting behavioral modifications in the rat," *Behavioral Neuroscience* 119 (2005): 1084–1096.

12. O. J. Bosch, "Maternal aggression in rodents: brain oxytocin and vasopressin mediate pup defense," *Philosophical Transactions of the Royal Society B* (2013): 368, http://dx.doi.org/10.1098/rstb.2013.0085.

13. K. G. Lambert, "The life and career of Paul MacLean: a journey toward

neurobiological and social harmony," *Physiology and Behavior* 79 (2003): 343–349; P. MacLean, *The Triune Brain in Evolution: Role in Paleocerebral Functions* (New York: Plenum, 1990).

14. J. P. Lorberbaum, J. D. Newman, A. R. Horwitz, J. R. Dubno, R. B. Lydiard, M. B. Hamner, D. E. Bohning, and M. S. George, "A potential role for thalamocingulate circuitry in human maternal behavior," *Biological Psychiatry* 51 (2002): 431–445.

15. P. Kim, L. Strathearn, and J. E. Swain, "The maternal brain and its plasticity in humans," *Hormones and Behavior* 77 (2015): 113–123.

16. P. Kim, P. Rigo, L. C. Mayes, R. Feldman, J. F. Leckman, and J. E. Swain, "Neural plasticity in fathers of human infants," *Social Neuroscience* 9 (2014): 522–535.

17. M. Bardi, M. Eckles, E. Kirk, T. Landis, S. Evans, and K. G. Lambert, "Parity modifies endocrine hormones in urine and problem-solving strategies of captive owl monkeys (Aotus spp.)," *Comparative Medicine* 64 (2014): 486–495; A. Garrett, V. J. Capri, N. Torrey, S. Evans, A. Hughes, C. H. Kinsley, and K. G. Lambert, "Parenting experience enhances spatial learning in common marmosets (*Callithrix jacchus*)," poster presented at Mother and Infant Conference, Montreal, Canada, 2003.

18. A. S. Ivy, K. L. Brunson, C. Sandman, and T. Z. Baram, "Dysfunctional nurturing behavior in rat dams with limited access to nesting material: a clinically relevant model for early-life stress," *Neuroscience* 154 (2008): 1132–1142.

19. S. Dhungel, "Effect of maternal deprivation on growth of wistar rats in preweaning period," *Kathmandu University Medical Journal* 5 (2007): 210–214.

20. K. G. Noble, S. M. Houston, N. H. Brito, H. Bartsch, E. Kan, J. M. Kuperman, and E. R. Sowell, "Family income, parental education and brain structure in children and Adolescents," *Nature Neuroscience* 18 (2015): 773–778.

21. K. Jednorog, I. Altarelli, K. Monzalvo, J. Fluss, J. Dubois, C. Billard, G. Dehaene-Lambertz, and F. Ramus, "The influence of socioeconomic status on children's brain structure," *PLoS One* 8 (2012): e42486.

22. Y. Bhattacharjec, "The first year," *National Geographic* (January 2015): http://ngm.nationalgeographic.com/2015/01/baby-brains/bhattacharjee-text.

23. L. Buchen, "In their nurture," *Nature* 467 (2010): 146–148.

24. M. Hartley and A. Commire, *Breaking the Silence* (New York: G. P. Putnam's Sons, 1990).

25. A. Velando, H. Drummond, and R. Torres, "Senescent birds redouble reproductive effort when ill: confirmation of the terminal investment hypothesis," *Proceedings of the Royal Society B* 273 (2006): 1443–1448.

26. "Brown rat removing young," ARKive, http://www.arkive.org/brown-rat/rattus-norvegicus/video-09d.html.

27. C. A. Nelson, N. A. Fox, and C. H. Zeanah, *Romania's Abandoned Children* (Cambridge, MA: Harvard University Press, 2014).

28. E. Marshall, "An experiment in zero parenting: a controversial study of Romanian orphans reveals long-term harm to the intellect," *Science* 345 (2014): 752–754.

29. Nelson, Fox, and Zeanah, *Romania's Abandoned Children*.

30. Marshall, "An experiment in zero parenting," 752–754.

31. A. S. Hodel, R. H. Hunt, R. A. Cowell, S. van den Heuvel, M. R. Gunnar, and K. T. Thomas, "Duration of early adversity and structural brain development in post-institutionalized adolescents," *NeuroImage* 105 (2015): 112–119.

32. J. C. Simpson, "It's all in the upbringing," *Johns Hopkins Magazine* (April 2000): http://pages.jh.edu/jhumag/0400web/35.html.

33. J. B. Watson and R. Rayner, "Conditioned emotional reactions," *Journal of Experimental Psychology* III (1920): 1–14.

34. J. B. Watson and R. R. Watson, *Psychological Care of the Infant and Child* (New York: Norton, 1928), 81–82.

35. J. B. Watson, *Behaviorism* (rev. ed.) (Chicago: University of Chicago Press, 1930), 82.

36. C. Smirle, "Profile of Rosalie Rayner," in *Psychology's Feminist Voices Multimedia Internet Archive*, ed. A. Rutherford, 2013: http://www.feministvoices.com/rosalie-rayner/.

37. M. Hartley and A. Commire, *Breaking the Silence* (New York: G. P. Putnam's Sons, 1990).

38. N. Joyce and C. Faye, "Skinner Air Crib," *Observer* (2010): 23, http://www.psychologicalscience.org/index.php/publications/observer/2010/september-10/skinner-air-crib.html.

39. H. Rohrs, "Maria Montessori," *Prospects: The Quarterly Review of Comparative Education*, Paris, UNESCO: International Bureau of Education, 1994.

40. Ibid.

41. A. Lillard and N. Else-Quest, "Evaluating Montessori education," *Science* 313 (2006): 1893–1894.

42. C. S. Dweck, *Mindset* (New York: Random House, 2006); "The secret to raising smart kids," *Scientific American* (2015), http://www.scientificamerican.com/article/the-secret-to-raising-smart-kids1/; "Carol Dweck revisits the 'growth mindset,'" *Education Week* (2015): http://www.edweek.org/ew/articles/2015/09/23/carol-dweck-revisits-the-growth-mindset.html.

43. C. Dickson, "America's recidivism nightmare," *Daily Beast* (2014), http://www.thedailybeast.com/articles/2014/04/22/america-s-recidivism-nightmare.html.

44. Judge Francis, his staff, and the participants of the Drug Court Program, personal communication, December 16, 2014, Dallas, TX.

45. Ibid.

46. N. Khan, "Crime and punishment is looking a lot different in tough-on-

crime Texas," *Al Jazeera America* (2014): http://america.aljazeera.com/articles/2014/5/30/texas-criminal-justiceprisonreform.html.

47. Judge Francis, his staff, and the participants of the Drug Court Program, personal communication, December 16, 2014, Dallas, TX; Khan, "Crime and punishment is looking a lot different in tough-on-crime Texas."

48. Khan, "Crime and punishment is looking a lot different in tough-on-crime Texas."

49. Ibid.

50. Judge Francis, his staff, and the participants of the Drug Court Program, personal communication, December 16, 2014, Dallas, TX.

Chapter Eight. Calculating Effective Strategies for Treating Mental Illness

1. S. Nasar, *A Beautiful Mind* (New York: Simon and Schuster, 2001).

2. K. G. Lambert and C. H. Kinsley, *Clinical Neuroscience: Psychopathology and the Brain* (New York: Oxford University Press, 2011).

3. C. Rampell, "The half-trillion dollar depression," *New York Times*, July 2, 2013, http://www.nytimes.com/2013/07/02/magazine/the-half-trillion-dollar-depression.html?_r=0, accessed July 15, 2016.

4. Lambert and Kinsley, *Clinical Neuroscience*.

5. K. G. Lambert, "The clinical neuroscience course: viewing mental health from neurobiological perspectives," *Journal of Undergraduate Neuroscience Education* 3 (2) (2005): http://www.funjournal.org/downloads/Lambert.pdf.

6. K. Lambert and S. O. Lilienfeld, "Brain stains," *Scientific American Mind* (October/November, 2007): 46–53.

7. Ibid.

8. Sheri J. Storm, personal communication, 2016.

9. T. Ban, "The role of serendipity in drug discovery," *Dialogues in Clinical Neuroscience* 8 (2006): 335–334.

10. Lambert and Kinsley, *Clinical Neuroscience*.

11. E. Castren, "Is mood chemistry?," *Nature Reviews Neuroscience* 6 (2005): 241–246.

12. R. Whitaker, *Mad in America* (New York: Perseus Publishing, 2002).

13. T. V. Padma, "The outcomes paradox," *Nature* 508 (2014): S14–15.

14. Ian Birky, personal communication, June 2016.

15. M. M. Merzenich, T. M. van Vleet, and M. Nahum, "Brain plasticity-based therapeutics," *Frontiers in Human Neuroscience* (2014): 1, https:doi.org/10.3389/fnhum.2014.00385.

16. M. Fisher, C. Holland, M. M. Merzenich, and S. Vinogradov, "Using neuroplasticity-based cognitive training to impact verbal memory in schizophrenia," *American Journal of Psychiatry* 166 (2009): 805–811; M. Merzenich, *Soft-wired* (San Francisco: Parnassus, 2013).

17. R. C. Kessler, M. Petukhova, N. A. Sampson, A. M. Zaslavsky, and H. U.

Wittchen, "Twelve-month and lifetime prevalence and lifetime morbid risk of anxiety and mood disorders in the United States," *International Journal of Methods in Psychiatric Research* 21 (2012): 169–184; J. S. Kaplan and D. F. Tolin, "Exposure therapy for anxiety disorders," *Psychiatric Times* (2011): http://www.psychiatrictimes.com/anxiety/exposure-therapy-anxiety-disorders; M. Olfson and S. C. Marcus, "National patterns in antidepressant medication treatment," *Archives of General Psychiatry* 67 (2010): 1265–1273; C. B. Nemeroff and M. J. Owens, "Treatment of mood disorders," *Nature Neuroscience* (supplement 5) (2002): 1068–1070; K. Lambert, *Biological Psychology* (New York: Oxford University Press, 2018).

18. S. D. Hollon, R. J. DeRubeis, R. C. Shelton, J. D. Amsterdam, R. M. Salomon, J. P. O'Reardon, M. L. Lovett, P. R. Young, K. L. Haman, B. B. Freeman, and R. Gallop, "Prevention of relapse following cognitive therapy vs. medications in moderate to severe depression," *Archives of General Psychology* 62 (2005): 417–22.

19. Kaplan and Tolin, "Exposure therapy for anxiety disorders."

20. E. Anthes, "Depression: a change of mind," *Nature* 515 (2014): 185–187; Hollon, DeRubeis, Shelton, Amsterdam, Salomon, O'Reardon, Lovett, Young, Haman, Freeman, and Gallop, "Prevention of relapse following cognitive therapy vs. medications in moderate to severe depression."

21. D. M. Price, "For 175 years: treating mentally ill with dignity," *New York Times*, 1988), http://www.nytimes.com/1988/04/17/us/for-175-years-treating-mentally-ill-with-dignity.html?pagewanted=print.

22. D. R. Anderson, J. Bryant, A. Wilder, A. Sanbnero, M. Williams, and A. M. Crawley, "Researching blues clues: viewing behavior and impact," *Media Psychology* 2 (2000): 179–194.

23. N. S. Jacobson, C. R. Martell, and S. Dimidjian, "Behavioral activation treatment for depression: returning to contextual roots," *Clinical Psychology: Science and Practice* 8 (2001): 255–270.

24. R. N. Carleton, M. K. Mulvogue, M. A. Thibodeau, R. E. McCabe, M. M. Antony, and G. J. G. Asmundson, "Increasingly certain about uncertainty: intolerance of uncertainty across anxiety and depression," *Journal of Anxiety Disorders* 26 (2012): 468–479.

25. S. Westlund, *Field Exercises* (British Columbia: Gabrioloa Island, 2014).

26. American Psychological Association, "Brain training reduces dementia risk across 10 years," (2016): http://www.apa.org/news/press/releases/2016/08/brain-training-dementia.aspx.

27. L. L. Carpenter, P. G. Janicak, S. T. Aaronson, et al., "Transcranial magnetic stimulation (TMS) for major depression: a multisite, naturalistic, observational study of acute treatment outcomes in clinical practice," *Depression and Anxiety* 29 (2012): 587–96; C. Ciobanu, M. Girard, B. Marin, A. Labrunie, and D. Malauzat, "rTMS for pharmacoresistant major depression in the clinical setting of a psychiatric hospital: effectiveness and effects of age," *Journal of Affective Disorders* 150 (2013): 677–681.

28. M. Koenings, E. D. Huey, M. Calamia, V. Raymont, D. Trand, and J. Grafman, "Distinct regions of prefrontal cortex mediate resistance and vulnerability to depression," *Journal of Neuroscience* 28 (2008): 12341–12348.

29. L. Schulze, S. Wheeler, M. P. McAndrews, C. J. E. Solomon, P. Biacobbe, and J. Downar, "Cognitive safety of dorsomedial prefrontal repetitive transcranial magnetic stimulation in major depression," *European Neuropsychopharmacology* 26 (2016): 1213–1226; N. Bakker, S. Shahab, P. Giacobbe, D. M. Blumberger, Z. J. Daskalakis, S. H. Kennedy, and J. Downar, "rTMS of the dorsomedial prefrontal cortex for major depression: safety, tolerability, effectiveness, and outcome predictors for 10 Hz versus intermittent theta-burst stimulation," *Brain Stimulation* 8 (2015): 208–215.

30. A. Vedeniapin, L. Cheng, and M. George, "Feasibility of simultaneous cognitive behavioral therapy (CBT) and left prefrontal rTMS for treatment resistant depression," *Brain Stimulation* 3 (2010): 207–210.

31. T. Christensen, L. Jensen, and E. V. Bouzinova, "Molecular profiling of the lateral habenula in a rat model of depression," *PLoS One* (2013): https://doi.org/10.1371/journal.pone.0080666.

32. P. M. Baker, S. E. Oh, K. S. Kidder, and S. J. Mizumori, "Ongoing behavioral state information signaled in the lateral habenula guides choice flexibility in freely moving rats," *Frontiers in Behavioral Neuroscience* (2015): https:doi.org/10.3389/fnbeh.2015.00295.

33. B. Li, J. Piriz, M. Mirrione, C. D. Prulx, D. Schulz, F. Henn, et al., "Synaptic potentiation onto habenula neurons in the learned helpless model of depression," *Nature* 470 (2011): 535–539.

34. S. Lecca, F. J. Meye, and M. Mameli, "The lateral habenula in addiction and depression: anatomical synaptic and behavioral overview," *European Journal of Neuroscience* 39 (7) (2014): 1170–1178.

35. A. D. Craig, *How Do You Feel? An Interoceptive Moment with Your Neurobiological Self* (Princeton, NJ: Princeton University Press, 2015).

36. R. Sprengelmeyer, J. D. Steele, B. Mwangi, P. Kuman, D. Christmas, M. Milders, and K. Matthews, "The insular cortex and the neuroanatomy of major depression," *Journal of Affective Disorders* 133 (2011): 120–127.

37. M. Kent, M. Bardi, A. Hazelgrove, K. Sewell, E. Kirk, B. Thompson, K. Trexler, B. Terhune-Cotter, and K. Lambert, "Profiling coping strategies in male and female rats: potential neurobehavioral markers of increased resilience to depressive symptoms," *Hormones and Behavior* (forthcoming).

38. C. L. McGrath, M. E. Kelley, P. E. Holtzheimer, B. W. Dunlop, W. Craighead, A. R. Franco, D. C. Craddock, and H. S. Mayberg, "Toward a neuroimaging treatment selection biomarker for major depressive disorder," *Journal of American Medical Association* 70 (2013): 821–829.

39. R. Veit, V. Singh, R. Sitaram, A. Caria, K. Rauss, and N. Birbaumer, "Using real-time fMRI to learn voluntary regulation of the anterior in-

sula in the presence of threat-related stimuli," *Social Cognitive and Affective Neuroscience* 7 (2011): 623–634.

40. "Toward a new understanding of mental illness," a TED talk by T. Insel, posted in 2013, http://www.ted.com/talks/thomas_insel_toward_a_new_understanding_of_mental_illness.

41. A. Regalado, "Why America's top mental health researcher joined Alphabet," *MIT Technology Review* (2015): https://www.technologyreview.com/s/541446/why-americas-top-mental-health-researcher-joined-alphabet/, accessed July 31, 2016.

Chapter Nine. Getting Down to Business

1. Judy Cochrane Gilman-Hines, personal communication, July 2016.
2. E. S. Jackson, *Mr. Cochrane's Overnite* (Richmond VA: William Byrd Press, 1989).
3. Ibid.
4. Ibid.
5. Gilman-Hines, personal communication; Jackson, *Mr. Cochrane's Overnite*.
6. Jackson, *Mr. Cochrane's Overnite*.
7. Ibid.
8. Jackson, *Mr. Cochrane's Overnite*.
9. Ibid.
10. M. Buckingham and C. Coffman, *First, Break All the Rules: What the World's Greatest Managers Do Differently* (New York: Simon and Schuster, 1999), 48.
11. Ibid., 71.
12. "Passing on the Crown," *Economist* (November 4, 2004): http://www.economist.com/node/3352686/print.
13. C. O'Conner, "Inside an $8 billion family feud: who poisoned the Orkin fortune?," *Forbes* (2014): http://www.forbes.com/sites/clareoconnor/2014/09/29/inside-the-3-billion-feud-tearing-georgias-rollins-family-apart/#fd315b638ab7.
14. G. Stalk and H. Foley, "Avoid the traps that can destroy family businesses," *Harvard Business Review* (January–February 2012): https://hbr.org/2012/01/avoid-the-traps-that-can-destroy-family-businesses; C. Fernandez-Araoz, S. Iqbal, and J. Ritter, "Leadership lessons from great family Businesses," *Harvard Business Review* (April 2015): https://hbr.org/2015/04/leadership-lessons-from-great-family-businesses.
15. Stalk and Foley, "Avoid the traps that can destroy family businesses."
16. Ibid.
17. Fernandez-Araoz, Iqbal, and Ritter, "Leadership lessons from great family businesses."
18. E. R. Hendry, "7 epic fails brought to you by the genius mind of Thomas Edison," Smithsonian.com, 2013, http://www.smithsonianmag.com/innovation/7-epic-fails-brought-to-you-by-the=genius-mind.

19. D. Grossman, "Secret Google lab 'rewards staff for failure,'" BBC Newsnight, January 24, 2014, http://www.bbc.com/news/technology-2588 0738.

20. D. B. McKim, A. Niraula, A. J. Tarr, E. S. Wohleb, J. F. Sheridan, and J. P. Godbout, "Neuroinflammatory dynamics underlie memory impairments after repeated social defeat," *Journal of Neuroscience* 36 (2016): 2590–2604.

21. A. F. T. Arnsten, "Stress signaling pathways that impair prefrontal cortex structure and function," *Nature Review Neuroscience* 10 (2009): 410–422; B. S. McEwen, C. Nasca, and J. D. Gray, "Stress effects on neuronal structure: hippocampus, amygdala, and the prefrontal cortex," *Neuropsychopharmacology Reviews* 41 (1) (2016): 3–23.

22. S. Caspers, S. Heim, M. G. Lucas, E. Stephan, L. Fischer, K. Amunts, and K. Zilles, "Dissociated neural processing for decisions in managers and non-managers," *PLoS ONE* 8 (2012): e43537.

23. A. Lawrence, L. Clark, J. Nicole, J. N. Labuzetta, B. Sahakian, and S. Vyakarnum, "The innovative brain," *Nature* 456 (7219) (2008): 168–169; S. Kotler, "Training the brain of an entrepreneur," *Forbes* (March 15, 2012): http://www.forbes.com/sites/stevenkotler/2012/05/14/training-the -brain-of-an-entrepreneur/#56f3f64a3b3d; M. Gladwell, "The sure thing: how entrepreneurs really succeed," *New Yorker* (2010): http://www.new yorker.com/magazine/2010/01/18/the-sure-thing).

24. M. Zollo, "The innovative brain," *MIT Management* (2013): http:// mitsloanexperts.mit.edu/the-innovative-brain-maurizio-zillo/.

25. C. De Young, "The neuromodulator of exploration: a unifying theory of dopamine in personality," *Frontiers in Human Neuroscience* (2013): https: doi.org/10.3389/fnhum.2013.00762.peters.

26. T. E. Robinson and K. C. Berridge, "Beyond Wise et al.—neuroleptic-induced 'anhedonia' in rats: pimozide blocks reward quality of food," in *Brain and Behaviour: Revisiting the Studies*, ed. B. Kolb and I. Whishaw (Washington, DC: Sage, 2017).

27. J. D. Salamone and M. Correa, "The mysterious motivational functions of mesolimbic dopamine," *Neuron* 76 (2012): 470–485.

28. C. M. Stopper and S. B. Floresco, "Dopaminergic circuitry and risk/ reward decision making: implications for schizophrenia," *Schizophrenia Bulletin* 41 (2015): 9–14.

29. J. Robbins, "Reversing course on beavers," *New York Times* (October 27, 2014): http://www.nytimes.com/2014/10/28/science/reversing-the-course -on-beavers.html.

30. S. F. Owen, J. L. Berl, and J. W. Edwards, "Raccoon spatial requirements and multi-scale habitat shelter within an intensively managed central Appalachian forest," *American Midland Naturalist* 174 (2015): 87–95.

31. K. Kennedy, "Forest-preserve raccoons seeking food, water in city," *Chicago Tribune* (August 8, 2005).

32. S. Humphries and G. D. Ruxton, "Bower-building: coevolution of display traits in response to the costs of female choice," *Ecology Letters* 2 (1999): 404–413.

33. D. Thompson, "A world without work," *Atlantic* (July/August 2015): 50–61.

34. K. G. Lambert, *Lifting Depression: A Neuroscientist's Hands-on Approach to Activating Your Brain's Healing Power* (New York: Basic Books, 2008).

35. M. B. Crawford, *Shop Class as Soul Craft* (New York: Penguin Books, 2009).

36. Thompson, "A world without work."

37. U.S. Office of Strategic Services (OSS), training film (circa 1944): https://www.youtube.com/watch?v=Z8TfP7W5ex8.

Chapter Ten. Stretching the Contingency Limits

1. R. Ader and N. Cohen, "Behaviorally conditioned immunosuppression," *Psychosomatic Medicine* 37 (1975): 333–340.

2. K. Q. Thomas, "The mind-body connection: Granny was right, after all," *Rochester Review* (1977): https://www.rochester.edu/pr/ReviewV59N3/feature2.html.

3. J. Marchant, *Cure: A Journey into the Science of Mind over Body* (New York: Broadway Books, 2016).

4. S. Metalnikov and V. Chorine, "The role of conditioned reflexes in immunity," in *Foundations of Psychoneuroimmunology*, ed. S. Locke, R. Ader, H. Besedovsky, N. Hall, G. Solemon, and T. Strom (New York: Aldine, 1926), 263–267; Marchant, *Cure*.

5. K. Lambert, *Lifting Depression* (New York: Basic Books, 2008).

6. M. Schedlowski and G. Pacheco-Lopez, "The learned immune response: Pavlov and beyond," *Brain, Behavior, and Immunity* 24 (2010): 176–185; S. Vits, E. Cesko, P. Enck, U. Hillen, D. Schadendorf, and M. Schedlowski, "Behavioral conditioning as the mediator of placebo responses in the immune system," *Philosophical Transactions of the Royal Society B* 366 (2011): 1799–1807.

7. R. Jutte, "The early history of the placebo," *Complementary Therapies in Medicine* 21 (2013): 94–97.

8. M. J. Niemi, "Placebo effect: a cure in the mind," *Scientific American Mind* (2009): http://www.scientificamerican.com/article/placebo-effect-a-cure-in-the-mind/.

9. J. W. Langston and J. Palfryman, *The Case of the Frozen Addicts* (New York: Pantheon Books, 1995).

10. A. Katsnelson, "Why fake it?," *Nature* 476 (2011): 142–144.

11. I. Kirsch, "Antidepressants and the placebo effect," *Zeitschrift für Psychologie* 22 (2014): 128–134.

12. Katsnelson, "Why fake it?"; P. A. Clark, "Placebo surgery for Parkinson's

disease: do the benefits outweigh the risks?," *Journal of Law, Medicine and Ethics* 30 (2002): 58–68.

13. K. Lambert, *The Lab Rat Chronicles: A Neuroscientist Reveals Life Lessons from the Planet's Most Successful Mammals* (New York: Perigee, 2011).

14. J. Panksepp, "Can PLAY diminish ADHD and facilitate the construction of the social brain?," *Journal of Canadian Academy of Child Adolescent Psychiatry* 16 (2007): 57–66.

15. A. Collins and E. Koechin, "Reasoning, learning, and creativity: frontal lobe function and human decision-making," *PLoS Biology* 10 (2012): e1001293, https:doi.org/10.1371/jounal/pbio.1001293.

16. Panksepp, "Can PLAY diminish ADHD and facilitate the construction of the social brain?"

17. B. M. Cooke and D. Shukla, "Double-helix: Reciprocity between juvenile play and brain development," *Developmental Cognitive Neuroscience* 1 (2011): 459–470.

18. G. A. Vicino and E. S. Marcacci, "Intensity of play behavior as a potential measure of welfare: a novel method for quantifying the integrated intensity of behavior in African elephants," *Zoo Biology* 34 (2015): 492–496.

19. G. M. Burghardt, "The comparative reach of play and brain: perspective, evidence, and implications," *American Journal of Play* (Winter 2010): 338–356.

20. H. C. Bell, S. M. Pellis, and B. Kolb, "Juvenile peer play experience and the development of the orbitofrontal and medial prefrontal cortices," *Behavioural Brain Research* 207 (2010): 7–13; B. T. Himmler and S. M. Pellis, "Juvenile play experience primes neurons in the medial prefrontal cortex to be more responsive to later experiences," *Neuroscience Letters* 556 (2013): 42–45.

21. S. M. Pellis, V. C. Pellis, and H. C. Bell, "The function of play in the development of the social brain," *American Journal of Play* (Winter 2010): 278–296.

22. P. D. MacLean, *The Triune Brain in Evolution* (New York: Plenum Press, 1990).

23. J. Lind, M. Enquist, and S. Ghirlanda, "Animal memory: a review of delayed matching-to-sample data," *Behavioural Processes* 117 (2015): 52–58; S. T. Yang, Y. Shi, Q. Wang, J. Y. Peng, and B. M. Yi, "Neuronal representation of working memory in the medial prefrontal cortex of rats," *Molecular Brain* (2014): 7, http:www.molecularbrain.com/content/7/1/61.

24. M. Petit, "The problem of raccoon intelligence in the behaviourist America," *British Journal for the History of Science* (2010): https:doi.org/10.1017/S0007087409990677.

25. Ibid.

26. P. Sengupta, "The laboratory rat: relating its age with humans," *International Journal of Preventative Medicine* 4 (2013): 624–630.

27. J. K. Finn, T. Tregenza, and M. D. Norman, "Defensive tool use in a coconut-carrying Octopus," *Current Biology* 19 (2009): R1069–R1070.

28. J. A. Endler and L. B. Day, "Ornament colour selection, visual contrast and the shape of colour preference functions in great bowerbirds, Chlamydera nuchalis," *Animal Behaviour* 72 (2006): 1405–1416.

29. S. Liu, H. M. Chow, Y. Xu, M. G. Erkkinen, K. E. Swett, M. W. Eagle, D. A. Rizik-Baer, and A. R. Braun, "Neural correlates of lyrical improvisation: an fMRI study of freestyle rap," *Scientific Reports* 2 (2012): 834, https:doi.org/10.1038/srep00834.

30. S. M. Ritter, R. B. van Baaren, and A. Dijksterhuis, "Creativity: the role of unconscious processes in idea generation and idea selection," *Thinking Skills and Creativity* 7 (2012): 21–27.

31. A. Faust-Socher, Y. N. Kenett, O. S. Cohen, S. Hassin-Baer, and R. Inzelberg, "Enhanced creative thinking under dopaminergic therapy in Parkinson disease," *Annals of Neurology* 75 (2014): 935–942.

Epilogue

1. "Champagne bubbles: it's all in the glass," *Guardian* (2012): https://www.theguardian.com/lifeandstyle/the-womens-blog-with-jane-martinson/2012/dec/31/champagne-bubbles-in-the-glass.

2. J. J. Gibson, "The theory of affordances," in *Perceiving, Acting, and Knowing: Toward an Ecological Psychology*, ed. R. Shaw and J. Bransford (Hillsdale, NJ: Lawrence Erlbaum, 1977).

3. F. Averill and D. M. Bernad, "Review of perceiving the affordances: a portrait of two psychologists," *Cognitive Systems Research* 4 (2002): 385–389.

4. E. J. Gibson, *Perceiving the Affordances: A Portrait of Two Psychologists* (New York: Taylor and Francis Group), 160.

5. B. F. Skinner, *Science and Human Behavior* (New York: Free Press, 1953), 41.

Index

Page numbers in *italics* refer to illustrations.

academia, 29, 60, 62, 76–78, 101, 102, 108, 117, 118, 171, 186, 193, 217; awards, 105; suicide and, 112–114, 117

acetylcholine, 55–56

action-outcome contingencies, 17, 24, 107

addiction, 2–3, 256

Ader, Robert, 234–236, 239

adoption, 168–170

adrenaline, 56

Adrian, Edgar, 57

affluenza, 103–104

affordances, 257–259

aggression, 48, 154; maternal, 157

Aldine, Giovanni, 54

Alphabet Life Sciences, 209

Alzheimer's disease, 16, 199, 200

amygdala, 52, 53, *53*, 75, 116, 146, 157

analytics, 140–143

animal models, 2, 14–16, 17, 28, 29–35, 38, 43–46, 48, 51, 52, 54–61, 64–66, 78–84, 87–92, 143–166, 203–204, 207, 225, 235, 239, 250–252; coping styles, 147–149; enriched environments, 143–145, *145*, 146–147; foraging behavior and, 43–45; neurogenesis, 58–60; optimism and, 119–121; parenting, 150–152, *152*, 153–158, 161–166; rat mazes, 78–84, 155–156, 222. *See also specific animals*

anterior cingulate, 88, 116

antidepressants, 192–195, 202, 243–244

antihistamine, 191

anxiety disorders, 16, 99, 113, 184, 186, 192, 193, 199, 204, 227

arrogance, 123, 124

art, 60, 68, 253

asset bubbles, 1–2, 3, 4; emotional, 3, 4, 5

associative learning, 31

astronomy, 35

asylums, 192, 196

attention deficit/hyperactivity disorder, 23, 192, 193, 245

Attention Restoration Theory, 146

Australian National University, 85

autism, 69

automated response, 40–42

awards, 97, 104–108

axons, 57–58

baboons, 61

backstory, 78–80

bacteria, 237

Bardi, Massi, 146, 162

Barrie, J. M., *Peter Pan*, 98

basal ganglia, 40–42, 116; habitual behavior and, 40–41, *41*, 42

baseball, 19, 142

Bastian, Amy, 20

BBC, 99

Beautiful Mind, A (biopic), 21, 183

beavers, 225, 252

Beer, Jennifer, 123, 126

behavior, 2, 13, 15–20, 26–47, 49; animal, 29–35, 38, 43–46, 78–84, 87–92, 143–166; brain and, 26–47, 52–54; creative, 249–254; distortion of contingency filters and, 95–121; foraging, 43–45, 155–156, 161, 225; genetics and, 16–17; habitual, 39–41, *41*, 42–43; innovative responses, 33–36; mental health and, 15–20; mental illness and, 182–210; optogenetics, 89–92; parenting and, 150–181; play, 244–245, *246–247*, 248–249; rat mazes, 78–84, 155–156, 222; reflexive, 15, 26–28, 40, 41; science of, 26–47, 170–173; understanding, 36–39; work, 211–231

behavioral activation therapy (BAT), 198–200, 202, 208, 209

behaviorism, 2, 13–14, 19, 26–47, 90, 103, 170–173, 217, 235, 250, 259; dirty little secrets of, 31–36; history of, 27–31; parenting and, 170–173; radical, 30, 35; of Skinner, 13, 17, 30–33, 81, 172–173; of Watson, 170–172

Bell, Heather, 249

biology, 12, 29

birds, 59–61, 165–166, 225, 248, 252

Birky, Ira, 192–193

Bjorkland, Anders, 242

"blank slate" strategy, 94

blood, 13, 122

Blue's Clues (TV show), 197–198

booby birds, 165–166

boredom, 23

bowerbirds, 225, 252

brain, 1–5; areas involved in depression, 204–205, *205*, 206–208; basal ganglia and habitual behavior, 39–41, *41*, 42–43; behavior and, 26–47, 52–54; bubbles, 11, *11*, 23, 47, 94, 118, 122, 182, 183, 189, 193, 195, 203, 204, 211, 221, 222, 224, 229, 232–233, 255–257; building cognitive capital, 85–89; building contingency circuit for, 73–94; bumps, 51; chemical imbalance, 191–194; comedians and, 124–128; contingency calculators, 6–25, 78, 122–149; creative, 249–254; decision-making and, 74–77, *77*, 78–80, 92–94; decoding, 11–14; development, 101, 244, *245*; distortion of contingency filters and, 95–121; dopamine and, 132–136, 224; electrical sparks, 54–58; failure and, 128–132; functions, 14–18, 48–72; habits, 39–41, *41*, 42–43; hemispheres, 68, 223; hidden treasures of, 60–69; imaging, 29, 37, 38, 49–54, 158–162, 169, 207, 223, 252; inner workings of, 48–72; lateralization, 68; localization of function, 52–53, *53*, 54; mental illness and, 182–210; neuroeconomics of parenthood and, 162–166; neurogenesis, 58–60; optimism and, 117–121; parenting and, 150–181; placebos and, 240–244; play and, 244–245, *246–247*, 248–249; privilege and poverty, 100–104; religion and, 108–111; size, 60–69, 164, 266*n*35; soup, 63; stain, 49, 50, 188, 189; stress and, 221–224;

suicide and, 112–117; triune, 160, *160;* tumors, 199; well-grounded, 122–149; whispering, 203–208; work and, 221–231. *See also specific regions of the brain*

brain-derived neurotrophic factor (BDNF), 204, 248

"Brain Stains" (Lambert and Lilienfeld), 188–189

brainstem, 63

breast cancer, 109

Breland, Keller, 33

Breland, Marion, 33

Brundin, Lena, 115

Bucharest Early Intervention Project (BEIP), 168–169, 174, 175

Buckingham (Marcus) and Coffman (Curt), *First, Break All the Rules,* 216

Buffett, Warren, 3

Burrell, Brian, *Postcards from the Brain Museum,* 54

Bush, George W., 92–94; Presidential Library and Decision Points Theater, 92–94

business, 211–231; brain and, 221–231; contingency calculators, 211–231; evolution of, 224–227, *228;* failure, 221; family, 219–221; stress, 221–224; success, 212–219

Byron, Lord, 54

Cajal, Santiago Ramon y, 49, 50

California deer mouse, 157

camouflage, 18–20; contingencies, 18–20

camphor, 236–237

cancer, 14, 109, 233–234, 241

Caporeal, Linnda, 110–111; "Ergotism: The Satan Loosed in Salem?," 110

career, 23, 24, 76–78, 100, 137, 211–231; brain and, 221–231; contingency calculators, 211–231; evolution of, 224–227, *228;* family

business, 219–221; lack of, 226–227; spy, 229–230; stress, 221–224; success, 212–219

Carillo, George, 242

Carlsson, Arvid, 191

Carr, Harvey, 250

Carson, Johnny, 125–126

cats, 29–30, 248

caudate nucleus, 222

Ceausescu, Nicolae, 167

celebrity, 3–4, 6, 46, 97, 98–100, 256

cerebellum, 63, 66, 118

cerebral cortex, 31, 66, 101, 266*n*32

champagne, 256

Champagne, Frances, 165

chemical imbalance, 191–194

chemistry, 28, 29

chemotherapy, 237

Chenery, Chris, 136, 137

Chenery, Penny, 136–139

children, 18, 24, 32, 33, 58, 95–97, 99, 149, 197–198, 228; abuse, 99, 115, 187, 189; academic performance, 101–102; awards, 104–108; behaviorism and, 170–173; birth of, 24; contingency distortion and, 95–97; exploration, 134; institutionalized, 167–171; Montessori method, 173–175; mortality rates, 14, 42; movement disabilities, 134–135; neglected, 168–170; next-generation leaders, 219–221; parenting and, 150–181; play and creativity, 244–245, 248, 250, 251; privilege and poverty, 100–104; Romanian orphans, 167–170; socioeconomic status and, 162–166

chimpanzees, 4, 22, 34, 61, 67, 98

chlorpromazine, 191

Christmas, 95–97

Church, George, 17

cingulate cortex, 52, 53, *53,* 88, 94, 159

CLARITY, 52

Clark University, 80

classical conditioning, 28, 33, 45
Clinton, Bill, 7–8
cocaine, 154, 156, 253
Cochrane, Harwood, 212–216, 218
coffee, 172
cognition, 22–23, 44, 61, 194
cognitive-behavioral therapy (CBT),
    92, 148, 195, 197, 198, 200, 202,
    207, 208
cognitive capital, building, 85–89
Cohen, Nicholas, 235–236, 239
Coke vs. Pepsi study, 38–39, 75
Columbia University, 29, 100, 137,
    165
comedians, 124–128
communication, 60
conditioned canine therapy, 189, *190*
conditioned fear, 171
conditioned taste aversion, 32
consciousness, 12–13, 29
consequences, 30
contingencies, 6–25, 46, 66, 67; action-
    outcome, 17, 24, 107; awards,
    104–108; boot camp, 15–16, 83–84;
    building cognitive capital, 85–89;
    calculators, 6–25, 78, 122–149;
    camouflaged, 18–20; capital, 9;
    circuit, 73–94; comedians and,
    124–128; conundrum, 24–25,
    122–149, 258; coping styles,
    147–149; creative, 249–254;
    decision-making and, 74–80, 92–94;
    distortion, 95–121; dopamine and,
    132–136; enriched environment
    and, 143–145, *145*, 146–147;
    experience and, 9–11, 78–80; failure
    and, 128–132; fine-tuning, 122–149;
    make-believe, 24; mental illness
    and, 182–210; neural-immune,
    233–240, 241–242; next generation
    and, 219–221; optimism and,
    117–121; optogenetics, 89–92;
    parenting and, 150–181; passive-
    response, 9–10, *10*; placebos and,

240–244; play, 244–245, 246–247,
    248–249; prisons and, 175–181;
    privilege and poverty, 100–104; rat
    mazes, 78–84, 155–156, 222;
    religion and, 108–111; response-
    outcome, 17, 21, 31, 89, 107, 111,
    124, 149, 180, 249; statistics and,
    140–143; stretching limits of,
    232–254; success and, 136–139;
    suicide and, 112–117; terminology,
    6, 20; well-grounded brain and,
    122–149; work, 211–231
Cool, Nadean, 184, 185, 188
coping styles, 147–149, 207
corpus callosum, 53, *53*, 67–68
cortex, 51, 63–67, 70, 76, 77, *77*, 91,
    94, 170; thickness, 100–101
corticosterone, 84
cortisol, 146
Couch, Ethan, 103–104
Craig, Bud, 206
Crawford, Matt, 227; *Shop Class as Soul
    Craft*, 227
creativity, 24, 68, 97, 146, 218, 224,
    233, 249–254
crime, 176–181
Cuban, Mark, 7
curiosity, 233, 249–254
cyclophosphamide, 239
Czerski, Helen, 255–256

Dale, Henry, 55, 56
Danckert, James, 23
Da Vinci, Leonardo, 68
Davis, Herbert, 251
death, 3, 14, 42, 238; suicide, 112–117
decision-making, 37, 51, 53, 67, 74–77,
    78, 79–80, 92–94, 101, 123, 125,
    132, 141, 142, 194, 206, 257; cold
    vs. hot, 222–223; George W. Bush
    and, 92–94; rat mazes, 78–84,
    155–156, 222; statistics and,
    140–143; work and, 221–231
deep brain stimulation, 201, 206

Dellu-Hagedorn, Francoise, 88
delusions, 21, 182, 191, 253
demonic spirits, 110–111
dendritic spines, 157
dentate gyrus, 58–59
depression, 14, 16, 17, 23, 46, 83, 112,
    148, 149, 181, 182, 191–201, 204,
    205, 227, 278n27, 279n29; brain
    whispering and, 203–208; paternal,
    161; placebo effect and, 243–244;
    therapies, 191–208
Descartes, René, 5, 27, 36
De Young, Colin, 134
DHEA, 84
Dhungel, Shaligram, 163
diabetes, 210
Diamond, Marion, 144
Dismukes, Key, 42; The Multitasking
    Myth, 42
displacement behavior, 46
Disseroth, Karl, 52
distortion, 95–121, 123, 127; awards,
    104–108; optimism and, 117–121;
    privilege and poverty, 100–104; of
    reality, 6–7, 11, 95–121, 182, 211,
    232; religion and, 108–111; suicide
    and, 112–117
divorce, 185, 186
DNA, 8, 132
dogs, 9, 17, 28, 33, 45–46, 235, 237,
    248, 250, 251, 265n29; therapy, 189,
    190
dolphins, 33, 61, 68, 135–136, 266n36
Donders, F. C., 35
dopamine, 40, 57, 132–136, 191, 204,
    224, 242–243, 248; creativity and,
    253
dorsal cingulate cortex, 141
dorsolateral prefrontal cortex, 76, 77,
    77, 130, 279n29
dorsomedial prefrontal cortex, 201,
    252
Double Decision, 199
Downar, Jonathan, 201

driving, 39–40, 40, 89, 124–125, 226
drug rehabilitation programs,
    176–181
drugs, 2–3, 6, 18–19, 21, 24, 46,
    99–100; industry, 55, 57, 208, 209,
    242; placebos and, 240–244; prison
    and, 176–181; for psychiatric
    illnesses, 191–195, 210; psycho-
    active, 2–3, 6, 18–19, 21, 24, 46,
    99–100, 184, 186, 188, 191–195,
    209, 210; recreational, 154, 156,
    253
Dry Land Maze, 81, 84, 155, 156
dualism, mind-body, 5
Dweck, Carol, 175

economics, 37–39; housing bubbles, 2,
    118, 255
Edison, Thomas, 221
education, 29, 76–78, 100, 101, 217;
    Montessori method, 173–175;
    socioeconomic status and, 100–104
Edwards, Jerri, 199
effort-based reward model, 15–16, 83
Einstein, Albert, 61
electricity, 54–58
electroconvulsive shock therapy, 191,
    192
electroencephalogram (EEG), 169
elephants, 61, 248, 283n18
elevated-plus maze, 80
embarrassment, 69
Emory University, 188
emotions, 2, 4, 17, 23, 49, 53, 67, 69,
    75, 117, 204, 206, 222, 256; abuse,
    46; asset bubbles, 3, 4, 5; mental
    illness and, 182–210; parenting and,
    150–181. See also specific emotions
empathy, 151
encephalization quotient (EQ), 61–62
energy, 87, 155
Engber, Daniel, 80
enriched environment, 143–145, 145,
    146–147

environment, 2, 9, 15, 22, 23, 24–25, 35, 58, 65–66, 79, 85, 123, 143–147, 184, 198, 217, 257; enriched, 143–145, *145*, 146–147; genetics and, 164–165; toxins, 101; work, 211–231

epigenetics, 164–165

Equilibrium Theory, 21

ergotism, 110–111

errors, 20, 76, 86–89; correction, 20; prediction, 74, 83, 89, 118, 199, 207

Ese-Quest, Nicole, 174

evolution, 8, 15, 16, 22, 23, 43, 52, 58, 152–153, 155, 166, 248, 259; of work, 224–227, *228*

experience, 9–11, 78–80, 124, 216, 257–258; backstory, 78–80; contingencies and, 9–11, 78–80; Montessori method, 173–175; rat mazes, 78–84, 155–156, 222; work, 211–231

exploration, 134

exposure therapy, 195

facial recognition, 68

failure, 18, 20, 112, 114, 128–132, 224; business, 221; learning from, 20, 128–132; value of, 128–132

family business, 219–221

fathering (paternal behavior), 153, 161, 165–166

fear, 28, 52, 75, 206, 208; conditioned, 171

Fechner, Gustav, 35

Felten, David, 236

Ferris, Craig, 154

Few Good Men, A (movie), 158

Fields Medal, 108

filgrastim, 237–238

financial markets, 1–2, 59, 118; crashes, 1–2, 3, 118, 255

fire, discovery of, 64

fish, 59, 60, 61

flexibility, 61, 115, 148–149

float response, 148

Floresco, Stan, 224

Focalin, 193

food, 2, 3, 16, 22, 24, 28, 71, 74–75, 162, 168; cooked, 64; decision-making and, 74–76; foraging behavior, 43–45, 155–156, 161, 225; poisoning, 32; reward, 15–16, 29–30, 32, 45, 79–84, 88, 90–92, 105, *106*, 119, 155, 161, 198; weight loss and, 98

football, 20

foraging behavior, 43–45, 155–156, 161, 225

fos, 248

foster care, 168–170

Fox, Nathan, 167

foxes, 44

France, 164, 191, 221

Francis, Robert, 176–181

freestyle rapping, 252

free will, 46–47

Freud, Sigmund, 13

Frey, Bruno, 107

frogs, 54, 55, 56

frontal lobe, 133

frontal lobotomy, 19, 190–191, 194

functional magnetic resonance imaging (fMRI), 29, 38, 51, 52, 109, 130, 159, 207, 223, 252, 279*n*39

GABA, 114–115, 133

Gach, John, 49

Galen, 27

Gall, Franz Joseph, 51

Gallup Organization, 216–219, 226

Galvani, Luigi, 54

galvanism, 54–55

Garcia, John, 31–32

genetics, 7–11, 15, 86, 184, 201, 259; behavior and, 16–17; beyond, 7–11; environment and, 164–165; mental illness and, 16–17; sequencing, 7–8

genome, 7–11, 15, 16–17, 259; beyond, 7–11; sequencing, 7–8
Germany, 65, 221
germs, fear of, 182
Gibson, Eleanor, 258
Gibson, James, 257, 258
glia, 63–65
Glimcher, Paul, 37, 75
global economy, 221
glucose, 207
glutamate, 115
Godbout, Jonathan, 222
Goldberg, Rube, 9; "Self-Operating Napkin" invention, 9–10, 10
Golgi, Camillo, 49, 50
Golgi stain, 49, 50
Goodnow, Frank, 170
Google, 209
Google X, 221
gorillas, 61, 64
Graybiel, Ann, 40
Great Britain, 1; South Sea Company crash, 1–2
Greece, ancient, 12, 15, 27, 54–55
Greenspan, Alan, 2, 255
grooming, 84
groundhog predictions, 131–132
growth mind-set, 175
guilt, 69, 178, 179
guinea pigs, 237
gut feelings, 86–87

habits, 39–41, 41, 42–43, 79, 249
Hale, John, 111
Hall, Monty, 140
hallucinations, 21, 182, 191, 253
happiness, 117, 206
Harlow, Harry, 34–35, 172
Hartley, Mariette, 172
Harvard University, 17, 30, 31, 52, 64, 115, 167, 172, 243
Harvey, William, 12–13
health care costs, 184
hearing, 52

heart, 12–13, 14, 15, 18, 56; disease, 13, 14, 23, 209, 210; rate, 56
hedonic hotspots, 133
helplessness, 83–84, 205–206
Herculano-Houzel, Suzana, 62–65
hippocampus, 52, 53, 53, 58, 59, 60, 63, 116, 157, 164, 170, 208
Hippocrates, 12, 49
Hof, Patrick, 69
Hoffa, Jimmy, 214
Holleran, Madison, 112–113, 116
homosexuality, 68
hope, 180
hormones, 154; reproductive, 154; stress, 84, 146, 162
horses, 136–139
housing bubbles, 2, 118, 255
hunches, 86–87
hunger, 43–45, 48, 52, 154
Hunter, Walter, 250–251
Hurricane Katrina, 93
Hurt, Hallum, 164
Hutcheson, Archibald, 1
hypnotherapy, 186–189, 190
hypothalamus, 153–155, 159, 161

imagination, 24
imaging, brain, 29, 37, 38, 49–54, 109, 130, 158–162, 169, 207, 223, 252; history of, 49–54
immune system-neuro connections, 233–240, 241–242
Implicit Association Test, 115
income, 100–104
independence, 171, 174
India, 192
inflammation, 115
innovative responses, 33–36
insects, 18, 219
Insel, Thomas, 14, 208–209
insomnia, 185, 186
Institute of Pennsylvania Hospital, 196
insula, 67, 204, 205, 206–208

insular cortex, 67, 69
intelligence, 44
International Behavioral Neuroscience
    Society, 63
interoception, 206–207
invariants, 257–258
ions, 14, 57
Iowa Gambling Task, 85–88
iproniazid, 191
Iraq War, 93
isotropic fractionation, 63–64, 66

Jackson, Michael, 4, 6, 98–100, 103
Jacobson, Neil, 198
Jakob the Liar (movie), 112
James, William, 28; *Psychological
    Principles*, 28
Japan, 65
Jefferson, Thomas, 240–241
Johns Hopkins University, 20, 29, 135,
    136, 170, 171, 172, 250
Johnson, Spencer, *Who Moved My
    Cheese*, 73–74, 79, 249
*Journal of Undergraduate Neuroscience
    Education*, 185
joy, 117, 206
just noticeable difference, 35

Kahneman, Daniel, 36, 76, 78
Kempermann, Gerd, 58–59
Kent State University, 69
Kentucky Derby, 137, 138
Kesner, Ray, 81
Kinsley, Craig, 127, 151, 154, 155,
    158, 159
Kirk, Emily, 91
Kirkbride, Thomas, 196
Kirsch, Irving, 243–244
Klein, Gary, 140, 141
Kohler, Wolfgang, 34
Kolb, Bryan, 249
Krakauer, John, 135–136
Krebiozen, 241

labor unions, 214
Lab Rat Chronicles, The (Lambert), 156,
    245
Lacey, Mike, 124, 127
Ladd, Diane, 137
Lamictol, 193
Langston, Bill, 242
language, 52, 65, 68, 164
Lashley, Karl, 31, 34
latent learning, 78–79
lateral habenula, 204–205, 205, 206,
    208, 279n32, 279n33
lateral intraparietal cortex, 75, 77, 77
lateralization, 68
Law of Consequences, 30
Law of Effect, 30
lawyers, 76–78
learned helplessness, 83–84, 205, 206
learned persistence, 84
learning, 52, 58, 61, 118, 157, 170;
    latent, 78–79; Montessori method,
    173–175; rat mazes, 78–84,
    155–156, 222
left-handedness, 68
Lehigh University, 192
Leno, Jay, 124–128, 137, 149; *Leading
    with Your Chin*, 124
Lent, Roberto, 62–65
Let's Make a Deal (TV show), 140
leukemia, 14
Lewis, Michael, *The Big Short*, 118
Lexipro, 193
Lichtman, Jeff, 52
life expectancy, 10
lifestyle, 3–4, 5, 9, 23, 95–121, 210,
    254; awards, 104–108; distortion
    of contingency filters and, 95–121;
    mirrors, 97–100; privilege and
    poverty, 100–104; religious,
    108–111; suicide, 112–117
Lifting Depression (Lambert), 238
Lillard, Angeline, 174
limbic system, 158

lipopolysaccharide (LPS), 165
Little Albert, 171
lizards, 14–15, 26
lobotomy, 19, 190–191, 194
Loewi, Otto, 55, 56
Lorberbaum, Jeffrey, 158–161
Los Angeles Times, 127
lungs, 14, 18

MacLean, Paul, 158–160, 249; *The Triune Brain*, 249
Massachusetts General Hospital, 128–130
mathematics, 20–22, 49, 108, 175, 183
mazes, 78–84, 155–156, 222
McGill University, 165
McHenry, Jenna, 91
Meaney, Michael, 165
media, 103, 112, 113, 120
medial prefrontal cortex, 75, 77, 77, 251, 252
medial preoptic area, 154
Medical School of South Carolina, 158
memory, 31, 52, 58, 157, 164, 170, 281n20; working, 101, 251
mental illness, 9, 13–14, 23, 181, 182–210, 257; behavior and, 15–20; brain whispering and, 203–208; contingency void in psychiatric therapies, 189–196; damaging treatments, 184–189; depression therapies, 191–208; drug therapies, 191–195, 210; effective strategies for treating, 182–210; genetics and, 16–17; merging magnetic and contingency-building fields, 201–203; respect for, 196; surgical therapy, 190–191
Merzenich, Michael, 193–194, 208, 209
Metalnikov, Sergey, 237
mice, 52, 73–74, 91–92, 157, 222, 249, 251–252

Michigan State University, 115, 247
microscope, 116, 203
Milgram, Anne, 142
Miller, Arthur, *The Crucible*, 111
mind-body dualism, 5
mirrors, 97–100
mistakes, 128–130
MIT, 40
Moneyball (movie), 142
monkeys, 34–35, 38, 64, 65, 67, 75, 194; parenting, 161–162
Montague, Read, 38–39, 130–131
Montessori, Maria, 173–174
Morrell, Joan, 156
Morris Water Maze, 80, 82
mortality rates, 14, 42
mothering (maternal behavior), 150–181; contingencies and, 150–181; helicopter, 104, 154; in rats, 150–152, 152, 153–158, 162–164, 166
motivation, 154
Mount Sinai School of Medicine, 69
movement, 52, 53, 66; disabilities, 134–135
movie theaters, 26, 27
MRI, 100, 169
multiple personality disorder, 184, 186–189, 190
multiple sclerosis, 210
multitasking, 42
music, 253
Myers-Briggs personality test, 211

NASA, 42
Nash, John, 21, 183
Nash Equilibrium Theory, 183
National Institute of Mental Health, 14, 209
National Institutes of Health (NIH), 17
neglect, 168–170
Nelson, Charles, 167–169
neocortex, 39

nervous system, 7, 36; central, 36, 56;
    electrical nature of, 54–58; immune
    connections, 233–240, 241–242;
    parasympathetic, 56; peripheral, 56;
    sympathetic, 56
neural-immune contingencies,
    233–240, 241–242
neuroeconomics, 17–18, 37–39, 45,
    74–80, 162–166, 206; decision-
    making, 74–80; of parenthood,
    162–166
neurogenesis, 58–60
neurons, 50, *50*, 51, 52, 57, 58, 62–66;
    electricity and, 54–58; networks,
    79; sensory, 35, 36; von Economo,
    69, *70*
neuroscience, 12, 13, 15, 31, 48, 74,
    90, 109, 170, 259
neurotransmitters, 57, 114–115,
    132–136, 191, 224, 242–243
New England Journal of Medicine, 129
New York City, 120, 121
New York Times, 95
New York University, 37
Next-generation leaders, 219–221
Nicholson, Jack, 158
Nobel, Alfred, 107
Nobel Prize, 13, 21, 28, 36, 49, 56–57,
    76, 107–108, 183, 191, 237
Noble, Kimberly, 100
Nock, Matt, 115
non-Hodgkin's lymphoma, 233–234,
    241
noradrenaline, 204
Northeastern University, 154
nucleus accumbens, 40, 130–131, 132,
    154
Numan, Michael, 154

Obama, Michelle, 3–4
obsessive-compulsive disorder (OCD),
    17, 46, 181, 182
odor-outcome situations, 88
Ohio State University, 221–222

Oldfield, Kenneth, 102
Olson, Kenneth, 184–189
O'Neill, Jessie, *Golden Ghetto: The
    Psychology of Affluenza*, 103
operant conditioning, 30–31, 34
opioids, 133
opsin proteins, 89–92
optimism, 117–121, 124
optogenetics, 89–92, 201
orbitofrontal cortex (OFC), 88–89, 94,
    123, 159, 161
Orkin, Otto, 219
outcomes paradox, 192
outer cortex, 65, 66
Overnite Transportation, 213–216, 218
owl monkeys, 65, 161–162
owls, 44
oxytocin, 57, 154

pain, 204
Panksepp, Jaak, 245
parenting, 35, 42, 95–97, 149, 150–181,
    228–229; behaviorism and, 170–173;
    contingency distortion and, 95–97;
    helicopter, 104, 154; in monkeys,
    161–162; Montessori method,
    173–175; neuroeconomics of,
    162–166; prisons and, 175–181;
    privilege and poverty, 100–104;
    in rats, 150–152, *152*, 153–158,
    162–164, 166; Romanian orphans,
    167–170; scanning recalculations in,
    158–162; snow plow, 104; socio-
    economic status and, 162–166
Parkinson's disease, 16, 210, 242–244,
    253
parrots, 61
passive-response contingencies, 9–10,
    10
Pavlov, Ivan, 13, 17, 28, 29, 32, 34, 36,
    37, 45, 170, 235, 237, 250
Pellis, Sergio, 249
Pellis, Vivien, 249
Personal Genome Project, 17

personality, 79, 211–212
pessimism, 116
PET scan, 207
philosophy, 12, 27, 28, 29
phobias, 195
phrenology, 51, 77
physics, 29, 49
physiology, 28, 29
Pidcoe, Peter, 134
pigeons, 17
pigs, 33, 147
Pittman, Laniqua, 180
pizza rat, 120–121
placebo effects, 24, 194, 233, 239,
     240–244, 282n6
Plato, *The Republic*, 245
play, 97, 233, 244–245, 246–247,
     248–249, 283n18, 283n20
pleasure, 132
Polish Academy of Sciences, 119
politics, 6, 93, 141–142
Pollack, Seth, 101
Posit Science, 194, 199
posterior parietal cortex, 38, 39, 75,
     77, 77
posttraumatic stress disorder (PTSD),
     46, 199
potassium, 57
Poulter, Robert, 114–115
poverty, 6, 24, 46, 97, 100–102, 163,
     164, 168, 256
predators, 44, 205
prediction, 131–132, 142; errors, 74,
     83, 89, 118, 199, 207; groundhog,
     131–132
prefrontal cortex, 39, 53, 53, 67, 86,
     88, 114, 146, 159, 161, 170, 201,
     208, 222, 223–224, 249
pregnancy, 101, 143, 150, 151, 156,
     167
prenatal care, 101
presidential decision-making, 92–94
presidential elections, 141–142
primates, 60, 61, 64, 161

Princeton University, 21, 183
prisons, parenting of, 175–181
privilege, 6, 24, 97, 102–104, 221, 233
probability, 17–18, 75, 118
problem-solving, 43–45, 78, 91, 116,
     118, 146, 197
Proffitt, Dennis, 87
progesterone, 154
prolactin, 154
Prometheus, 54–55
propofol, 99
prosperity, 4–5, 7; redefining, 255–259
proteins, 16; opsin, 89–92
Prozac, 192
psychiatric illnesses, 46, 50, 69, 112,
     149, 181, 182–210, 257; brain
     whispering and, 203–208; contin-
     gency void in psychiatric therapies,
     189–196; damaging treatments,
     184–189; depression therapies,
     191–208; drug therapies, 191–195,
     210; effective strategies for treating,
     182–210; merging magnetic and
     contingency-building fields,
     201–203; surgical therapy, 190–191
psychiatry, 12, 13, 184–185
psychoactive drugs, 2–3, 6, 18–19, 21,
     24, 46, 99–100, 184, 186, 188,
     191–195, 209, 210
psychology, 12, 13, 28, 46, 78;
     behavioral, 26–47, 170–172
psychoneuroimmunology, 234–239
Puritanism, 110–111
Putnam, Ann, 111
puzzle boxes, 29, 32

Quakers, 196, 200
quinolic acid, 115

raccoons, 33, 65–66, 70, 225, 281n30;
     creativity, 250–251; von Economo
     neurons, 69, 70
race, 101
Radial Arm Maze, 155, 156

Randolph-Macon College, 136, 138
randomization of subjects, 168
Rat Gambling Task, 88
rats, 15–16, 30, 32, 52, 60, 64, 65,
    73–74, 87–92, 127, 171, 176, 194,
    199, 200, 204, 207, 212, 224, 225,
    235, 239; contingent-trained,
    15–16; coping styles, 147–149;
    creativity, 250–251; in enriched
    environment, 143–145, *145*,
    146–147; mazes, 78–84, 155–156,
    222; optimist, 119–121; optogenet-
    ics, 89–92; parenting, 150–152,
    152, 153–158, 162–164, 166; pizza,
    120–121; play, 245, *246–247*, 249;
    primary rewards, 105–106, *106*; tail
    length, 163–164
Rayner, Rosalie, 170, 171, 172
reading, 101
real estate bubbles, 2, 118, 255
reality, 6–7, 23; distortion of, 6–7, 11,
    95–121, 182, 211, 232; optimism
    and, 117–121; religion and,
    108–111; stretching contingency
    limits and, 232–254
recovered-memory therapy, 186–189
reflexive response, 15, 26–28, 40, 41
religion, 6, 28, 29, 97, 108–111
reptiles, 14–15, 26, 59, 60, 152, 160,
    248
respect, 196
response engineering, 31
response-outcome contingencies, 17,
    21, 31, 89, 107, 111, 124, 149, 180,
    249
reward, 15–16, 29–30, 32, 33, 35, 37,
    38, 45, 75, 79–84, 88, 90–92, 105,
    106, 119, 130, 132, 154, 155, 159,
    161, 198, 204, 207, 224; awards,
    104–108; dopamine and, 133, 135,
    224; effort-based, 15–16, 83; pri-
    mary, 105–106, *106*; rat mazes,
    78–84, 155–156, 222
Rhaganti, Mary Ann, 69

rhesus monkeys, 34–35, 38, 67
Riener, Cedar, 87
Ring, David, 128–130
risk, 224
Rolling Stone, 99
Rollins, Gary, 219, 220
Rollins, Glen, 219–220
Rollins, Wayne, 219
Romanian orphans, 167–170
Rome, ancient, 27
Royal College of Physicians of
    Edinburgh, 50
rTMS, 201–203
Rutgers University, 156
Rygula, Rafal, 119–120

Sahakian, Barbara, 222–223
Salamone, John, 132–133
Salem witchcraft trials, 110–111
saliva, 28, 235
Samford University, 27
"Santa on the Brain" (Lambert), 95–97
Schedlowski, Manfred, 239
schedules of reinforcement, 31
schizophrenia, 16, 21, 181, 182, 183,
    191, 192, 194, 224, 253
Schoenbaum, Geoffrey, 88, 89
Science, 110
Scientific American MIND, 188
Secretariat, 136–139
seizures, 191
self-awareness, 87
Self-Initiated Prone Progressive
    Crawler (SIPPC), 134–135
senses, 22, 35, 36, 53, 67, 88, 96, 173,
    194, 238
serotonin, 57, 114–115, 192, 204
serotonin-selective receptor inhibitor
    (SSRI), 192
Seroquel, 193
sex, 2, 13, 154
Shark Tank (TV show), 7
Sharot, Tali, 118
Shelley, Mary, 54–55; *Frankenstein*, 55

Shelley, Percy, 54
Shenger-Krestovnikova, N. R., 45
Sherrington, Charles, 36
shrews, 43–45, 61, 155
Silver, Nate, 141–142
Sinatra, Frank: "High Hopes," 121
60 Minutes (TV show), 184, 185
Skinner, B. F., 13, 17, 30–33, 36, 37,
    81, 103, 170, 172–173, 250, 259
Skinner Air Crib, 172–173
Skinner Boxes, 30–31, 38
Slate, 80
sleep, 52, 204; problems, 99, 185, 192
Small, Willard, 80
smell, 88
snakeskin strategy, 141
Snow White and the Seven Dwarfs, 97
social media, 113, 114, 146
Society for Neuroscience, 49, 127
socioeconomic status (SES), 100–104,
    162–164
soda, 38–39, 75
sodium, 57
Southern Society for Philosophy and
    Psychology, 42
South Sea Company crash, 1–2
Sowell, Elizabeth, 100
Spheramine, 242–243
spiders, 195
spinal cord, 36, 56
sports awards, 107
Spurzheim, Johann, 51
spy training, 229–230
Stanford University, 52, 76, 175
statistics, 140–143
stem cell transplant, 234, 238, 241,
    242
Sterelny, Kim, 85
Stern, Benjamin, 7
stimulus response, 28–30, 33, 34, 38,
    178, 245
stomach, 14
Stony Brook University, 159–161
Strayer, David, 146

stress, 15, 23, 82–83, 101, 115, 129,
    203, 204, 225, 248, 257, 281n21;
    hormones, 84, 146, 162; PTSD, 46,
    199; response, 82–83, 91, 154, 155,
    165; work and, 221–224
stroke, 20, 135
Stuber, Garret, 91
substantia nigra, 242, 243
success, 9, 17, 18, 112, 114, 117, 126,
    130, 131, 136–139, 206, 212–219,
    257; contingencies and, 136–139;
    work, 212–219
suicide, 97, 112–117, 172; academia
    and, 112–114, 117
superstition, 19
surgery, 190–191; mistakes, 128–130;
    sham, 243–244
survival, 3, 8, 16, 17, 22, 23, 81, 104,
    152, 206, 227
Swain, James, 159–161
swimming, 148
synapses, 36–37, 192

talent, 217
Talking Heads, "How Did I Get
    Here?," 79
taste, 238
teachers, 76–78
technology, 226, 228, 258
teenagers, 7, 104, 156, 158; suicide,
    112–114
teeth, 64; brushing, 42
Tel Aviv University, 253
television, 7, 34, 120, 125–126, 140,
    167, 197
tensor diffusion imaging, 52
terminal investment hypothesis, 166
terrorism, 93
Texas prisons, 175–181
thalamus, 52, 53, 53, 91, 159
Thaler, Richard, 76–78; Misbehaving,
    76
Thompson, Brooke, 91
Thorndike, E. L., 13, 29–30, 32, 37

time out, 173
Tolman, Edward, 78–79
Tonight Show, The (TV show),
    125–126
touch, 172
transcranial magnetic stimulation
    (TMS), 278n27, 279n29
trepanning, 11–12
Triple Crown, 137, 138
triune brain, 160, *160*
trucking industry, 213–216
Tuke, J. Batty, 49–51; *The Insanity of
    Over-Exertion of the Brain*, 49–51
Tversky, Amos, 76, 78

UCLA, 100
uncertainty, 46, 74, 85, 110, 199; Iowa
    Gambling Task, 85–88
unconscious, 13
Union Pacific, 214–215
University College London, 118, 256
University Federal of Rio de Janeiro,
    62
University of Alabama, Birmingham,
    236
University of Bordeaux, 88
University of British Columbia, 224
University of California, Berkeley,
    31–32, 78, 144
University of Cambridge, 222
University of Chicago, 76, 80, 154,
    250
University of Connecticut, 132
University of Illinois, 102
University of Lethbridge, 249
University of Maryland, 88
University of Minnesota, 134
University of North Carolina, Chapel
    Hill, 91
University of Pennsylvania, 112, 113
University of Richmond, 136, 151
University of Rochester, 234, 236
University of Texas, Austin, 123

University of Toronto, 201
University of Utah, 81, 146
University of Virginia, 87, 174
University of Washington, 198
University of Waterloo, 23
University of Western Ontario,
    114–115
University of Wisconsin, 101, 174
University of Zurich, 107

vagus nerve, 56
Vanderbilt University, 62
Veenema, Alexa, 247
ventral tegmental area, 75
Virginia Commonwealth University,
    134
Virginia Tech Carilion Research
    Institute, 38
vision, 38, 52
vocabulary, 101
von Economo neuron, 69, *70*
vos Savant, Marilyn, 140

walking, 20
Watson, John B., 13, 29, 80, 103,
    170–172, 173, 250; parenting and,
    170–172; *The Psychological Care of
    Infant and Child*, 171; "Psychology
    as the Behaviorist Views It," 29
weather forecast prediction, 131–132
weight loss, 98
well-grounded brain, 122–149;
    comedians and, 124–128; coping
    styles, 147–149; dopamine and,
    132–136; enriched environment
    and, 143–145, *145*, 146–147; failure
    and, 128–132; statistics for,
    140–143; success and, 136–139;
    terminology, 122
Westlund, Stephanie, 199
whales, 61
white matter, 52, 67
Williams, Robin, 112

Willocks, Peggy, 243
witchcraft, 110–111
work, 23, 24, 76–78, 100, 211–231;
    brain and, 221–231; contingency
    calculators, 211–231; evolution of,
    224–227, 228; family business,
    219–221; lack of, 226–227; spy
    training, 229–230; stress, 221–224;
    success, 212–219

World Health Organization, 14
World War I, 57
Wrangham, Richard, 64
Wright, Mr., 241
Wundt, Wilhelm, 28–29

Yerkes, Robert, 251

Zeanah, Charles, 167